Curing the Colonizers

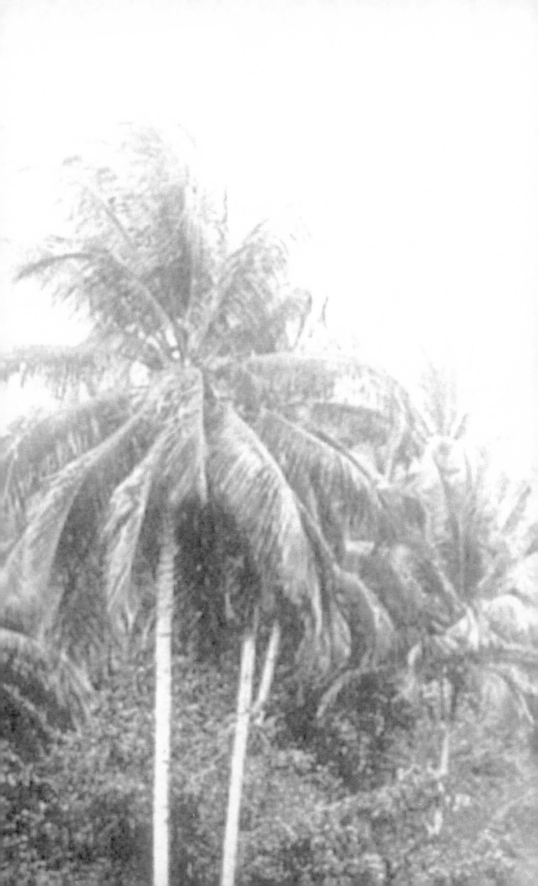

Curing the *Colonizers*

HYDROTHERAPY,
CLIMATOLOGY, AND
FRENCH COLONIAL SPAS

Eric T. Jennings

Duke University Press
Durham and London   2006

© 2006 Duke University Press

Printed in the United States of America
on acid-free paper ⊗
Designed by Heather Hensley

Typeset in Fournier by Tseng
Information Systems, Inc.

Library of Congress Cataloging-in-
Publication Data appear on the last
printed page of this book.

*Duke University Press gratefully acknowledges the support of Victoria College at
the University of Toronto, which provided a Victoria Senate Research Grant toward
the distribution of this book.*

For Tina, who knows why

Contents

Preface and Acknowledgments

The importance and pervasiveness of colonial hydrotherapy dawned on me while I was researching my previous book on the colonial politics of the Vichy regime. The town of Vichy's longstanding colonial function, its countless imperial connections, including its missionary house, its colonial associations, and its hospital that had catered to colonial troops since the invasion of Algeria all begged for explanation. Similarly, in Madagascar under Pétainist rule, I observed how colonials stranded in the colony and denied their regular furloughs back to France — a minor inconvenience of global war — thronged to the highland spa of Antsirabe, which they took for an ersatz home. At this "Vichy of Madagascar" they sought not merely leisure, but also cures for malaria and colonial "anemia," reinvigoration, reimmersion in clement climes, and revitalization through a potent mineral water cure. How did Vichy itself and Antsirabe in Madagascar emerge as sites of colonial *villégiature?* What was their role in the French colonial matrix? How did hydrotherapy come to be seen as the method of choice for treating or even avoiding colonial ills? These questions drove me to undertake this book, whose ramifications soon extended beyond Vichy and Antsirabe to encompass spas in Réunion Island, Guadeloupe, and Tunisia.

Spa research and fieldwork, pleasant though it may sound, requires funding. I could not have immersed myself in colonial hydrotherapy without the support of the Social Science and Humanities Research Council of Canada, which funded major research trips to Aix-en-Provence, Madagascar, and Guadeloupe. Subsequent research at Vichy and in Norway's missionary archives was made possible thanks to grants from the Associated Medical Services/Hannah Institute for the History of Medicine. A Victoria College Senate Research Grant enabled me to undertake the research for chapter 3 on Réunion Island. The University of Toronto's Joint Initiative in German and European Studies funded Paris- and London-based research on acclimatization. The Department of History and the Faculty of Arts and Science at the University of Toronto generously provided me with a term off to focus on writing. Victoria College covered map-making and indexing costs.

I am indebted to the staffs of several archives and libraries for their assistance: the National Library of Medicine in Maryland, the Académie de Médecine in Paris for their help with the Ninard collection, the Wellcome Institute for the History of Medicine in London, the Bibliothèque nationale de France in Paris, the Institut Pasteur in Paris, the Bibliothèque Schoelcher in Martinique, the National Archives of Madagascar, the Archives départementales de la Guadeloupe, the Archives départementales de la Réunion, the Centre des Archives d'outre-mer in Aix-en-Provence, the Norwegian Missionary Society Archives in Stavanger, Norway, and in Isoraka Antananarivo, the Archives diplomatiques in Nantes (which covers the protectorate of Tunisia), the library of the Maison du Missionnaire in Vichy, Vichy's municipal archives, the Médiathèque de Vichy, and the University of Toronto's Sablé Centre.

Portions of chapter 3 previously appeared in an article form in the *Social History of Medicine* 15:2 (August 2002). I wish to thank the editors and Oxford University Press for their permission to reprint these sections.

At Duke University Press, Valerie Millholland showed enthusiasm for this project from the start. My thanks as well to Mark Mastromarino who shepherded the book through production and book designer Heather Hensley. Outside the press, Natalie Hanemann designed the maps, Larry Kenney copyedited the manuscript, and Celia Braves compiled the index.

I owe a special debt of gratitude to Pascal Chambriard for providing me with Vichy-related iconography. I am profoundly thankful to Lawrence Jennings for sharing materials relating to Guyana that I use in chapter 1 and that he has been collecting for his forthcoming study on settlement attempts in Mana. I wish to acknowledge Ellen Furlough's kindness for pointing out to me a special issue on spas in *L'Afrique du nord illustrée*, which I cite at the beginning of chapter 2. My thanks to Caroline Douki for volunteering information on Polish exiles seeking to take French waters between 1830 and 1840. I am deeply thankful to Tina Freris for offering to help me research in Antananarivo, Stavanger, and Fort-de-France.

Skilled and dedicated research assistants at the University of Toronto provided valuable contributions to this book. Rosita Marcel and Rikke Andreassen translated documents relating to the first part of chapter 5, from Malagasy and old Norwegian, respectively. Deborah Neill, a fellow traveler in the history of French colonial medicine, patiently scoured numerous newspapers and journals searching for spa references. Nick Bentley researched spa legilsation in the *Journal officiel de l'Indochine française* at Cornell University's Kroch Library.

I wish to thank Graham Bradshaw and Richard Landon of the University of Toronto Libraries for ordering microfilmed journal and newspaper collections as well as rare hydrotherapy manuals that yielded a wealth of information. As always, Jane Lynch and her colleagues at interlibrary loan succeeded in tracking down invaluable tomes in distant collections.

My thanks to Tyler Stovall and John Merriman for their very careful readings and insightful suggestions. Susanna Barrows, Alison Bashford, Chantal Bertrand-Jennings, Ritu Birla, Julia Clancy-Smith, JP Daughton, Tina Freris, David Higgs, Linda Hutcheon, Jennifer Jenkins, Lawrence Jennings, Michael Lambek, Michelle Murphy, John Noyes, Cliff Rosenberg, and Peter Zinoman all improved chapter drafts or versions thereof with their very helpful comments and ideas. I gratefully recognize the comments offered by members of the Stanford French History Group; by those in attendance at a workshop in French history at Berkeley in 2005; by members of an international symposium entitled "Postcolonialism Today," held in Toronto in September 2002; by Leonard Smith and his Oberlin seminar in 2005; by the University of Toronto's History and Philosophy of Science and Technology symposium; and by those in attendance at several meetings of the Society for French Historical Studies, the American Association for the History of Medicine, and the Modern Language Association. Finally, I am thankful to Robert Aldrich, Monique and René Balvay, Claude Bavoux, Chantal Bertrand-Jennings, Pascal Chambriard, Isabelle Cochelin, Ellen Furlough, Albert Jauze, Amélie Ah-Koon, Pier Larson, Philippe Nun, Yannick Portebois, Scott Prudham, and Andrew Walsh, for tips, finds, and leads that took me in fruitful new directions. All translations from French are my own, unless otherwise specified.

Introduction

THROUGHOUT THE FRENCH COLONIAL EMPIRE, SPAS
thrived in the nineteenth and twentieth centuries. *Villes
d'eaux* (literally, "water towns") and *villes d'altitude*
("high-altitude resorts") were widely believed to serve
vital therapeutic, curative, even prophylactic functions
against tropical disease and the tropics themselves. They
were seen as critical to the well-being of the colonizers.
Hydrotherapy (*thermalisme* or *crénothérapie*), the branch
of medicine dealing with mineral water cures, and climatology (*climatologie, climatisme*), the branch concerned
with altitude therapy, constituted two interconnected
centerpieces of French colonial and tropical medicine between 1830 and 1962.

Water cures, often combined with altitude cures, became, like the ubiquitous cork helmet, mainstays of the
colonial regimen. The Ministry of the Colonies published
bulletins accrediting a host of spas thought to treat tropical ailments, ranging from malaria to yellow fever and
amoebic dysentery. Specialized guidebooks dispensed advice on the best spas for *colonialites* (literally, "colonial
ills"). Administrators were granted regular furloughs to
take the waters back home. In the colonies themselves,
highland hydromineral resorts became so vital that they

often emerged as seats of colonial power, as in Guadeloupe, Réunion, and Madagascar.

In the colonies, spas served as potent reminders of home for the colonizers. Teams of scientists compared the chemical composition of overseas and metropolitan spas, seeking clones of Vichy, Vittel, or Plombières. Spa towns themselves became evocative symbols of colonial power. Their modernist architecture, quaint "metropolitan" villas, and segregated bathhouses were intended as much to remind settlers of home as to impress and distance the colonized. Most important, spas re-created oases of France, where settlers could overcome homesickness through *ressourcement* (literally, "reimmersion"). This empire rested at least partly on baths—even claiming to emulate ancient Rome in this regard.

How did this pervasive reliance on water cures come about? Hydrotherapy and climatology answered profound, long-standing anxieties over colonial settlement. In his memoirs, written in 1927, Serge Abbatucci reflected widespread beliefs when he wrote, "European generations can only survive in the tropical zone in . . . artificial conditions."[1] This book is largely concerned with the justification, elaboration, and production of such an artifice. In the French case, colonial hydrotherapy and climatology represented prominent parts of this construction—as Abbatucci knew well, given his position as a leading French colonial hydrotherapist. Sometimes the artifice involved exploiting microclimates reminding colonials of home, sometimes it related to tapping spring waters akin to French ones, and at other times it simply featured the creation of an oasis of cultural Frenchness in the tropics. All three phenomena were usually interconnected in French colonial spas.

Colonial spas therefore illuminate some of the foundations of empire. They found their raison d'être in eighteenth- and nineteenth-century fears over the tropics. These fears were constantly recast and reformulated—around notions of climatic determinism and around the impact of milieu, heredity, racial purity, degeneration, and creolization. The link between these haunting fears on the one hand and colonial practices and policies on the other constitutes the focus of my opening chapter. Colonizers would not have resorted to hydrotherapy and a host of other preventative and curative agents had they not been struggling to understand European fragility and mortality in the tropics.[2] This is partly, therefore, a history of colonial anxieties and countermeasures.

My decision to examine spas in Guadeloupe, Réunion Island, Madagascar, and Tunisia warrants explanation. Simply put, these colonies boasted the most important *stations thermales* and *climatiques* ("hydrotherapeutic" and "climatic resorts") of the French empire. Sub-Saharan French continental Africa, the French South Pacific islands, and French colonial Indochina counted very few sites where previous or ongoing volcanic activity permitted the construction of a highland hydromineral spa. Settlers and administrators in these colonies instead thronged to metropolitan spas catering to colonial ills. Admittedly, Algeria and Martinique also possessed noteworthy colonial spas that were deemed both *stations climatiques* and *thermales*. Unfortunately, however, very few materials on Algeria's and Martinique's spas are present in colonial-era archives. As for Vichy, my choice of spas in metropolitan France, it was widely recognized to be the "port of call of colonials everywhere"—the top spa to treat colonial ills.[3] Its role as a de facto imperial hydrotherapeutic hub made it an obvious case study (see chapter 7). Finally, the geographical diversity of my five case studies, situated in the Indian Ocean, the Caribbean, Africa, and France, makes for broad and rich comparisons. Indeed, these colonies reflect different waves of French imperialism—Guadeloupe and Réunion having been claimed by France in the seventeenth century, while Tunisia and Madagascar entered the French imperial orbit in the late nineteenth century (1881 and 1896, respectively). And yet, one discerns remarkable continuities and parallels between these case studies, a fact that underscores the endurance of climatic and thermal logics and their remarkable capacity for reinvention.

Based upon extensive, original primary research on three continents, this book contributes to the studies of empire, tourism, leisure, and medicine. If colonialism was essentially a struggle over geography, as Edward Said asserts, then these purportedly healthful sites of leisure and power were certainly at the very heart of the French empire.[4] While historians have begun to explore some of the networks of imperial power (ranging from freemasonry to imperial clubs and colonial schools)[5] and geographers and historians have analyzed the function and workings of British colonial hill stations,[6] the case of French colonial hydrotherapy has until now garnered no historical attention whatsoever.

To be sure, historians of medicine have shown how hydrotherapy and related sciences were utilized in a host of other medical sectors, from dermatology to gynecology. The business aspect of French hydrotherapy, its emergence as a bona fide science, its position as a state-sponsored sector, and its status as a bourgeois activity have likewise elicited historiographical interest.[7] And again, there is no shortage of studies of British colonial hill stations, sites where the British practiced climatic, rather than hydrotherapeutic or mixed cures. To date, however, the powerful connection between French spas and empire has been utterly ignored.[8] And yet French colonial spas were more than mere imperial curiosities. The connection between hydrotherapy and empire has profound repercussions that extend well beyond the history of medicine. Indeed, this book stands at the crossroads of the histories of empire, leisure, tourism, power, culture, and medicine.

I propose six interventions straddling these fields. First of all, recent scholarship has demonstrated how European medicine used the colonies as testing grounds, how doctors controlled indigenous bodies, and how indigenous populations reacted to Western medicine.[9] Megan Vaughan's impressive book *Curing Their Ills: Colonial Power and African Illness* is emblematic of the second of these approaches. She demonstrates how "in British colonial Africa, medicine and its associated disciplines played an important part in constructing 'the African' as an object of knowledge, and elaborated classification systems and practices which have to be seen as intrinsic to the operation of colonial power."[10] My book, while equally centered on questions of colonial power, suggests that we cannot lose sight of the centrality of European health to colonial medicine. Colonial hydrotherapy and climatology evolved out of a nebula of racial theories, climatic and environmental determinism, and degeneration paradigms, concentrated as much, if not more, on the colonizers as on the colonized, as we shall see in chapters 1 and 2. In this same vein, colonial medicine's mix of control and regulation over indigenous peoples is often couched in the understanding that European scientists established their medicine as normative and African medicine, for instance, as either backward or superstitious. While I would not for an instant call into question this bias in European medical thinking, the prevalence in a purportedly Cartesian culture of hydrotherapy and climatology for curing colonial ills certainly underscores its intrinsic contradiction.

Second, the temptation when thinking of colonial tourism is to conjure up film-induced clichés of mythical treks to Angkor Wat, of big game hunts, or of daring automobile rallies across the Sahara. And yet, far from seeking the exotic, the French colonial tourists I study (considerably more numerous than the big game hunters, Angkor visitors, or Sahara rally enthusiasts) actually craved the familiar at sites of leisure and medicine created in the image of the metropole. Students of colonialism persuaded of exoticism's hegemonic sway have too often overlooked this evocative lateral or internal tourism.

Third, the elaboration of what Dane Kennedy has called "islands of white," "pinnacles of power," and "magic mountains" — and their configuration in this instance around high-altitude mineral springs — reveals the inherent dystopianism of this French colonial project.[11] French colonial spas were not only conceived as an artifice; they constituted an attempt at achieving a colonial tabula rasa, involving the strategic cloning of a slice of France in the tropics. Here colonialism is laid bare: gone is the pretense of altruistic colonization — of colonizing to build bridges, aid, to elevate and improve colonized populations. Around these spas, the colonizers hoped to achieve regeneration, maintain strength, and cultivate difference.

Fourth, colonial spas shed light on everyday colonial practices and colonial sensibilities. While the intimate, the sartorial, and the experimental, to give only three examples, have all recently come into sharper focus in colonial settings, much work remains to be done on the relationship between colonial epistemologies, sensibilities, medicine, and practices.[12] Whereas Michel Foucault's writings on power and governmentality have been repeatedly projected onto the colonial sphere, fewer attempts have been made to apply either his studies on medicine, or for that matter the methodologies of Alain Corbin, Georges Vigarello, or Michel de Certeau, to colonial practices.[13] Yet both everyday medical practices and colonial sensibilities open windows onto the mechanisms, foundations, and functioning of empire. Here I invert or, rather, historicize Kristin Ross's contention that in the 1950s and 1960s the colonial situation was suddenly infused into the "everyday life" of the "metropolitan existence."[14] French colonial spas, then, offer many glimpses into the workings of empire: they served as military bases, rest stations, seats of colonial power, replicas of home, way stations for preseasoned arrivals, antechambers of the tropics, and detoxification centers. They not only acted as the interface between metropole and colony, but were also believed to make empire possible.

Fifth, colonial spas constituted sites where colonial margins and identities themselves were negotiated around multiple and complex power relations.

These included the kind of internal fractures identified by Ann Stoler in other contexts.[15] Quarrels between settlers and administrators, rival spa promoters and clients, and recent settlers and Creole populations as well as tensions over the status and role of missionaries all spring out from an analysis of colonial spas. Vaster imperial fault lines are also revealed. Metropolitan and colonial spas soon entered into competition. But at the same time, spas like Vichy also permitted vastly different colonial constituencies to meet and mingle. Vichy, and to a lesser extent spas in the colonies, enabled lateral contact among administrators and other colonial agents from every corner of the French empire. Spas therefore reveal some of the complex traffic patterns of French colonialism.

On a related identity matter, colonial doctors systematically elided precolonial uses of hydromineral springs by indigenous peoples, so as to postulate their Frenchness. By labeling Antsirabe a piece of France in Madagascar, by virtue of its supposed chemical affinity to the spring at Vichy, French colonial medicine was able to lay a symbolic claim over the site. Paradoxically, in the end, the line between colony and metropole, between Réunionais, Guadeloupean, and French spas, became both culturally and even chemically blurred. The very project intended to carve out a piece of France in the colonies arguably ended up hazing the lines of home. "Are we really in the colonies?"[16] asked a journalist about Madagascar's spa, Antsirabe. And, at a metropolitan French spa like Vichy, the unexpected blurring would take on a different form, when colonized elites began frequenting the resort, bringing the empire home to the French provinces.

Sixth, such considerations lead one to ponder the encounters and more generally the relations between the French medical establishment, *baigneurs*, and *curistes* (spa practitioners) on the one hand and indigenous or colonized peoples on the other. How, if at all, did precolonial Arawak or Carib practices in Guadeloupe, maroon practices in Réunion, Betsileo and Merina practices in Madagascar, and Ottoman and Maghreb practices in Tunisia spill over onto French perceptions and uses of mineral springs? Medical literature systematically denied any influence of the Tunisian *hammam* or of Malagasy religious and cultural meanings on "proper" French scientific uses of mineral waters. Such denials were far from uniquely French: Michael Fisher has shown how nineteenth-century British doctors appropriated the Turkish Bath, claiming it "as an aboriginal British tradition."[17] But in this case, as in the British one, the reality was manifestly more complex, as indigenous elites, Creoles, and colonials all jockeyed for influence at the very sites which settler society was actively seeking to define as inherently French.

Colonial spas sprang out of a complex firmament. At these spas, concepts of human bioengineering and of racial and moral regeneration stood cheek by jowl with the notion of human rootedness, with the idea of tropical toxicity, and with the growing ritualization of colonial conduct. Before turning to how colonial hydrotherapy and climatology were practiced — first in the colonies themselves, then back home at Vichy — I will therefore begin by tracing the genesis and rationalization of French colonial hydrotherapy itself. The certainty that water and altitude cures could stave off or even cure the nefarious impact of the tropics is sufficiently foreign to us today to warrant thorough explanation.

CHAPTER I

Acclimatization, Climatology, and the Possibility of Empire

HOW DID FRENCH SCIENCE COME TO PRESCRIBE water and altitude cures to combat the influence of the tropics? The answer lies in some of the epistemological foundations of French overseas hygiene and medicine. Geographers, historians of science, and others have traced the emergence of moral climatology, tropical geography, and taxonomies of climes over the course of the eighteenth and nineteenth centuries. Similarly, a number of studies have examined how the tropics were constructed as a "putrid" and "unhealthy" space, or more generally how European science understood disease as climatically determined.[1] The connection between these "sciences" and the sensibilities and practices of the colonizers, however, has yet to be thoroughly investigated. By focusing on debates over human acclimatization, this chapter traces the link between the production and practice of colonial knowledge in the field of tropical hygiene.

If altitude and water cures came to be seen as essential to detoxify, recalibrate, or otherwise heal the constitutions, organs, even the blood composition of French people who had spent time in "hot climes," then the said climes must indeed have been considered highly noxious. Nowhere is the anxiety over colonial settlement and over the inherent toxicity of the tropics more apparent than in the interminable debates over human acclimatization, which weighed considerably on modes of European behavior in the colonies.

To Acclimatize or Not to Acclimatize?

It is difficult to reconstruct the importance of climate in eighteenth- and nine-teenth-century scientific discourse. Many Enlightenment philosophes oper-ated within a framework of climatic determinism, descended from Hippoc-rates. Indeed, the Hippocratic legacy, centered as it was on "Airs, Waters and Places," lies at the root of three sciences treated in this book: climatology, hydrotherapy, and *mésologie*.[2] In his monumental study of the idea of nature in eighteenth-century France, Jean Ehrard notes the philosophical complicity between geographical and climatic determinism and the Enlightenment: each married the sensual with the material while providing an experimental confir-mation of Spinozism.[3] Admittedly, climate occupied a more central place for some philosophes than for others: it appears virtually insignificant to David Hume, for example, while being paramount to J. G. Herder.[4]

Denis Diderot's and Jean le Rond d'Alembert's *Encyclopédie* (1777) reveals that tropical weather was believed to render indigenous women oversexed, to the point that men traveling to these climes were advised to wear chastity belts.[5] Similarly, Baron de Montesquieu asserted, the only reason European women need not have been "locked up" was because northern climes guaranteed "good mores."[6] These widely held ideas were reiterated by Count Georges Louis Le-clerc Buffon in his famous eighteenth-century *Histoire naturelle*. In a stereotype descended from antiquity, nymphomania was time and again associated with the tropics.[7]

Climate did more than affect the humors and sexuality. It was thought to lie at the very origin of behavioral and cultural differences—themselves grossly distorted to legitimize European dominance. Montesquieu, in particular, ex-pounded upon the tyranny of climate. His *De l'Esprit des Lois* (1748) imputed sati in India, daughter selling in China, and even the decline of ancient Rome to differences of temperature.[8] In fact, to Montesquieu the main difference be-tween Europeans and "savages" resided in the fact that the latter "were al-most entirely dominated by climate and nature."[9] The degree and novelty of

Montesquieu's climatic determinism have been called into question, however. Some deem it perhaps the least original aspect of his oeuvre.[10] While conceding that climatic determinism was so widespread at the time as to be unavoidable, others view Montesquieu as breaking from the more cautious appraisal Abbé François-Ignace d'Espiard articulated in his *Essais sur le génie et le caractère des nations* (1743), which treated climate as one variable among countless others.[11] The harshest interpretation holds that for Montesquieu "climate explains vice and virtue, industry and indolence, sobriety and drunkenness, 'monachism' and [even] the British constitution."[12]

Still, none of the philosophes questioned the possibility or the desirability of Europeans traveling to the tropics or settling there. If anything, the eighteenth-century settlement objective involved achieving a state of acclimatization—seasoning Europeans, so that they might best withstand the local environment and hence disease. It follows, therefore, that many a prescriptive guide written in the late eighteenth century and the early nineteenth dispensed advice on how to win the battle against climate. Some suggested sexual abstinence, others recommended frequent baths. Some counseled the consumption of wine, others warned against the dangers of alcohol.[13] There was no shortage of advice on how to soften the transition to living in the colonies.

Montesquieu concluded that Europeans were intensely vulnerable in faraway lands: "Those who wish to settle [in tropical colonies] cannot take on the local lifestyle under such different climes; they are forced to bring all the commodities of everyday life from the country whence they came."[14] Here, medicine and commodity culture met the practice of everyday colonial life. Colonizers, Montesquieu argued, would have to re-create Europe in the tropics in order to prosper. This was considered one front in a titanic war against the overriding impact of climate. In the words of the historian Anthony Pagden, "Try as they might to remain Frenchmen or English or Spaniards in the tropics, sooner or later the environment would reclaim its empire, and re-establish things in their proper order."[15] The emergence of a Creole identity, however, ultimately belied this belief. For French scientists, the process of becoming Creole seemed double-edged: it signaled a gradual loss of Europeanness but might hold the promise of acclimatization. Acclimatization, in turn, might prove medically invaluable for those contemplating long stays or even permanent moves to the tropics.

In the nineteenth century, acclimatization and creolity underwent profound reassessments in France. A century prior, the philosophes had certainly stressed the dominance of climate over constitutions. But most also recognized that acclimatizing and becoming Creole were necessary steps toward living elsewhere. In the nineteenth century this cosmopolitan view was first called into question and then utterly rejected by a growing number of scientists, who would reinvent creolity and acclimatization into pathologies. The trajectory to making acclimatization deviant was by no means straightforward. A host of early influences shaped the process. The physician Pierre-Jean-Georges Cabanis's *Rapports du physique et du moral de l'homme* (1802) established the connection between climate—defined as the "totality of physical circumstances attached to each locality"—and morality and mental capacities.[16] Cabanis's school, known as the Ideologues for their science of ideas, was not alone in auguring an initial shift circa 1800. Around the same time, the famous naturalist Georges Cuvier was likewise charting a course toward a "deterministic, physicalist interpretation of the capacities and potentials of the diverse races."[17] Although they anticipated the later nineteenth-century hardening of determinisms, these sources displayed nowhere near the same rigidity.

Martin Staum has shown how races were not yet considered fixed in the second half of the eighteenth century: the Dutch anatomist Petrus Camper even speculated that after a thousand years, whites in the tropics could turn black—precisely the opposite of what the German anthropologist Rudolf Virchow would assert a century later, namely that whites could not even survive in the tropics, let alone morphologically adapt to them.[18] And William Cohen has observed how an avowed racist like the medical doctor Julien Joseph Virey, writing in 1801, still allowed for the possibility that environment could trump race. Race, in other words, was not yet immutable, the way it would soon become for hard-line "scientific racists" later in the nineteenth century.[19] Most important, pathologies were not heavily racialized, as they would so markedly become in the second half of the nineteenth century.[20] By 1888, Joseph Onésime Orgeas, who had served at a colonial hospital in Cayenne (Guyana), concluded from clinical evidence that "human races differ no less in their pathological characteristics than in their physical ones . . . Pathological differences, themselves derived from physical variations, have vast and profound consequences: a race lives and prospers where another dwindles and goes extinct."[21]

I would argue that such determinism itself, be it climatic, environmental, hereditarian, or racial, would reach its zenith in the second half of the nineteenth century, when strands of European science would posit, without regard for paradox, the fixity of race, the immutability of national cultures, and the impossibility of migration. Indeed, each of these threads soon became intertwined with the theories of so-called scientific racists, which asserted that climate conditioned racial degeneration, fragility, or supremacy. Interestingly, fragility and supremacy frequently ended up inscribed in the same equation — even within the same variable of a given equation. One contradiction in particular lay at the heart of the anti-acclimatization position. Humankind and other organisms were believed to rapidly transform — or degenerate — in the tropics. But this transformation could only work in one direction and resulted in a fixed, immutable outcome.

According to Mark Harrison, the second half of the nineteenth century marked the rejection of the very possibility of European acclimatization and settlement in the so-called torrid zones — an obvious irony if one thinks of this era as the zenith of European overseas expansion. Whereas it had been held in the eighteenth century that Europeans "could adapt physiologically to their new environments," the very idea of acclimatization was now called into question by some racial doctrines: "This new [nineteenth-century] conception of difference stressed heredity and the innate, unalterable characteristics of the 'races' of Mankind." [22] Anne-Marie Moulin has been even more chronologically specific, situating the shift in the 1860s. She writes,

> All the naturalists raised the crucial question of the survival of French people in the tropics. Transformative logic provided the theoretical axis for a very pragmatic line of questioning. Schematically speaking, until the 1860s, doctors were optimistic, guided by theories of acclimatization. Different races or variants of a single species (monogenism) could easily adapt to new climes. This optimism was maintained in spite of the terrifying morbidity of the French in Algeria [after 1830] . . . But, in a second phase, pessimism emerged vis-à-vis the colonization of Africa and Asia. Doctors, more than naturalists, henceforth weighed in with considerations of "race." [In this view] natives had a natural advantage, being hereditarily adapted to their milieu. [23]

Although the precise timing of the shift can be debated — I would suggest that pessimism toward acclimatization was already on the rise in the 1830s, and that in any event the battles over acclimatization played themselves out over several decades[24] — Moulin's model provides an extremely helpful map of changing French views of "warm climes" in the nineteenth century.

There can be no doubt that the growing rigidity of racial models over the course of the nineteenth century both enabled and sharpened beliefs in immutable essences, whether racial, regional, or climatic. Karl Linnaeus or the Enlightenment more generally should not be saddled with the transformations popularized later by the likes of Arthur de Gobineau and Hippolyte Taine. Neither can they be held accountable for the increasing rejection of the very possibility of productive hybridity and mixity. As Moulin suggests, this trend accompanied the intensification of the debate over the unity of humankind: monogenists, like promoters of acclimatization, found themselves very much on the defensive by the mid-nineteenth century (American polygenist ethnographers like Samuel George Morton weighed in heavily on this conflict).[25] The polygenism versus monogenism debate was inextricably connected to that over acclimatization. In 1861, the French anthropologist Eugène Dally drew a direct line between the two: "It seems to me that if it were demonstrated that mankind is not cosmopolitan, that our European races, for example, cannot acclimate to other lands where other races thrive, that would provide strong proof in favor of the multiplicity of human species."[26]

In this sense, although climate had admittedly played an important role in framing and delineating the non-European "other" since ancient times, it was in the nineteenth century that battle lines were drawn over climate's teleological impact on race.[27] In the nineteenth century, French scientists thus recast the primacy of climate in a crucial question: should Europeans even attempt to acclimate to the tropics? In other words, should the uphill struggle against climate even be waged? Such anxieties were widely shared. The same internal debate was occurring simultaneously at the heart of the world's other colonial superpower. Alan Bewell has remarked, "[The nineteenth-century British] medical literature on tropical invalidism was intrinsically a reflection on the feasibility of empire."[28] In France, two schools of thought battled over the viability of migration and empire over the course of the nineteenth century: one was increasingly racially and climatically deterministic, while the other found itself defending the very possibility of acclimatization, even over the long term. At stake were quite simply the cosmopolitanism and oneness of humankind and the feasibility of empire.

Which Tropics?

The notion of the tropics itself came under intense scrutiny in the nineteenth century. The tropics, to borrow the geographer David Livingstone's expression, fell victim to "negative environmental stereotyping" on a pan-European scale.[29] This had not always been the case, and some significant exceptions remained. These included paradisical islands, in the Pacific and Indian oceans most notably, where tropical influences were said to be attenuated by breezes or other factors. The image of tropical Edens, emblematized in its romantic version by Bernardin de Saint-Pierre's *Paul et Virginie*, proved resilient even as the tropics were being pathologized.[30] In Derek Gregory's analysis, the tropical nature of excrescence coexisted — and actually became entangled with — that of tropical nature as abundance.[31] This helps in part to explain the stubborn quest for a salubrious tropical microclimate within the increasingly demonized tropical zone. It also accounts for the generally positive outlook cast on the isle of Réunion, which I will come to in chapter 4.

Still, as environmental determinists coded the tropics as increasingly dangerous sites, tropical Edens were gradually confined to the realm of the exceptional. Indeed, the stain associated with the tropics spread to warm, nontropical climes. Algeria and Tunisia illustrate this point. The heavy losses incurred during and after the French conquest of Algeria in 1830 cast serious doubts on the region's healthfulness to Europeans, doubts that endured for the remainder of the century. In 1841, a French general, Franciades-Fleurus Duvivier, famously pronounced, "Cemeteries . . . are the only flourishing colonies in Algeria."[32] Two decades later, one Dr. Vital, a physician posted in the Constantinois region of Algeria reported, "European children are mercilessly leveled [by the local climate]." In 1863, the anthropologist Jean Boudin related the story of some twelve northern French peasants who had emigrated to a purportedly healthful part of Algeria: even there, only one survived his new climes.[33] During the conquest of Tunisia in 1881, a quarter of the French expeditionary force was felled by disease (typhoid fever in this case).[34] I will return shortly to the conviction that climate, rather than disease, killed. Here I wish to stress that Algeria and Tunisia, like sub-Saharan Africa, South Asia, and Southeast Asia, had established murderous reputations in nineteenth-century France. If anything, far from being circumscribed as the nineteenth century progressed, the "tropical menace" was seen as spreading over onto liminal climates. Indeed, French scientists most often referred to a generalized peril of *pays chauds* ("warm climes"), lumping together all French colonies save Saint-Pierre and Miquelon.

The Acclimatization Camp and the Feasibility of Empire

The historian Michael Osborne has described *acclimatation* as "the essential science of [French] colonization." [35] Certainly the popularity of French acclimatization societies, zoos, and gardens tends to confirm this view (though these institutions were largely concerned with animal and botanic rather than human acclimatization). *Acclimatation*, the amorphous concept popularized by the naturalist Isidore Geoffroy Saint-Hilaire (1772–1844) and influenced by Jean-Baptiste de Monnet Chevalier de Lamarck's (1744–1829) theories of physiological adaptability, transformation, and subsequent transmission, was gaining broad currency in the early nineteenth century. [36] Its gist has been broadly defined as "a rationally forced adaptation to new environments." [37] While certainly ascribing a dominant role to environment, at its very core acclimatization involved *facilitating*, rather than hindering, the settlement of people or indeed species from one climate to another. Beneath its naturalistic surface lay some deep universalistic and cosmopolitan currents. Warwick Anderson has observed that acclimatization theories seem to have gained greater favor in France than elsewhere, Britain particularly. [38] Even though they drew considerable criticism from some quarters after 1830, "human acclimatization" theories would continue to shape French colonial policy and practices long after. As for the anti-acclimatization turn launched in earnest in France in the 1830s, it would arguably prove all the more virulent in France than elsewhere, precisely because it first needed to loosen acclimatization's grip.

Antoine Joseph Dariste's guide for Europeans traveling to the colonies, written in 1824, belongs to the first wave of enthusiasm for the potential of human acclimatization. It demonstrates how powerful an ideal acclimatization had become in French colonial medicine and practice. Focusing on the case of yellow fever, he wrote,

> Acclimatization is achieved by habit, which offsets the actions that the agents of yellow fever have on our organs. I base this theory on: 1) The fact that natives of the Caribbean, as well as Europeans acclimated there, lose the privilege of accli-

matization when they have lived for some time in cold climes. 2) That among the small number of Creoles who have fallen ill with yellow fever without having left the colony, one finds only inhabitants who live in higher elevations where the temperatures are cooler. They then came to areas where yellow fever was rampant, and fell victim to the disease. 3) That among those who, previously acclimated, left the colony for cooler climes, it was the young who lost the privilege of acclimatization the fastest.[39]

Dariste, who had served as a doctor in Martinique in 1794, clearly strove to "creolize" Europeans in the colonies.[40] The role of French medicine, he argued, was to accelerate and smoothen the process of adaptation by any way possible, through bleedings or the consumption of potions, for example.[41] Here, resolutely premodern medical practices were pressed into service to achieve the ideal of acclimatization.

Dariste's views were echoed by many French doctors familiar with the colonies. N. Huillet's *Hygiène des blancs, des mixtes et des Indiens à Pondichéry* (1867) reached the same conclusion concerning the desirability of creolization: "The body's economy undergoes, gradually, an organic transformation which allows it to indigenize itself, to borrow the wonderful phrase of Dr. Celle's *Hygiène pratique des pays chauds*, or if one prefers, to creolize itself. In other words, the body achieves a mixed temperament, halfway between that of the European and the native. That is the Creole temperament, the only one compatible with tropical regions . . . [As for] escaping diseases brought on by tropical climes . . . that is the domain of practical hygiene."[42] Here, Huillet grafted the emerging discipline of tropical hygiene studies upon Dariste's earlier goal of achieving a measure of indigenization within a humor- or temper-based paradigm. In Huillet's view, creolization, combined with the proper hygienic practices, could help stave off disease.

Although under sustained attack by the end of the nineteenth century, the acclimatization ideal had not vanished altogether; instead, tropical hygienists had absorbed and appropriated its residual elements. In fact, the growing field of French tropical hygiene defined its very existence as tributary to the aims of acclimatization. A commission formed in 1893 to popularize hygienic principles, concluded as much: "If we were to define the 'colonial settler' as one who settles definitively or spends very long periods of time in foreign lands, even tropical ones, then we would eliminate the need for the present study altogether, since in these cases, acclimatization is already resolved. Indeed, colonial hygiene's goal is to achieve this acclimatization, while preventing the unfortunate side effects of transiting from one climate to another, and adapting to new and unfamiliar surroundings."[43] The compatibility of the creolization ideal, based upon telluric and humor logics, with recently invented hygiene studies suggests surprising continuities in French colonial science. Such continuities seem largely counterintuitive in view of the breakthroughs of the nineteenth century, in the realm of germ medicine most notably.

Among the modern backers of acclimatization, none defended the notion more resolutely than the famed tropical hygienist George Treille. His *De l'acclimatation des Européens dans les pays chauds* (1888) depicted a deeply polarized French scientific community: in one camp ethnographers denying the possibility of acclimatization, and in the other camp hygienists like himself arguing that rational, modern hygiene could overcome the admittedly daunting challenge of tropical climate. Treille presented the divide as follows: "Anthropology is not favorable to the migration of whites to the tropics." Ethnographers, he wrote, "take a philosophical approach, where [they] assume as a given the extinction of the race after two or three generations, if it is not regularly reinforced by immigration."[44] In contrast, the role of the tropical hygienist was not to question the merits of settlement, but to rationalize and regiment its forms. In his words, "I said that hygiene is not concerned with the anthropological study of the decline of the race, and that its only goal should be to improve the conditions of the settler and his family. Nevertheless, in order to draw up rules of conduct for the settler to live in this new climate, hygiene must find inspiration from the examples of acclimatization furnished by the historical geography of our planet."[45] Treille hoped, in other words, to use modern hygiene to overcome both climatic barriers and gradual racial degeneration. Treille and his fellow hygienists kept acclimatization relevant, after leading scientists—anthropologists in particular—had questioned the very possibility of successful colonial settlement.

Colonial Experimentation: The Example of Guyana

The acclimatization debate did not occur in a vacuum. Data on European morbidity rates in the colonies fueled metropolitan scientific discussions about the wisdom of tropical migration and settlement. The example of French colonial

Guyana suggests that the 1820s and 1830s already witnessed a gradual shift in French thinking about acclimatization.

In August 1820, a debate within the French colonial office over settlement possibilities in Guyana pitted optimists against skeptics. All agreed at least that the question had been hanging in suspense for some time. The minutes read as follows: "The possibility of establishing white farmers in this colony has been contested by some, admitted by others; it is a controversy that has been lasting for years, and it is only on location and through experimentation that we will be able to learn if a settlement by white farmers is possible." [46] Guyana was thus considered a laboratory of French acclimatability. In 1826, the interim governor of Guyana, Joseph Burgues de Missiessy, wrote of "immigrants destined to sacrifice themselves, so as to find a solution to the problem of acclimatization and to the question of settlement by European farmers." [47] Settlers were explicitly presented as acclimatization guinea pigs.

During the debate of 1820, the minister of the Navy and the Colonies cut to the heart of the matter: "The fundamental question in fact is that of settlement: is it possible to transplant to this colony Europeans, who might acclimate there and dedicate themselves to cultivating the lands?" [48] The language of development derived from that of acclimatability. And in turn acclimatization remained well within the realm of possibility — reflected in the optimism of one Catineau-Laroche, an influential figure in the colonial administration. Better yet, acclimatization was still considered desirable, indeed a vital necessity if any potential migrant was to survive in Guyana.

Still, previous settlement fiascoes tempered even Catineau-Laroche's enthusiasm. Precautions would need to be taken, first and foremost with the locations chosen for settlement. Highlands would be selected partly for their "pure air," but mostly because "only there can whites acclimate and dedicate themselves to land cultivation." [49] Microclimates reminiscent of Europe or other "exceptional milieus" already loomed large as acclimatization facilitators.

By 1825, the first results, drawn mostly from a settlement attempt at Mana, were anything but rosy. Governor Pierre Bernard, Baron de Milius wrote to the minister of the Navy and the Colonies, "Only blacks seem able to withstand the fatigue and live in the heart of these deleterious miasmas that decimate Europeans." [50] The politics of unfree labor certainly weighed heavily in this debate. But it is on the closely related French biopolitics that I wish to concentrate here. By 1831, the minister of the Navy and the Colonies, the Comte de Rigny, concluded, "Why continue . . . this chimera: the colonization of Guyana by Europeans? It is more than time that we abandon these ideas which experience has condemned once and for all." [51] A report of 1835 observed that in Mana "when examining the morbidity rates among black and white settlers, we found that fifteen out of one hundred whites had died, as opposed to only two blacks per hundred." The report noted bluntly, "If new dispositions are adopted, they will certainly not involve continuing the attempts of colonization by Europeans." [52] The acclimatization skeptics seemed vindicated. Successful or unsuccessful settlement in Guyana had been measured entirely through climate and race.

Acclimatization and Slavery

The battles over climatic determinism were anything but abstract. The politics of unfree labor, to which I have already alluded, weighed into the debate. Prior to abolition (1833–34 in Britain, 1848 in France, 1865 in the United States), slaveholders and their lobbies tapped into the rising anti-acclimatization tide to justify their position that whites were incapable of performing hard labor in warm climes and that such tasks befell those who were born in and were therefore racially favorably disposed to warm climes. Remove African slavery from the equation, they contended, and the sugar colonies would collapse because whites were simply unable to work the jobs to which blacks were predisposed. [53] Rigorous environmental determinism would of course have dictated that indigenous peoples, rather than African slaves, would have provided the most adapted forced laborers in the Americas. Indeed, in the eighteenth-century model, African slaves, like Europeans, were widely believed to require "seasoning" in the Americas, since this land was foreign to them. Seasoning of African slaves involved a host of rituals, including bathing and body scrubs, and was highly structured along several distinct stages. [54] The internal contradictions of climatic determinists lie beyond the scope of my study: I wish to show here how nineteenth-century opponents of abolition used racio-climatic arguments to buttress their position.

To be sure, the idea that native Americans or blacks were better suited to the heat than whites can be traced back to the Enlightenment and earlier. But as Mary Stewart has shown, in the mid-nineteenth century, slavery advocates, in this case in the American South, recast this older belief along polygenist lines, fusing climatism with racialism in the process. Stewart notes that in this new interpretation, "Africans did not have [the] ability [to survive and thrive in the South] because they had developed it in a long interaction with tropical climates; [instead] they had it because they were created differently." In sum, "acclimation was now evidence of permanent and immutable differences, rather than of a process of differentiation."[55] It was but a small step to making acclimatization tantamount to degeneration.

A Transitional Figure

Although no single doctor can embody the shift from acclimatization to racioclimatic determinism, Louis-Daniel Beauperthuy nonetheless represents an interesting transitional figure. In 1837, with acclimatization theory already under attack, Beauperthuy, the famed Guadeloupean physician sometimes credited with first suspecting yellow fever's mosquito vector, and even with anticipating germ theory, wrote his seminal thesis "On Climatology."[56] In it, he argued that "each land imprints its characteristics on the man who is born there, or lives there a certain amount of time; like plants, man is exposed to the laws and elements of nature"[57] — a position the white Guadeloupean-born doctor seems not to have fully thought through. Fortunately, wrote Beauperthuy, nature offers microclimates, notably vast plateaus, where "the inhabitant of the gentlest European climates transposed to the [tropics] can find a hospitable environment."[58] In the tropical lowlands, meanwhile, "extreme heat and humidity soften the sinews and fibers, and impair digestive and locomotive functions: the body becomes weighed down . . . the liver and the spleen swell, their indolence is extreme."[59] Hereditary immunities only comforted Beauperthuy's determinism. Very few Amazonian Indians, he wrote, are stricken with intermittent fevers.[60] Beauperthuy was obliged to concede, however, that yellow fever had decimated Guadeloupeans indiscriminately. "Creoles and Europeans alike," he recognized, had been stricken in an epidemic at Sainte-Rose, around the time of his birth in 1807.[61] And while he was convinced, for example, that a non-Arab would be intensely vulnerable — indeed condemned to — diseases if transposed to North Africa, he nevertheless came to consider acclimatization a kind of vaccination that could ward off the most pernicious effects of warm climes.[62]

The Anti-Acclimatization Turn and Its Impact

Some elements of the anti-acclimatization turn were certainly imported from across the English Channel. James Johnson's *The Influence of Tropical Climates on European Constitutions* (1813) marked an important turning point. Up to then, Alan Bewell argues, the prevailing colonial settlement doctrine had been to season European troops or settlers, so as to adapt them to the tropics. In the wake of Johnson's seminal text, "doctors began to speculate on a progressive deterioration of the European body in tropical regions."[63] By 1828, James Annesley was turning acclimatization on its head, suggesting that human races, like exotic plants, could not be successfully transferred to other climes. Acclimatization societies had once made precisely such botanical experiments their raison d'être. By 1870, concludes Bewell, the predominant view guiding British colonialism held that "lengthy stays in the tropics were to be avoided at all costs."[64]

In France, where acclimatization was by all accounts more deeply entrenched than in Britain, the anti-acclimatization backlash appears to have been all the more violent. Treille's remarks in 1888 speak to the chasm between pro- and anti-acclimatization camps in France. The 1860s and 1870s had signaled the rise of hereditarian theories at the expense of acclimatization.[65] The divide was as disciplinary as it was political. Soon, ethnographers armed with these theories as well as with new weapons like phrenology took aim at the once-dominant acclimatization model. In 1863, notes Osborne, the fourth president of the Société d'Anthropologie, Jean Boudin, bluntly rejected acclimatization in an article entitled "On the Non-Cosmopolitanism of Mankind." Boudin did so on racial grounds, persuaded of the connection between disease and ethnicity, but also for political motives, based on his hostility to Napoleon III's plans for settling Algeria with French pioneers.[66] Boudin's stance is symptomatic of what seems in retrospect a striking paradox. In the nineteenth-century French case, it was the opponents of colonial settlement, like Boudin and Donatien Thibaut, rather than the proponents, who were elaborating and promoting rigidly racist models. Gobineau, after all, claimed that ancient Rome had fallen because of imperial miscegenation. Paul Broca's *Société d'anthropologie* brewed a similar concoction, while adding a hint of preservationism to the broth.[67] Evidently, opponents of the new imperialism were anything but uniformly progressive.

Far from toppling the logic of climatic determinism, as one might have expected, the arrival of hereditary, germ, and racial theories in the nineteenth century distorted and accentuated it in complex ways. The historian David Arnold has underscored this paradox:

> The importance attached to climate and topography as determinants of disease, a theme so elaborately worked out and so authoritatively stated in the medical texts of the early nineteenth century, remained a remarkably powerful force in medical ideas in India for the rest of the century. Even when challenged by a new paradigm, the germ theory of disease, many old India hands still clung resolutely to climatic or environmental determinism or hastened to explain that microbes and germs provided no more than a partial explanation for the incidence and etiology of specific diseases.[68]

Livingstone has taken this verdict a step further, noting the endurance of moral climatology well into the 1950s.[69] Little wonder, then, that in the French case hydrotherapy, climatology, and modern tropical medicine could not just coexist, but actually entered into symbiosis throughout the nineteenth and twentieth centuries.

The nineteenth century saw no clear resolution to the ongoing acclimatization debate. In this sense, Livingstone, like Arnold, is correct in discerning continuities in the use of "moral climatology, in spite of the advent of the new parasitology of the nineteenth century."[70] One could speak even of an exacerbation. Starting in the 1830s, preexisting climatic theories came to be codified and polarized into immutable laws of toxicity and salubrity, through the synthesizing and popularization of racial thinking that established a taxonomy and hierarchy of races. Rather than acting solely upon "constitutions," "morality," "culture," or "character," climate was seen as determinant in the production of "race." What did this mean with respect to the ideal of acclimatization? Fears of racial degeneration brought acclimatization increasingly under attack. Indeed, many French scientists came to question the very possibility of achieving acclimatization without suffering the terrible cost of racial degeneration.

Degeneration, the haunting obsession of nineteenth-century European science, had been defined at mid-century by Bénédict Augustin Morel as a pathology that acted over generations, culminating in cretinism, idiocy, sterility, and death. The condition was thought to affect the spirit and the body in equal measure and increasingly came to be applied not merely to individuals and lineages, but also to peoples and races. "Physical degeneration," writes one historian, "could not but lead to eventual intellectual and moral collapse and vice-versa."[71] Some of the earliest degeneration theorists had speculated that milieu, along with heredity, could account for the condition.[72] It followed, therefore, that the tropics could induce and accelerate this pathology. Fears of degeneration further compounded the belief—which had already been gaining ground—that Europeans denaturalized in the tropics.

The acclimatization battles reached a fever pitch at mid-century. Decorum was tested in the chambers of the Société d'Anthropologie de Paris in July 1861, as an associate member, one Dr. Chaix of Geneva, dared challenge Boudin's contention concerning the impossibility of Europeans acclimating to warm climes. Chaix had pointed to British settlers in Australia and South Africa and to a small group of German pioneers in Texas as examples of successful white settlement in warm climes. Boudin conceded only one point: the Southern Hemisphere's warm climes appeared, on the surface at least, to be less deleterious than the north's (which might account for Australia and South Africa). But Boudin did not give an inch on his basic principle. "We know that in Algeria climate kills far more French soldiers than do Muslims' bullets," he contended. Fellow anthropologists rallied to Boudin's position. A certain Rameau opined, "Mr. Chaix completely misjudges the nefarious influence of climate." He invoked the Algerian province of Bouffarick, where Europeans had cleared marshes and trees and established very lucrative tobacco crops but still languished, as evidenced by the fact that their births lagged behind deaths.[73] In this view, humankind was even less cosmopolitan, less transferable, than plants. Chaix's humble reservation, that acclimatization, while difficult, might not be entirely impossible, had been roundly dismissed.

Likewise concentrating on Algeria, Thibaut's *Acclimatement et colonisation: Algérie et colonies* (1859) repudiated the possibility of human acclimatization altogether. Thibaut wrote, "Acclimatization, as it is generally understood in

France, especially, is a fiction. It seems to be the starting point for countless deplorable errors, ruinous for our country, since our systems of colonization rest on a misunderstanding of matters of hygiene.[74] For all those who have thought about it, the condition of the acclimated in hot countries is synonymous with impotence, incapacity, and inaptitude for the work of colonization. Everyone is in agreement that whites in the torrid zone, once broken by the influences of climate, are reduced to physical and moral weakness."[75] Race was clearly the prime mover for Thibaut. He lashed out against the naïveté of French abolitionists and philanthropists: "White-skinned French people — I specify because philanthropists have imagined black ones — will never be able to live with impunity in the Antilles or Algeria." "Nature," he insisted, "would not permit such infractions to its immutable laws."[76] Worse than transgressing the laws of nature, acclimatization was tantamount to degeneration and loss of Frenchness: "If a Frenchman has become acclimated in Algeria or the Antilles . . . then he has become Arab or Creole."[77] Thibaut did not stop there: "If, in order to colonize Algeria, French settlers must transform themselves into Arabs so as to perpetuate themselves in that land, then why are we busily trying to transform Arabs in our image?"[78] Striking at both France's purported "civilizing mission" and the colonial lobby's Algerian settlement policies, Thibaut elaborated a terrifying model of degeneration and déracinement.

Thibaut buttressed his arguments with medical research. The acclimatization debate did not spring up ex nihilo; it had at its roots the undisputedly high mortality levels of Europeans in the tropics. Thibaut relied extensively upon J. A. Rochoux's work on yellow fever from 1828. Rochoux had described the process of acclimatization as follows: "Soon, the Frenchman changes [in the Caribbean]. He ceases to be himself; he loses the vivacity that is so familiar to us. Already his traits have changed, and it is soon noticed by all around him. One can then consider the subject acclimated, and his blood thinned."[79] To be sure, the medical language of the acclimatization debate would shift over time. But the debate would not die. In the second half of the nineteenth century, the unabatedly high mortality rates among settlers, soldiers, and administrators led many to question the possibility of successful acclimatization. Geographers and hygienists began to scramble for historical examples (settlement fiascos in Guyana, successes in the Indian Ocean, the Pacific, etc.) with which to establish some elusive medico-climatic coherence. In 1892, a naval doctor,

H. Gros, published his findings on the physiological changes undergone by a boatload of Bretons even in a "relatively salubrious" tropical environment, the Pacific Iles de la Société.[80] Could breezes and trade winds provide sufficient racial and medical protection? Could highlands be considered safe havens and if so, at what elevations? What other countermeasures could be used against the tropics? On each of these scores, hydrotherapy and climatology would be pressed into service by French medicine.

Anderson reminds us that "until the early twentieth century, medicine was as much a discourse of settlement as it was a means of knowing and mastering disease."[81] French colonial and tropical medicine was thus intimately implicated in the process of colonization, indeed in the actual choice of which areas to settle. Within the French "colonial lobby" the questioning of acclimatization meant that settlement colonies must be chosen carefully indeed. Here, historical patterns were introduced into evidence: had the French not chosen cool climes—that is, Québec—in which to settle permanently in large numbers? The defenders of acclimatization were forced to answer their critics by identifying proven salubrious oases in the tropics. In 1897, Treille declared,

> No doubt, braving high mortality rates . . . it is possible for some functionaries, and a handful of business people to stay for relatively long periods in inter-tropical climes—for perhaps three or four years. . . . But where the task becomes most laborious, where it is in fact mainly a futile attempt, is when trying to found a European-blooded family in countries with such climates. . . . Fortunately, there are several exceptions to these limitations to the European race's expansion in the tropics. . . . Everywhere, indeed, where nature has endowed equatorial lands a sufficient counter-influence to their humid heat, by giving them altitude (as in the Andes), or an atmosphere that is vigorously renewed by constant breezes (as in the Antilles or Polynesia), it has been possible for whites to settle, and generation after generation, gain some of the adaptation of the locals.[82]

At a time when the French pondered which of their territories were colonizable—in the same sense as Australia and North America were for the British—Guadeloupe's and Réunion's highland microclimates figured prominently in French scientific rationales. In this respect, French science was far from unique. In 1846, the Englishman Sir James Scott had already offered an elaborate mapping of global microclimates, ranking the salubrious and the insalubrious, in his seminal text *The Sanative Influence of Climate*.[83]

The impact of the anti-acclimatization turn was felt well beyond the politics of colonial settlement. It cut to the heart of questions of identity and race in the nineteenth century. In an influential hygiene manual written in 1895 for Europeans in the tropics, the naval doctor Just Navarre concurred with his colleague Thibaut: "The Caucasian race has not acclimated to inter-tropical lands . . . and nothing suggests that it will do so soon."[84] Navarre was singularly uncharitable to those whom a previous generation of doctors had considered acclimated. Of them, Navarre wrote, "These supposedly acclimated humans . . . are *minus habentes*, barely physiological . . . they are, in their vast majority, pathological subjects."[85] In short, Navarre saw himself as part of a vast scientific reaction against a naïvely cosmopolitan and egalitarian vision of humankind. "My conclusions," he wrote, "are shared by the international congress of colonial doctors, held in Amsterdam in 1883, where not a single doctor defended the idea of the cosmopolitanism of man."[86] This scientific backlash was so complete that between 1850 and 1900 it had overturned "the Enlightenment emphasis on the unity of the human race . . . allied to an Evangelical Christian belief in the family of man."[87]

In 1886, the naval doctor Joseph Orgeas wrote an anthropological study of "the pathology of human races," drawing from his experience in a Guyanese hospital. Orgeas, not coincidentally a dual specialist in racial degeneration in the colonies and climatological winter resorts at home, doubted the possibility of Europeans remaining racially unscathed for more than one generation in the tropics.[88] He affirmed that "the forces of climatic milieu on a race, are exponential . . . compounding the effects year after year."[89] This decline was inexorable: "A European residing in the tropics descends a slope at the end of which lies the disappearance of the individual and the extinction of the race. The slope is more or less steep, depending on the artificial conditions in which he finds himself."[90] For Orgeas, acclimatization was not merely a mirage, but a dangerous lie. "Acclimatization does not exist," he averred, "if by acclimatization one means . . . the process of adapting to a new climate." The only case in which the term had any meaning, he suggested, was in the Americas, where it could in some cases signal not so much a permanent alteration as a "passing, pathological change" (here Orgeas had in mind immunity from yellow fever).[91] In the rest of the world, Orgeas maintained, "an acclimated European can only be a . . . sick European."[92] In sum, wrote the award-winning naval doctor, "by staying in tropical climes, Europeans violate the laws of nature, much as one violates biological laws by trying to cultivate bananas or oranges in France."[93]

The same decade marked the publication of Alfred Jousset's oft-cited *De l'acclimatement et de l'acclimatation*. Jousset, a doctor and teacher at the school of naval medicine, was an expert on respiratory systems, physiology, and tropical pathology.[94] He began his magnum opus by bemoaning an increase in global migration and uprootedness, a diasporism he perceived as a harbinger of degeneration. Jousset's massive study then proceeds to catalog purported racial differences in everything from respiratory rates to sensibility to pain to genitalia sizes (both female and male) before concluding, "By comparing the temperate man to the tropical man, I have shown how nature modifies an emigrant's bodily functions, ultimately rendering them similar to that of the native. Breathing, blood circulation, body heat, in sum all the functions of life tend to adapt to one's new milieu . . . All races are obliged to . . . adapt the different components of their organisms to mesological conditions: individual acclimatization thus always precedes that of the race."[95] Here, acclimatization has become a buzzword for racial degeneration, by way of an accelerated and deterministic reading of Lamarck[96] (of Charles Darwin, too, although, as Harry Paul has shown, in the 1860s and 1870s Darwin had come under attack from French positivists, skeptical of his transformative model).[97] To be sure, Jousset recognizes that "man seems to resist the influence of milieu more than certain animal races." But, he adds "when circumstances are such that he cannot utilize his preventative faculties, or when the new milieu is too energized, then he falls victim to milieu much as animals do. Even adult humans can be singularly altered."[98] If cosmopolitanism was tantamount to errantry, race, on the other hand, seemed to bear the promise that it could be fixed, so long as outside influences and milieu remained static.

Mésologie, Race, and the Apogee of Anti-Acclimatization

By his own admission, Jousset relied upon a new science known as mesology, the study of how milieux influenced their inhabitants. The entry on *mésologie* in the *Dictionnaire encyclopédique des sciences médicales* (1873) was written by none other than the notorious inventor of anthropometry and cataloger of criminal types, Alphonse Bertillon. Interestingly, Bertillon's ideas caused him to break with some of his polygenist French contemporaries, for Bertillon, in a Lamarckian vein, held that milieu shaped individuals within a species, rather than the species itself.[99] The young Bertillon's example of how to apply this new science involved a stunning metaphor of anatomy and empire:

> The following should show the influence of milieu . . . upon one's hereditary properties. We know that the periosteum[100] has as a basic property the growth of a bony deposit on its surface. If one dips some periosteum cells into the mass of another living body, the periosteum continues to live there, first on its own terms, and covers itself in bony matter. But, gradually, in this new milieu, its own activity ceases, and is replaced by the eliminating and absorbing influence of surrounding tissues, so that the periosteum, after having grown for a time in this foreign body, now shrinks and disappears . . . This is precisely what happens to a European when he is transported to Egypt, Guyana, or Senegambia: at first he victoriously withstands the onslaught of climate; but gradually, his nutrition changes, his spirit declines, etc.

In order to catalog the overriding influence of one's milieu or environment on anatomy, Bertillon advocated that scientists launch an exhaustive investigation, comparing the size of livers and lungs among northern and southern peoples.[101] Acclimatization was not only illusory, argued Bertillon, but also ran contrary to the basic tenets of mesology.

In hindsight, *mésologie* represents the high-water mark of two trends. On one score, it constitutes the ultimate expression of environmental determinism, in which individuals, rather than a species, group, or race, could themselves undergo profound alterations from their environment within a generation. On another level, *mésologie* ascribed a pathological quality to the same *créolité* that had once been considered if not a virtue, then at least a necessary step toward acclimatization. Here the French person who migrated to Senegambia or Guyana was no longer on their way to acclimatizing, so much as to languishing and degenerating.

The German scientist Rudolf Virchow emerged as one of the most radical opponents of acclimatization — like Boudin, he used the language of anti-acclimatization to oppose colonial settlement, in this case the kaiser's plans for colonial expansion. In 1885, the widely circulated Parisian *Revue Scientifique* translated a lecture by this famed German doctor and ethnographer, demonstrating a European complicity and dialogue in tropical medicine at the time.[102] Virchow has long enjoyed a reputation as a political progressive and German republican.[103] Some have noted how he put his prestige on the line to oppose empire and to combat anti-Semitism. Others have suggested that he utilized cranial measurements to challenge facile connections between phrenology and race.[104] A recent study describes him plainly as a monogenist and an "anti-racist . . . in late nineteenth-century contemporary terms."[105] The fact that even Virchow should treat race as the prime mover — or rather as the prime impediment — behind colonization speaks volumes on how thoroughly embedded these concepts were in late-nineteenth-century thought.[106]

In this important but long-neglected piece entitled "De l'acclimatement des Européens aux colonies," Virchow asserted that higher concentrations of Aryan blood in northern over southern Europe explained why the French sustained greater loss of life in the Caribbean than the Spanish, and the British in turn more losses than the French. He argued, "The results of colonization in the [French] Antilles have always been disastrous for migrants from Europe, while in the Spanish Caribbean the results have been more favorable."[107] In Virchow's *Weltanschauung*, the Maltese and the Jews, as the "least Aryan" and most southern of Europeans, could be considered the best candidates for tropical colonization, precisely because they were the least white. Germans and Britons, conversely, were the most vulnerable in the tropics, paradoxically because of their "Aryanness":[108] "Compared to races where the Aryan element has maintained its purity, the races [in southern Europe], especially those who have drawn from Semitic origins, are incomparably more apt at acclimatizing and thriving in new conditions when they are transplanted to hot climes."[109] Virchow did not explicitly posit the superiority of Aryans; if anything he underscored their fragility in the tropics. But the acknowledged fragility of Europeans in the tropics had never precluded popular belief in European superiority. Acclimatization had been reinvented as a weakness. And it would be a small step to transform the image of the protean, acculturable, acclimatable Jew outlined by Virchow into that of the cosmopolitan, errant, and déclassé Jew contrasted by late-nineteenth-century racialists with the firmly rooted Aryan (to take it a step further, this model also set the stage for the idea that Germany should colonize only in Europe and that Jews could be shipped to Madagascar).[110]

The important point for our purposes is that in Virchow's distinctly post-Enlightenment view race trumped the ideal of acclimatization. Climatic relativism, already prominent in the Enlightenment, had given way to a form of racio-climatic determinism. Ultimately, Virchow concluded that even the French, less Aryan though they might be, were still incapable of long-term tropical settlement, given the implacable impediment of climate.

The issue of long-term settlement brought Virchow to the question of degenerational time. How many generations would it take for a family to go Creole? or to degenerate, if the two meant one and the same thing? Some incurable cosmopolitans, Virchow implied, had pointed to the case of old European families settled in the Indian Ocean and indistinguishable, to the naked eye at least, from other Europeans: "In order to convince us of the aptitude of the white race to settle in such or such a place, one needs more than isolated examples. There are admittedly, in the heights of the isle of Réunion, a small group of so-called *petits blancs*. . . . [But such] cases remind me of exotic plants that we transplant to our forests; a few may take root, and then become the object of boundless curiosity . . . All the same, they remain isolated examples."[111] Interestingly, Réunion island's *Créoles des hauts* ("highland Creoles") found themselves invoked as exceptions to the rule of racio-climatic determinism. The exception was no doubt owed to highland Réunion's reputation as a salubrious microclimate. Navarre, less certain than Virchow on this score, set about disproving the putative Réunion exception:

> Some have argued that old [European] families remain, Créoles in Mauritius and Réunion. This is true. But these families are neither numerous nor very ancient (none go back to more than four generations without racial mixing), and can one say that they are truly acclimated? No, they simply survive. Have these Creoles become true sons of the land? No, they neither till it nor hold it. The little whites of Réunion island, so often cited, are first of all more racially mixed than is acknowledged, and can moreover, only cultivate lands between 600 and 1600 meters, in other words in microclimates, whose conditions are much closer to those [of Europe].[112]

Even Réunion's white highlanders, Navarre asserted, were anything but racially sound. They merely clung to life, even in artificial conditions. Here, two subtly different readings of climatic impediments clashed: for the likes of

Navarre, spas, resorts, microclimates, and other artifices could only temporarily forestall degeneration. Still, for administrators (whose length of stay in the colonies varied but rarely surpassed ten years in a single post) and even permanent settlers and their descendents, forestalling no doubt seemed more appealing than the gloomy alternative of degeneration within a single generation—a possibility raised by the new science of *mésologie*.

Finally, Virchow repeated a classic tropical medical rationale to account for European disease and degeneration in the tropics. The sensitive European liver (again, more sensitive for Aryans than non-Aryans) lay at the root of most colonial ailments. Virchow explained: "It is precisely the liver that will first be affected by alterations, not only deriving from malaria, but also from ordinary diseases of acclimatization."[113] Here, Virchow hardly broke new ground. Jousset encapsulated the view of the entire French medical establishment when he wrote, "There is not a single European having lived some time in the tropics, whose liver is not abnormally swollen."[114] Given the primacy of the liver to nineteenth-century tropical doctors more generally and to French hydrotherapists as well, the French colonial hepatic obsession is hardly surprising. But what renders Virchow's analysis so striking is how it interwove ambient racial taxonomies and climatic determinism in a model that completely rejected *métissage* and acclimatization, while simultaneously pointing to the liver as the Achilles heel of Europeans in the tropics. In this long-forgotten worldview, the liver, its condition and treatment, constituted the key for the very survival of those whites who had already settled in the tropics.

Bertillon's and Virchow's theories would serve as touchstones, even influencing some advocates of colonial settlement. Jean Lémure, a doctor who analyzed the hygienic debacle incurred during the French conquest of Madagascar in 1895, wrote,

> The most striking example of [acclimatization] is provided by the Jewish type, which possesses a high degree of acclimatization potential. . . . To adapt to the torrid zone, given his point of departure, the Jew needs only to undergo what Mr. Bertillon calls "small acclimatization." To attempt "big acclimatization" to lands far removed from their place of origin, for instance to colder climes, Jews have been able to overcome these obstacles by moving gradually, over generations, from one town to another. In each station—settled over a long period of time—they let their descendents soak in the climate and some indigenous

blood, able to avoid misery through their industry, to avoid excesses through sobriety, to avoid dangers through their prudence.[115]

If the French were to succeed as settlers, they would have to draw from a supposed Jewish experience. They would have to not only settle gradually, inching from one climate to another over generations, but also follow a careful regimen, taking baby steps, small degrees of acclimatization, to guard against excess and degeneration. In this view, the regularizing and temperate influence of hill stations and hydromineral spas could facilitate settlement. Thanks to these sciences, French settlers would be faced with the more manageable "small acclimatization" process.

The Persistence of *Climatisme*

If any single tendency emerged from the acclimatization debates, it involved the hardening of climatic determinism. Placed on the defensive, even proponents of acclimatization, like hygienists, reformulated their role — in a revalorizing manner no less. Their mission now involved the elaboration of indispensable countermeasures against climate's overwhelming influence. The science dedicated to gauging, harnessing, and applying the lessons derived from climate's impact on humans became known in France as *climatisme*. In its most popular nineteenth-century form, it involved "reimmersing" patients into "clement" climes over the course of a standardized "cure." Once again, the objective was *ressourcement*, an untranslatable term connoting a return to one's place of origin, climate, milieu, or spring.

In France, the legacy of climatic determinism proved especially enduring. Indeed, *climatisme* held sway in France long after it had been utterly discredited elsewhere. Ronald Ross's formal connection of mosquitoes with malaria in 1897 signaled a major shift in thinking in Britain. It let climate off the hook in many scientific communities. While this news certainly reached France quickly, it did little more than alter the etiology of malaria. It failed, in other words, to topple or even begin to challenge climatic convictions. The renowned naval doctor and developer of the spa of Cilaos in Réunion, Jean-Marie Mac-Auliffe, is a case in point. News of Ross's findings reached him midway through the drafting of his book *Cilaos, pittoresque et thermal* (1902). He simply inserted an addendum into his earlier discussion of how "organic matters in the soil and waters engender, through decomposition . . . a series of chemically laden infections [that is, malaria]."[116] Ross's discovery of anophele mosquitoes as malarial vectors certainly did not prevent Mac-Auliffe from prescribing water and altitude cures as a means of both avoiding and curing malaria.

In Britain, the post-Rossian rupture was more immediate and profound. An article in the *Geographical Journal* in 1898 captured this moment. Its author, the Italian scientist Luigi Westenra Sambon, explained: "Those who believe that the heat of the tropics is noxious to Europeans, uphold their contention by stating that it induces diseases, and they mention anaemia, hepatitis, and sunstroke. At one time, undoubtedly, these diseases were attributed to the direct and sole agency of solar heat, just as malarial fevers were attributed to the moonshine. But now they have been inscribed deeply on the tablets of bacteriology, and certainly the demonstration that disease belongs to the domain of parasitism is the greatest advance that medical science has ever made."[117] With this breakthrough firmly established, the author went on to deduce a plausible — indeed, fascinating — explanation for the popularity and persistence of climatic explanations for disease: "The belief that white men cannot work in the tropics arose greatly from the advocates of coloured labour. It is certainly disproved by the facts."[118]

Sambon even responded to the Virchow thesis: "Now, if Aryans of remote immigration have not only been able to thrive, but have even absorbed semitic dwellers of India, why should the Aryan of today be unable to colonize even those parts of the great peninsula that have been called the 'English climates of India'?" Although Sambon used racial theories himself to dispute Virchow's, the thrust of his argument would nonetheless seem far more familiar to present-day scientists: disease, rather than climate, kills. And yet, in spite of the sea change brought about in 1897–98, the legacy of climatic determinism would prove remarkably influential in the colonial sphere, especially in the French case.[119]

Late-nineteenth-century scientific revolutions dented climatic determinism's hold, but only slightly.[120] Although parasitology and the French Pasteurian revolution identified the microbe as the new enemy, climate remained an important, if not the most important, pathological agent. Early-twentieth-century Pasteurians found themselves still preaching against the widespread belief that climate was to blame for European fragility in the colonies. Bruno

Latour cites a Pasteurian scientist who argued in 1908, "Even more than the heat, which is at most an unpleasant factor, fever and dysentery are the 'generals' that defend hot countries against our incursions."[121] But, as Latour notes, hygienists and Pasteurians, waging a perceived war on all fronts, tapped into their (often older) recipes, counsels, and formulae to deal with the bacterial menace: "Malaria or yellow fever were to be destroyed not with vaccines but by ordering the colonists and natives to build their houses differently, to dry up stagnant ponds, to build walls of different materials, or to alter their daily habits."[122] Everyday escape from tropical influences, in other words, remained the favored course of evasive action. Whether the precise threat stemmed from mosquitoes or miasmas seemed to matter little to the prophylactic method or to the curative process: segregation, hydrotherapy, and climatology remained the instruments of choice.

The endurance of climatic determinism in the twentieth century is especially apparent in guidebooks and how-to manuals to the tropics — veritable "hygienic" but also moral "catechisms."[123] In a 1938 prescriptive volume for French women considering colonial emigration, the doctor Serge Abbatucci stated matter-of-factly that "it is widely recognized that whites can only live as temporary hosts in the tropics, and then only if they abide by strict hygienic rules."[124] In the same tome, M. Diénert, the secretary general of the International Association of Hydrologers (or hydrotherapists), wrote of the importance of maintaining strict rules of behavior in the colonies: "At first, such precautions are very important, for there is a period of acclimatization during which European habits and tastes subsist; they have to be abandoned little by little, or at least accommodated to the necessities of climate."[125] Here, the notion of going Creole remained strong. Europeans, by virtue of living overseas, would eventually have to accommodate to climate, both culturally and racially. One of the best ways to achieve balance during this *accommodation*, or "small acclimatization," it was generally agreed, was to take a *cure thermale* or *climatique* — either back home if one could afford it or in the colonies themselves.

The effect of the acclimatization debate on preventative and curative practices like water and altitude therapies was profound. Climatology and hydrotherapy were enrolled to act directly on the body, by effecting a potent detoxification of fragile French organs. Some doctors recommended them for treating "colonial anemia," others to temper *cachéxie paludéenne*, a term designating the ongoing symptoms and consequences of malaria, and still others to deal with nagging amoebic infections. Some doctors justified the use of colonial spas more plainly as a way of achieving reimmersion in a French milieu. In a word, water and altitude cures seemed to hold out a way of maintaining Frenchness, of assuaging the effects of acclimatization in a tropical setting, and of forestalling degeneration or creolization. In the delicate balancing act of colonial settlement, highland resorts and spas would prove critical.

Negotiating and Applying Climatic Theories

Precisely how did the ebbs and flows of acclimatization theory affect colonial practices? Unlike Germany, where Virchow warned of the folly of colonial settlement as anathema to Aryan constitutions and where colonial expansion was limited, France had, since 1870, launched a massive new wave of colonial conquest. France established a protectorate over Tonkin in 1874. A year later, Savorgnan de Brazza began travels that would culminate in the claiming of large tracts of equatorial Africa (in and around Congo) for France. In 1880 and 1881, the French Third Republic annexed vast areas of the South Pacific. In 1881, it declared war in Tunisia with a view toward establishing a protectorate. In 1884, it annexed Cambodia and Cochinchina. Between 1888 and 1900, it launched its conquest of Dahomey and of western Sudan (Mali, Burkina Fasso, and Niger). In 1895, France invaded Madagascar.[126] This unprecedented surge of expansion involved several waves of migration to the colonies: first soldiers and sailors, then a substantial colonial administration, settlers, and entrepreneurs. Their families soon followed. As Philip Curtin and William Cohen have noted, the initial military conquests were undertaken at a considerable cost of lives, with French morbidity rates from disease ranging between 61 per thousand in the Tunisia campaign in 1881, 225 per thousand in the Sudanese campaign of that same year, and 332 per thousand in the Madagascar campaign of 1895.[127]

The concerns raised by biological racists who had opposed French colonial settlement in the nineteenth century seemed confirmed by these very high morbidity rates. If anything, as Cohen remarks, the rates were actually rising between 1870 and 1895, although Curtin cautions that less spectacular "barrack deaths" and peacetime deaths of European troops in the colonies declined in the second half of the nineteenth century.[128] As a result, the enthusiasm elicited by this wave of colonial expansion was tempered by profound fears. Even advocates of acclimatization like George Treille conceded that an elaborate regimen of hygienic commandments, countermeasures, and prophylaxes would need to be followed in order to guarantee the safeguard of the colonizers in the tropics. Unlike France's first great colonial experiment in the sixteenth and seventeenth centuries, largely conducted in colder climes, this second colonial wave, entirely directed at the tropical world, would be controlled and monitored by legions of hygienists and specialists of tropical medicine (though as Curtin argues they often proved incapable of applying recent medical breakthroughs in the field). A synthesis of sorts emerged out of the acclimatization debate. The difficulties of achieving acclimatization were acknowledged, but political imperatives, France's so-called civilizing mission, and its necessity to assert itself outside of Europe after 1870, outweighed those obstacles.[129] In this sense, the concerns raised by Thibaut and Boudin only served to heighten the medicalization of the French colonial enterprise.

Following successive waves of attacks on the ideals of creolization and acclimatability and the mounting loss of life among French troops in the colonies, climatic determinism had gained considerable ascendancy in the late nineteenth century — reinforced and recast in the late nineteenth century by new racial doctrines. Still, pragmatic considerations, especially France's colonial expansion after 1870, meant that a certain measure of accommodation, if not acclimatization, had to be inscribed into colonial medicine. The British faced a similar dilemma, described as follows by Thomas Metcalf: "Europeans took up residence in the tropics at their peril. Nevertheless, once committed to the rule of India, the British devised . . . strategies thought to insure a greater degree of survival in its climate."[130] In other words, while it was widely believed throughout Europe in the late nineteenth century that Europeans could not survive unaffected in the tropics, the hope remained that climatic oases or other "artificial environments" like hill stations or hydromineral spas might make longer stays possible. Such supposed cures could spell the difference between the manageable small and the more daunting big acclimatization.

To those still convinced of the possibility of settlement and acclimatization, microclimates and a strict regimen of precautions raised the possibility that

Boudin's, Thibaut's, and Virchow's extreme theories about the impossibility of tropical settlement could be disproved. Lémure held out hope for localized settlement even after the terrible mortality rates sustained by French troops during the conquest of Madagascar in 1895. Like Treille, Lémure based his cautious optimism on historical precedents: "Very near France, under a more temperate clime [than Madagascar's], we know the cost of the first phase of colonization. In Algeria, the possibility of acclimatization was questioned by Boudin [in his *Traité de géographie médicale* (1857)]. It took more than forty years for us to even hope. The aptitude of European races to live and proliferate in the more salubrious parts of Algeria was finally demonstrated on the day when general mortality amongst settlers diminished, and the number of births surpassed that of deaths."[131] Lémure relied on geoclimatic quirks—the potential offered by microclimates in the colonies—to disprove the racio-climatic contentions of Thibaut, Boudin, and Virchow.

The Logic of Colonial Hill Stations and Spas

Alexandre Kermorgant, an expert on health stations, encapsulated how the synthesis position colored colonial readings of topography. In 1899 he wrote, "Man is like a plant transported to a foreign soil, and the greatest pains must be taken in order to acclimate to that new soil. If hill stations are useful to the weakened in our own climes, how much more useful they are amongst victims of anemia in our overseas possessions."[132] A century-long debate was thus distilled. Humans were like a tropical plant, but acclimatization remained a remote possibility, especially if conditions could be doctored. In other words, regular immersion into an artificial environment, be it a hill station or a spa, could tilt the delicate balance back in favor of the feasibility of empire. Far from constituting a simple luxury, such cures were thus framed as absolute necessities in colonial settings. They rested squarely on a transformative mindset: if the colonial body could be altered by the tropics, then spas and microclimates could hopefully be marshaled to bring it back to normal.

Fin de siècle colonial doctors channeled the cult of temperateness into a quest for altitude in the tropics, contending that both spas and heights could combat pathologies associated with the "torrid zone." Curtin has dubbed this phenomenon "the panacea of seeking higher altitudes."[133] Again, these trends would carry over into the twentieth century. The volume *La vie aux colonies* (1938) suggested two ways of coping with the tropics: staying there as seldom as possible and "seeking, in tropical milieux, highland or seaside stations, capable of achieving climatic effects on the body, so as to remind it of temperate climes. Here, whites can take refuge during the hottest months."[134] As late as 1947, specialized guides for aspiring French colonialists admonished neophytes to acquire a colonial helmet (that great cork insulator against the tropics), to hire a team of domestics upon arrival, and to frequent hill stations, whose "pure air . . . cool nights, and waters will both help one regain good health and boost morale."[135] Free French General François-Joseph Jean Ingold learned the following lesson from the experience of the Second World War in Africa: "Non-essential personnel (women, children, NCOs) . . . must be sent to hill stations . . . There are too many children's graves in colonial cemeteries because we have not sufficiently followed this cardinal rule of general interest."[136]

Supposedly scientific findings about altitudinal immunity from malaria and yellow fever in particular had been instrumental in conditioning what could be called a scramble for altitude in the nineteenth century. But according to the colonial doctor Georges Dryepont, writing at the turn of the twentieth century, such a scramble was actually as old as colonialism itself: "Ever since the occupation of tropical lands by Europeans, we had remarked that some . . . regions enjoyed relative healthfulness. We strove to uncover what the causes of this privileged situation might be, in order to apply to other lands the fruits of this research, and in order to discover locales where one might find the same advantages."[137] Thus conceived as an element of common sense in a struggle for survival in settings for which the white race had not evolutionarily adapted, the quest for altitude became entrenched in the canon of tropical medicine.

Although the British had established as early as the 1830s the legendary hill stations at Simla and Ootacamund in India, the French combined the hill station model with the hydrotherapeutic spa (see chapter 2). The spas covered in this book are therefore both *villes thermales* and *climatiques* — in other words they claimed to provide both water and climate cures. To be sure, where warm springs and cool highlands failed to meet, French colonial doctors made do with one or the other. Hence the hill stations of Dalat, Tam-Dao, Bokor, and Sa-Pa in French Indochina and the high-altitude resorts of Ifrane in Morocco and Dschang in Cameroon bear greater affinities with the dry British Simla model. In Tunisia, lacking a high-altitude and mineral water resort, French colonial doctors utilized the seaside spring waters at Korbous near Tunis. Korbous, however, was still considered a station *climatique* and *hydrominérale*, because *climatisme* encompasses not just altitude but any variation in climate. As a seaside resort swathed in gentle Mediterranean breezes and soaked by a hydromineral spring, Korbous could still lay claim to both therapies. By the same token, Vichy qualified as a dual cure because to settlers in Africa it offered healthful springs *and* a temperate French climate.

Wherever possible, then, *climatisme* and *thermalisme* were combined. In the words of the malaria specialist Marcel Léger, writing in 1930, "*Crénothérapie* (hydrotherapy) . . . has a prominent place next to climate therapy in the treatment of malaria."[138] The twinning of climatology and hydrotherapy might seem surprising to readers unfamiliar with French medicine. But in France, *climatisme* and *thermalisme* (hydrotherapy, also known as *crénothérapie hydrologie* and *hydrothérapie*) were inseparable and remain so. The Institut d'hydrologie et de climatologie was founded in 1913 and served as a prestigious laboratory and graduate school in both sciences.[139] The *Commission permanente des stations hydrominérales et climatiques* was established in 1907 to advise the government on the creation and development of both high-altitude and mineral water resorts.[140] The main journal devoted to these sciences is still entitled *La presse thermale et climatique*, and the main hydrotherapy association is still known as the Fédération thermale et climatique française. George Weisz notes that between 1923 and 1933, the Institut d'hydrologie, a hydrotherapists' organization, equipped some twenty climatological stations.[141] Scientific congresses dealt with the two sciences in tandem. Ever since the nineteenth century, mineral water, altitude, and to a large extent beach cures were seen as complicit, if not actually synonymous.[142] Legitimized by two sciences, highland hydromineral spas sprang up wherever the colonial landscape provided the two necessary ingredients, spring water and cooler microclimates.

CHAPTER 2

Colonial Hydrotherapy

"YOU CAN'T BEAR IT ANY LONGER. THE AFRICAN CLI-
mate has been sapping you slowly. You need to reinvigorate yourself. Go to Vichy . . . Your blood is poisoned. It
is carrying enough toxins to mine your health and make
life miserable. Beware! Against the poison that is Africa,
there is but one antidote: *Vichy!*"[1] Far from inventing some
far-fetched new angle for Vichy waters, this 1924 magazine ad played upon widespread beliefs. The tropics, as we
saw in chapter 1, were still considered a climatic poison
well into the twentieth century. Already in the first half of
the nineteenth century, hydrotherapy had positioned itself
as one of the few countermeasures to their degenerative
and debilitating effects. The connection was so strong, the
equation of Vichy as antidote to the tropics so firm, that
the town of Vichy owed part of its rapid prosperity and
development to colonial expansion — much as La Rochelle
and Nantes had in centuries past. Indeed, as we shall see
in chapter 7, the rise of Vichy coincided with the conquest
of Algeria in 1830. In France, hydrotherapy thus emerged
as inseparable from empire. To trace this unexpected symbiosis, one must first decode some of the trappings of the
singular science known in France as *thermalisme*.

Hydrotherapy's Many Faces

The history of hydrotherapy is as long as it is virtually universal. Water cures and other rites tied to mineral waters have been practiced for centuries and in many cases millennia in cultures as different as Korea, England, Japan, Greece, Germany, Italy, New Zealand, and Turkey.[2] In seeking to establish *their* science of hydrotherapy in the colonies, the French encountered a variety of radically other indigenous beliefs tied to mineral springs. These ranged from different modes of balneology, or water immersion treatments, to the assignment of spiritual meanings to spring waters. In this sense, French colonial hydrotherapy represents merely one facet of a much broader practice.

I take French hydrotherapy to include more than merely *thermalisme*, which is, strictly speaking, the act of immersion in warm or hot waters. This book will consider hydrotherapy to encompass such bathing, of course, but also a host of other practices, including drinking mineral waters at the source (and to a lesser extent the bottled mineral water business, whose connections to hydrotherapy are manifest), mud baths and wraps, pulverizations and other intense shower devices, and a number of more intrusive practices (predominantly rectal and vaginal), broadly defined by the French as *douches ascendantes*.[3] Each of these — and a myriad of permutations on each practice — makes up the vast spectrum of French hydrotherapy. The hydrotherapy examined here, it will become readily apparent, bears very few affinities with the amorphous modern-day concept of the spa as beauty salon or new age relaxation center.

Beyond pure mechanics, the practice of French hydrotherapy in many ways eludes facile classification. It combines the roles of pilgrimage, sometimes taking on religious overtones (one thinks of parallels between Vichy and Lourdes), with an element of tourism, a social function, and, in its nineteenth-century French form, a quintessentially medicalized and structured regimen.[4]

The notion of return is vital to the ritualistic dimension of hydrotherapy. By this I mean not merely the idea of attracting return customers — which any resort seeks — but also that of taking a cure on a regular, extended, and repeated basis and in many cases of coming home for a cure or of making the site of a cure home. Cures, until recently, were believed to take a matter of weeks or months rather than days (new packages at Vichy and elsewhere are now breaking with this tradition, offering short fitness, wellness, and beauty treatments). For instance, the standard length of a Vichy drinking cure was fixed at twenty-one days.[5] This particularity sets *thermalisme* apart in the realm of tourism.[6] The *baigneur* or the *curiste*, as the French practitioner of hydrotherapy is known, sets down roots or in many cases actively seeks rootedness in an almost mystical return to the elements.[7] In 1935, the French Conseil national économique, noting the general resilience of hydrotherapy compared to the rest of France's tourist industry during the Great Depression, concluded, "The tourist is often a vagabond; on the other hand the bather who has tasted the benefits of a certain thermal cure, will return to find his same doctor, his same masseur, in a word, *his* spring."[8] The *curiste*, in short, was considered less fickle and more rooted than the average *touriste*. In the colonial context, hydrotherapy's promise of rootedness became all the more critical. Both on location in the colonies and back in the metropole colonials sought above all a reimmersion into France.

The inherent similarity of spa layouts only reinforced their perceived Frenchness in the colonies. In this respect, French spas projected a familiarity verging on uniformity, whether they were in Madagascar or the Pyrenees. Although architectural and decorative styles differed immensely, the overall plan of *villes d'eaux* and even of drinking and bathing facilities resembled variations of a single template, often Roman in inspiration. This uniformity increased markedly in the mid-nineteenth century as lodgings and balneological amenities were separated, and the spa inn was replaced by an imposing, though formulaic, public building. As early as 1840, Gustave Flaubert commented, "All spa establishments are alike: the drinking fountain, the baths, the eternal salon for balls, each can be found in every spa in the world."[9] In a colonial context, the production of the familiar would prove all the more critical. In the delicate balancing act between cosmopolitanism and particularism, spas seemed to offer both, reminding *curistes* of France under the arcades of a Moorish bathhouse, for example.

Nineteenth- and twentieth-century European spas had at their core a series of disciplining and regimenting functions. The rituals of drinking from standardized cups, of immersing oneself for prescribed lengths of time over a prescribed series of weeks, of subjecting the body to a number of painful intrusions, pulverizations, frictions, and other discomforts speak to *thermalisme*'s regularizing dimension. Douglas Mackaman shows that in the 1830s doctors began to control the prescription of waters, making it "virtually illegal" for anyone to bathe or drink at a spa without prior medical consultation. The doctor, in other words, drew up a line of conduct, a purportedly "sane and regular regime" for the would-be *curiste*.[10] Mackaman deduces from this extreme regimentation that French spas answered the desiderata of an emerging bourgeois sensitivity in the nineteenth century.[11] In a study of seventeenth-century French spas, L. W. Brockliss made a similar argument: the suffering, boredom, and formulary of water cures were endured by bathers because they were considered at once an essential regulating influence and a token of status.[12] I contend that in the nineteenth century, spas also found a strong resonance in colonial culture, specifically in settler and administrative circles. Expatriated as they were, their return to France—or to the closest replica thereof—could assume the triple values of structure, necessity, and leisure when the imperative of hydrotherapy was invoked. The collective nature of the mass seasonal migration, whether to Vichy or Vittel in France or to Korbous, Salazie, Dolé-les-Bains, or Antsirabe in the colonies, no doubt made the prospect of hydrotherapy all the more appealing.

George Weisz has stressed how in France "mineral waters constituted a quasi-public form of healing."[13] Mackaman, meanwhile, has cautioned that late-nineteenth- and twentieth-century French doctors sought precisely to individualize spa medicine—cloistering the body in highly segregated and rationalized compartments (not dissimilar from contemporaneous prison schemes).[14] The reason for this divergence lies at least in part in the mode of hydrotherapy under consideration: drinking cures involved days of queuing, strolling, and hence socializing, whereas bathing chambers were indeed highly compartmentalized after the mid-nineteenth century.[15] The spa town itself was a site of socialization unmatched in any other medical therapy. The medical geography of *villes d'eaux* made French spa towns alternately sites of networking, of camaraderie, and of constant "investigation of each other's social credentials."[16] Whether through competition or complicity, the colonial, like the bourgeois, actively defined himself or herself at spas. Local newspapers proudly announced new arrivals at the spa, and in the metropole local *Listes des étrangers* identified all spa newcomers (out-of-towners rather than foreigners as its title suggests) on a weekly or biweekly basis. As we shall see, petty quarrels dominated some aspects of life at French colonial spas. Nevertheless, the act of collectively setting out to take the waters in a conquered territory—or of collectively migrating back home for a cure—conflated by its very nature considerations of power and sociability.

In her analysis of the Italian spa of Salsomaggiore, Federica Tamarozzi has identified an important feature of spa towns. She notes the emergence of a " 'mythology of the quotidian,' the fruit of a particular conception of hydrotherapy, linked to the exceptional unity of the site and the actions inherent in the nature of water towns."[17] Nowhere is geography as relevant to medicine as in hydrotherapy. Mackaman speaks of the "didactics of milieu" in relation to spas.[18] In a sense, mineral springs were seen as exerting a kind of mesological impact on patients, conditioning them through their mineral contents. Indeed, hydrotherapy's restorative potential rested upon the ambient: ambient waters, ambient milieu, ambient climate, and so on. This is precisely why spas in the colonies were seen as presenting vast potential. If they featured the same chemical features as their metropolitan counterparts, then their effects must be similar. It followed that they must also share the same magnetic attraction, the same social dimension, and the same transformative qualities. In the words of the hydrotherapist Philippe Hérault, writing in 1899, "If the therapeutic value of waters is generally determined by the specific qualities of the waters, by climate, and by the temperature and the site where they emerge, it is mostly in the tropics that the influence of milieu becomes accentuated and takes on a capital importance for the treatment of patients."[19] In other words, if mineral springs could prove transformatively beneficial for French people in France, then they could assuredly perform even greater services for French settlers and administrators in the colonies. If properly administered, they could stave off degeneration, disease, and loss of Frenchness. So long as the surroundings could be controlled—and what more rooted, ritualized, and controlled a setting than spas?—then the colonizer's body could be saved.

The Dialectics of Tropical Hydrotherapy

How exactly were mineral waters understood to treat colonial bodies or constitutions? Weisz has outlined two basic ways in which mineral waters were believed to operate in twentieth-century France: "[They] could be seen as transforming the chemical composition of the internal fluids or organs or they could be thought of as a stimulus to the body's natural tendency to heal itself."[20] Both logics were indisputably present in colonial hydrotherapy. One more should be added, in relation to the treatment of tropical disease: the idea that a water cure could deliberately and calculatedly bring out latent malarial fevers or tropical dysentery. Hydromineral inducement was thought to operate as follows: "Amongst malarial patients, even those who have carried the disease for some time, even a short hydromineral treatment can bring out bouts of fever, in the form of a *crise thermale*. Quinine tends to alleviate them, and often they then disappear for good. This same temporarily reactivating action of a cure at Vichy can be turned to very good use in the case of latent, nagging dysenteries. Amoebae tend to reappear [through hydrotherapy] and the judicious use of the drug 'emietine' brings a complete and definitive cure."[21] As late as 1967 a doctor noted that the waters of Encausse-les-Thermes in the Pyrenees, used specifically to combat malaria, could likewise make latent malarial fevers resurface. But, he added, "it is certain that this bout of fever, provoked by the water treatment, will be the last. After one or at most two cures, no relapse will ever occur again."[22] And at the spa of La Bourboule, near Vichy, H. Verdalle held that "a La Bourboule cure often triggers one or two malarial fevers. . . . This is how the waters work against all troubles, traumas, or diseases. They awaken the latent malaria. But these fevers are, in general, mild. They are the last spasms of a defeated enemy."[23] The logic of this technique involved using potent mineral waters to bring pernicious tropical disease out of hiding for a direct and final confrontation with French medicine. The chronic, insidious, and nagging nature of many so-called colonial afflictions no doubt shaped the fantasy of harnessing the powers of mineral waters in such a manner. Mineral springs were imagined to be hounds that could drive the beast out of its lair, so that it might finally be slain.[24]

The more historically complete answer to how French hydrotherapy was believed to act upon tropical disease involves both a complex periodization and a constant: the certainty that specific waters were efficacious in treating colonial ills. Pre-nineteenth-century treatises on mineral water cures offer some general insights into the formation of hydromineral epistemologies. In particular, Sieur Cottereau du Clos's study in 1675, commissioned by the Académie royale des sciences, established a key concept, oft repeated afterward, namely, that mineral waters provided cures "for some otherwise resistant diseases, which do not respond to ordinary treatments." Where those "ordinary" remedies had failed, wrote du Clos, hydrotherapy promised to work through a "washing of the innards."[25] The purgative and cleansing logics to fighting colonial ills would last well into the twentieth century, as would the idea that hydrotherapy could function where other standard remedies had failed. This last notion would prove especially relevant in the treatment of diseases like malaria, whose workings remained largely mysterious until the turn of the twentieth century.

The nineteenth century saw some continuity, especially with respect to the questions of cleansing and alternative therapies for nagging and mysterious ailments. Auguste Durand de Lunel's treatise of 1862 on the use of Vichy waters in the treatment of "intermittent fevers," however, reveals a new approach. Durand de Lunel, the longtime doctor at Vichy's military hospital, was persuaded of Vichy's impact on sanguinity: "By comparing the analysis [of Vichy waters and blood], one finds a remarkable affinity between the inorganic composition of the two: carbon, phosphate, sodium chloride, iron oxide, lime, which gives blood serum its alkaline properties, as it does to Vichy water. And lo and behold, this sodium is predominant in Vichy waters. Well, the result is that as soon as the mineral water proves more alkaline than blood serum, it will, upon being absorbed by the body, reinforce in the blood serum the inherent properties of the sodas and particularly their alkaline virtues."[26] Durand de Lunel then proceeded to explain that Vichy's waters possessed two powers derived from their alkaline nature: physical and chemical powers, able, respectively, to emit an electric charge on the body and to penetrate organic tissues.[27] Delivered to their target in this manner, mineral waters could enter into a kind of symbiosis with blood. If one could find mineral waters capable of remedying or replacing the very elements sapped by the tropics, then it stood to reason that such waters could combat tropical ailments. And, Durand de Lunel argued, Vichy's fit the bill.

One of Durand's anonymous colleagues, writing in 1859, arrived at similar conclusions but enlarged the scope of Vichy's hydromineral purview. "Mineral waters," he wrote, "represent a marvelously adapted medicine to [tropical ills]." He noted three distinct ways in which they could recalibrate European bodies: "by reconstituting the blood, by reestablishing digestive activity and functions, and by resolving abdominal engorgement."[28] In 1857, Max Durand-Fardel explained in his *Traité thérapeutique des eaux minérales* how Vichy waters acted upon "engorgement of the liver resulting from intermittent fevers or malarial miasmas, or the *cachéxie paludéenne* that one often sees in those who return from the Levant, from India, North, or West Africa."[29] The liver constituted the central fetish of colonial hydrotherapists. And as we shall see, Vichy soon became known throughout Europe as the prime spa for the treatment of hepatic symptoms.

In the 1860s, the second facet of Durand de Lunel's theory was gaining favor as an explanation for the efficacy of mineral waters. By 1878, Durand-Fardel deemed that "only electric phenomena can explain the molecular changes brought about by Vichy waters."[30]

In many respects, these nineteenth-century codes, criteria, and concerns proved remarkably enduring in the twentieth century, seemingly unaffected by the Kochian, Pasteurian, and Rossian turns. J. Gandelin's account (1911) of the reasons for Vichy's efficacy against tropical disease speaks to these continuities. He wrote, "Vichy's alkaline medication is clearly a stimulant . . . It is a reconstituting and tonic agent. It combats through a substantive action passive or chronic engorgement of the liver, and engorgements of the spleen in colonials living in the tropics. [After a Vichy cure] the circulation of blood is more intense, the capillary veins are dilated. The blood is more alkaline and more fluid. Exchanges are more active in the structure of tissues."[31] Vichy water was still believed to condition the blood and decongest the liver through a tonic stimulation.

Paradigm shifts often hide some very basic recycling of key concepts, like the purgative or cleansing theory of mineral water ingestion. In 1908, Edmond Vidal returned to the classic seventeenth-century explanation of Vichy water's cleansing potential. He refined his hypothesis, bringing it up-to-date as follows: "Vichy water, absorbed after fasting, passes from the intestine into the valve. . . . This hypertension is transmitted to the organ tributary to the said valve, namely, the liver, whose irrigation is increased, and function is regularized. Thanks to its isotonic qualities, Vichy waters, whose salinity are of approximately 7 grams per liter, penetrate under pressure into cells, where they undertake a veritable cleansing, taking with them toxins . . . which after having entered the liver, circulated throughout the bloodstream."[32] If anything, modern cleansing theories seem to have successfully drawn upon previous humor-based or purgative models. Thus as late as 1924, Augustin Alquier, a colonial military doctor practicing at Vichy explained, "A Vichy cure is the treatment par excellence for . . . malaria. . . . First of all, rest and a return to France are necessary. One must modify the humeral system through a hydromineral cure, and that is when one should go to Vichy. . . . The cure at Vichy works through a complex mechanism — a cyto-cleansing or literally a laundering of our organs and our humors, rendered possible by the isotony of Vichy's waters."[33] Here, well into the twentieth century, ancient humor paradigms intertwine with complicated and largely unexplained theories involving the hydrotherapeutic purging of toxins. George Vigarello reminds us of the dually archaic and modern qualities of a related phenomenon, bottled mineral water. That which purifies in such a manner, writes Vigarello, harkens back to humoral bleeding or purging, while simultaneously relying on modern biochemistry.[34]

One more continuity should be stressed: the timing and justification for choosing hydrotherapy over other treatments. Du Clos's observation that *thermalisme* proved effective where all the other healing arts had failed finds special resonance in the modern French colonial context. Water cures were sometimes used as a primary treatment, sometimes as an adjuvant for another therapy, and sometimes as a last resort. The case of novelist Marguerite Duras's father fell into this last category. Henri Donnadieu was diagnosed with a severe gastrointestinal disorder, attributed to his many years of teaching in Indochina. He was repatriated to France alone in April 1921, then treated in Marseille's military hospital after the monthlong sea voyage to the metropole. In Marseille, he underwent a slew of unsuccessful treatments, whereupon medics decided to send him to Plombières, the spa specializing in gastrointestinal ills associated with the tropics. He perished there in December 1921 — and the spa's failure to issue a death certificate to his family left behind in Indochina would become the basis for the Duras family's misfortune.[35]

In other instances, one sees marked changes in the explanations for precisely how mineral waters delivered their curing effects to the body. Each generation of doctors seems to have set about explaining Vichy's efficacy against tropical pathologies through the latest scientific formulae — even while recycling older theories and grafting new models upon them. The principle of hydrotherapeutic effectiveness itself was rarely, if ever, called into question. Experimentation, in other words, skirted a single certainty: the efficacy of water cures. Over time, wildly different explanations were introduced to explain it: humor and bile changes, cleansing effects, chemical alterations, alkalinity, electricity, salinity, and soon radioactivity.

In this way, even when new variables, paradigms, and therapies gained favor in the twentieth century, they seemed only to confirm preexisting conclusions about the efficacy of hydrotherapy in combating tropical pathologies. Radio-activity was thus called upon to account for the effectiveness of some waters in treating tropical diseases. In 1913, only three years after Marie Curie isolated radium, the Pasteur Institute in Madagascar began speculating on the connections between radiation, mineral waters, and healthfulness. Its report for that year notes, "The waters of Antsirabe, through their abundant rare gasses, are rich in radio-active emanations. . . . This explains: A) the general attenuation of 'imported' microbes, and the total absence of bacteria in Antsirabe's waters. B) the efficacy of the *cure d'air* in these regions, rich in radio-active emissions, and at Antsirabe in particular. C) the very real efficacy of immersion in baths at Antsirabe against gout, rheumatism and so on." [36] A decade later, Paul Gouzien and Charles Moureu again marveled at the high levels of radioactivity emanating from Antsirabe's mineral waters. [37] This budding new science conferred the same panacean qualities to mineral springs as had previous sciences. This time, the explanation for efficacy came from an all-encompassing agent, radioactivity. Radioactivity, reasoned the authorities at Madagascar's Pasteur Institute, could account for the success of both *thermalisme* and *climatisme* (identified above as *cure d'air*). If anything, far from discrediting a practice descended from the early modern humor paradigm, new sciences like radio-activity seemed to confer newfound legitimacy upon it.

Cures for Colonials

Naturally, not all waters were believed to treat colonial ailments. By the nine-teenth century, hydrotherapy had become highly specialized, to the point that individual spas in France and in the colonies catered to diverse tropical patholo-gies, not to mention nontropically specific ones like gout, diabetes, dermato-logical ailments, and so on. [38] Today, French spas are branching out into new and revealing sectors like automobile accident recovery (Lamalou-les-Bains) and obesity (Brides-les-Bains, Châtel-Guyon, and Capvern-les-Bains). The target of cures seems to reflect the zeitgeist. It should therefore hardly come as a surprise that at the apogee of empire, spa promoters took aim at tropical diseases. Certain spa entrepreneurs certainly found it lucrative to do so. The French spa industry also featured many directly state-operated *thermes*.[39] At Vichy, the state leased the management of the main springs to a *compagnie fermière*, whose astute managers began targeting colonials in the early nineteenth century. Although it dominated the sector, Vichy was not alone in expanding into the tropical disease business in the nineteenth century. In 1851, Constantin James identified a series of other *stations thermales* specializing in what he termed revealingly "the diseases of Algeria." These included La Bourboule and Vittel on the French mainland and Orezza in Corsica.[40] All would maintain strong colonial connections well into the twentieth century, vying to draw customers away from Vichy.

In their remarkable guide to spas for colonials (*Le bréviaire thermal des coloniaux*, 1923), Serge Abbatucci and J. J. Matignon, practitioners of both tropical medicine and hydrotherapy, explained that Frenchmen in the tropics faced three menaces: "the ethnic threat, the pathological threat, and the climate's threat." Hydromineral spas, French doctors argued, could answer all three perils. Since the eighteenth century, medical treatises had grappled with achieving a "fundamental balance" for whites in the colonies.[41] The liver, the enduring fixation of French medicine, was understood as the key to regulating this balance. Nowhere was this organ supposedly more damaged than in the tropics; nowhere was it allegedly better cured than at Vichy. Admittedly, at one level, doctors were of course responding to perfectly real diseases: malaria did ravage the French colonial corps, and modern medicine confirms that malaria circulates via the liver after having entered the bloodstream.

A medical syllogism contributed to conferring legitimacy on French colonial hydrotherapy. Its popular expression was plainly summarized by Abbatucci and Matignon: "Vichy = Liver; Liver = Colonies; Vichy = Colonies."[42] In order to fully grasp the implications of this syllogism, one should remember that the liver, already the fetish of French medicine, was viewed from the eighteenth century as the organ most vulnerable to the tropics.[43] This theory had not found its way just into popular colonial culture; it was also firmly embedded in the mantra of modern tropical science. An important tropical medical manual, written in 1938 by the Belgian colonial doctor Clément Chesterman, still insisted, "As a rule, one should always think of the possibility of an amebic infection of the liver in white patients who have seen a marked decline of their health in the tropics."[44] Abbatucci and Matignon shared this belief: "Each malarial fever outbreak affects the liver and spleen: this is why these two organs must be carefully supervised in any malarial patient."[45] From this assertion, it was but a small step to endorsing hydrotheraputic *cures*—most notably Vichy's, which were seen as having especially beneficial effects upon the liver. Soon, colonial mimesis took over, and scores of spas in the colonies themselves came to be seen as analogous to Vichy. Abbatucci and Matignon prescribed an immediate water cure for any liver ailment resulting from tropical disease, for "the more one waits, the more difficult it will be for the liver to respond favorably to the action of hydrotherapy."[46] Thus legitimized by early-twentieth-century medicine, hydrotherapy, like altitude therapy, seemed to promise a heretofore elusive remedy against diseases contracted in the colonies.

The need for colonials to take water cures soon became as entrenched in the French colonial imagination as the quest for highland breezes and the importance of the ubiquitous colonial helmet.[47] This normalization is revealed once again by Abbatucci and Matignon. They listed three prescriptive treatments for whites in the tropics: "a proper diet, and a moderate and temperate climate. But the very best course of action, by far, is to take a hydromineral cure."[48] A detailed list of recommended spas followed, including La Bourboule in central France for malaria, Vichy for afflictions of the liver, and Plombières for gastrointestinal ailments linked to the tropics. Although spas in the colonies were not on the same scale of grandeur and comfort, the two doctors did deign to list many of them. Roughly half of their study is dedicated to spas in North Africa, Madagascar, Réunion, and the Caribbean. In 1938, Abbatucci concluded that the tropics represented an actual "climatic poison," one best cured at Vichy. Though Vichy was "by far the spa most frequented by colonials,"[49] it was certainly not the only spa to claim this specialization—a specialization that was becoming increasingly lucrative in the age of empire.

Balancing Twin Therapies and the European Context

In the nineteenth century, the French were not alone in utilizing water and altitude cures to combat malaria, although they seem to have clung to this therapy longer than others. A Belgian doctor wrote in 1865 of alleviating "intermittent fevers" through hydrotherapy at the military hospital in Brussels.[50] One Dr. Dobieszewski, a Polish doctor at Marienbad, then in the Austro-Hungarian empire, boasted in 1889 of his spa's efficacy against malarial fevers. In his lecture to the Société de médecine pratique in Paris in 1889, Dobieszewski asked a fundamental question about the balance between climatic and hydrotherapeutic therapies in the treatment of malaria. He began with a mesological postulate: in order to stem malarial fevers, one had to leave the place where one had contracted malaria. He then pondered: "Is it sufficient to place the [malarial] patient in a mountainous climate, without any additional treatment, to cure malaria? My observations on this subject lead me to answer that a stay in the mountains in and of itself is never sufficient to completely overcome malaria, and especially its side-effects."[51] The complementary treatment he advocated was, of course, hydrotherapy, specifically in waters containing soda and magnesium — both present in high levels at Marienbad, not surprisingly. Far from constituting some homeopathic curiosity, the combined action of hydrotherapy and climatology was thus considered one of the main weapons of the European medical arsenal against malaria.

One of the case studies Dobieszewski presented suggests that late-nineteenth-century French colonial patients traveled beyond the confines of France and its empire in search of hydrotherapeutic cures to their colonial ills. A certain Hubert V. had first contracted malaria when he had been posted as an attaché to the French embassy in Constantinople. He suffered a major recurrence in his next post, in Tonkin (northern Indochina). After returning to Paris, he was sent to Marienbad by a Doctor Faur-Miller. There, doctors found that his liver had swollen by three centimeters. His spleen was likewise engorged. After four weeks of mud and water baths, he was "completely cured." His organs had all returned to their normal size, and he had in fact been stationed back in the colonies, to Algeria more precisely. If he could survive in this malarial zone without recurrence, reasoned his doctor, then his cure at Marienbad must have been thoroughly effective.[52] Still, Marienbad could not count on British or French colonial customers alone, especially after the Great War. And as malaria was gradually controlled in continental Europe, Marienbad's malarial purview waned; in France, conversely, one registers the meteoric rise of imperial/tropical hydrotherapy with the new post-1870 imperial élan.

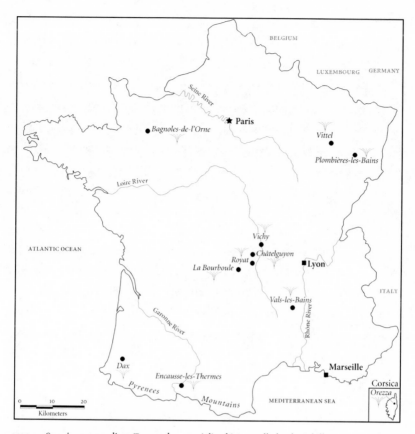

MAP 1. Spas in metropolitan France that specialized in so-called colonial ills.

Mandating, Classifying, and Prescribing Spas in France and the Empire

Mineral water cures were not taken lightly. The French colonial administration went to amazing lengths to both codify and rationalize spa treatments and to ensure that its functionaries were able to find *ressourcement* and *cures* at spas on a regular basis. In southern French Indochina (Cochinchine) between 1892 and 1896, the administration, facing the impracticality of sending patients to distant French spas, sent sick colonial officials to take the waters in Japan.[53] Hydrotherapy was thus seen not just as necessary, but vital, for French colonials. Where it proved difficult or absent, as in Indochina, it would have to be sought elsewhere—even, if need be, in culturally alien surroundings where hydrotherapy was practiced quite differently.

The spa market was as open as it was competitive. Not only did spas in the metropole and the colonies vie for business from colonial administrators, but French and foreign spas also competed for "colonial" clients, as the examples of Japan and Marienbad suggest. In the twentieth century, legislation was introduced to govern different types of cures: on the one hand repatriation cures to take the waters at Vichy, Vittel, La Bourboule, Encausse-les-Thermes, or other accredited spas in France proper, and on the other hand shorter leaves for the purposes of taking the waters or rest in the highlands on location in the colony. In 1924, Paul Gouzien summarized some of the commercial tensions pitting French against foreign spas and, increasingly, metropolitan against colonial ones: "We must try, on the one hand, to favor by all possible means, the exodus of foreigners and wealthy natives from our empire to our metropolitan thermal stations, thereby bringing to us part of the clientele that . . . used to frequent the 'Kurhaus' palaces . . . of central Europe. On the other hand we must not neglect our colonial thermal domain that is henceforth part of our national heritage, and it is now necessary to encourage scientific investigations of spas that seem so promising in these new distant Frances."[54] Internal competition was equally fierce. In 1909, in an effort to woo colonials and branch out into a new sector, Dax's *station thermale* in southwestern France began offering significant discounts to colonial administrators: free cures and food at the Grands Thermes, free consultations at the Baignots establishment, and discounts at the Graciot Hotel, upon presentation of the Ministry of the Colonies document authorizing their cure.[55] In 1929, Dax officials were forced to roll back all but one of these privileges — complimentary bathing and drinking.[56] Doctors became passionate advocates of their specific thermal spas as well as their country's. As one historian of French hydrotherapy has observed, the field ascribed the role of propagandist to its practitioners.[57]

Better than any professional historian, the novelist Erik Orsenna has captured the spirit of hydrotherapeutic competition over colonial customers. Two pages of his novel *L'Exposition coloniale* (1988) chronicle a petty feud between Vichy and nearby Châtelguyon. Louis, the failed colonial, tells his son Gabriel of a "miserable commercial strategy aimed at stealing Vichy's colonial clientele." Louis takes up Vichy's defense, drafting paragraphs that are anything but fictional, as they are borrowed verbatim from Gandelin's *Vichy pour les coloniaux et habitants des pays chauds*: "Vichy is the ideal sanatorium where colonials and patients from warm climes must come to find health, to regain their strength, and cure their afflictions contracted in the tropics." As well as underscoring internal French competition over colonial customers, Orsenna identifies international tensions. He rightly situates World War One as a turning point, after which French colonial patients were dissuaded from frequenting Marienbad, whose efficiency in the treatment of malaria had hitherto been widely recognized. Instead they were henceforth directed to Vichy, Châtelguyon, La Bourboule, or Vals-les-Bains.[58]

To govern the exploding domain of colonial hydrotherapy, grand rules and regulations were gradually established for all French colonial officials — rules that in a small and admittedly elitist way nonetheless anticipated some of the more universal coverage features of the welfare state. The *Journal Officiel* (French register of laws) listed numerous decrees, first accrediting, then mandating the duration, location, and reimbursement modalities of different spas for colonial officials. Thus, to give only one example, Indochina's public works bulletin, the local information sheet for colonial engineers, listed each new metropolitan spa to be recognized by the Ministry of the Colonies. Recognition was vital, for it meant that administrators could be treated for free and be reimbursed for their repatriation costs. In October 1923, the bulletin announced the recognition of the spa at Orezza, in Corsica, as "one of the *villes d'eaux* where functionaries of colonial services can be sent for treatment." In part perhaps because of Corsica's disproportionately high involvement in the colonial administration, Orezza would soon become one of the seven main metropolitan spas to cater to colonials (the others being Vichy, Vals-les-Bains, Encausse-les-Thermes, Vittel, Plombières, and La Bourboule).[59] Two months later, the bulletin announced the recent accreditation of the tiny spa of Sermaize-les-Bains in the Marne. Declared eligible for treatment there were administrators from every colony as well as ship personnel based in Le Havre, Nantes, Bordeaux, and Marseille who had spent time in the colonies. In October of the following year, it listed Bagnoles de l'Orne as a newly admissible spa for colonial functionaries.[60]

On the eve of World War One, H. Verdalle, a doctor based at La Bourboule and Cannes, expressed satisfaction that La Bourboule was now ranked as an "administrative cure" for colonial officials. This proved, according to this physician, that in "high places" authorities had agreed with his assessment, according to which "La Bourboule offers hydrotherapeutic resources for colonials that are well superior to those offered by other official spas."[61] Getting added to this elite list of official spas recommended by the Ministry of the Colonies was no small accomplishment. The increasing recognition and reimbursement of French and French colonial spas in the interwar period also served an obvious nationalist and protectionist purpose, by ensuring that colonial patients frequented French establishments rather than foreign ones, specifically the German, Austrian, and Czech Kurhauses mentioned by Gouzien.[62]

The French administration was not always so magnanimous to colonials seeking to take the waters in the metropole. As shown in chapter 7, administrators, military personnel, missionaries, and other categories of colonial society operated on different hydrotherapeutic benefit scales. Some, like settlers or foreigners, could claim no benefits at all. These problems of categories were posed early on. When in 1837 Polish political refugees who had found a safe haven in Algeria wrote Paris for authorization to take the waters in the Pyrenees, they were initially turned down on the grounds that they posed a political threat in the metropole (by virtue of the statute of refugees of 1832, these foreigners required permission to move within France and between France and its colonies). They were finally allowed to undertake the trip on health grounds, but were made to pay for their treatment and travel.[63] In July 1840 Polish refugee Hippolyte Wysocki likewise pleaded from Algeria with the administration to allow him to take the waters in Corsica.[64]

By the twentieth century, discretionary power over spa leaves had dwindled, and such leaves had indeed become hyperlegislated — a sure sign of their popularity. Regulations dated 1928 stipulated that requests for mineral water cures be addressed to the colonial administration, which was in turn to forward them to the military health division of the region where the patient was seeking to take a water cure. No colonial official was to receive hydrotherapeutic treatment "if he failed to present to the head of the spa establishment an authorization signed by the director of his health services, and the proper medical certificates."[65] The Ministry of the Colonies manifestly tapped into military channels when it came to water cures. The two ministries (War, Colonies) negotiated joint agreements with a number of *compagnies fermières*, or spa operating companies. Such arrangements sometimes created the equivalent of modern-day blackout dates and destinations. Thus between 1925 and 1930, the spas of Plombières, Châtel-Guyon, Mont-Dore, and Royat were temporarily removed from the Ministry of the Colonies' accredited list, due to their popularity. Vichy, conversely, remained available to those who booked early: It featured the most openings and rotations for military and colonial ministry personnel alike, thanks to the sheer size of its military hydrotherapy establishment.[66]

In addition to governing, mandating, and controlling access to individual spas in the metropole, the colonial administration classified the actual frequency of health furloughs according to colony. Thus, legislation in 1919 and 1920 stipulated that administrative leave would be awarded to administrators every two years in continental Africa and in French Guyana, every three years in Indochina, Madagascar, the small Indian colonies, and the New Hebrides, and every five years in other colonies.[67] Interestingly, until 1897, Creole colonial functionaries had received leaves only to return to their colony of origin, not to the metropole; a decree of December 23, 1897, allowed them to join their metropolitan colleagues on leave at Vichy, Royat, or Vals-les-Bains in the metropole.[68] These elaborate grids illustrate, first, how noxiousness was again determined by climatic variations and, second, how susceptibility to this noxiousness was conditioned by ethnicity. The ultimate antidote, of course, involved a trip home to Vichy or some other spa.

Spas in the colonies themselves were given ample consideration as well, although early on metropolitan spa promoters worried that spas in the colonies might draw patients away. As early as the 1830s, a *commission des eaux minérales* (commission on mineral waters) within the prestigious Académie de Médecine—whose purpose was to advise the government on public health matters—pronounced medical verdicts on spring water samples sent to it. These verdicts constituted veritable medical stamps of approval. In a single week in 1836, the commission answered two inquiries: one from the proprietors and operators of the spa at Barbotan in the Gers, seeking confirmation of the "goodness of their waters," the other from a certain Doctor Cavenne, who had sent samples of mineral water from the French Caribbean island of Martinique. After bemoaning that one of the bottles had been opened by customs, the members of the commission proceeded to describe in detail the contents of the remaining sealed bottles. They concluded that the mineral-induced effects of these French Caribbean spring waters should prove "most salutary against digestive diseases, a precious asset in a warm country like Martinique."[69]

By the twentieth century, access to mineral water spas for colonial officials came to be seen as more of a right than a privilege. In 1915, the colony of Réunion took a grievance to the Ministry of the Colonies, requesting that it be forwarded all the way to the Conseil d'état. The grievance involved a request to exempt Réunion's hydromineral spas from taxes and to allow administrators settled on location to obtain an even lower flat rate to take the waters than that enjoyed by functionaries from France.[70] Neither suggestion was accepted, the Ministry of the Colonies deeming that it supported the local spa industry sufficiently as it was by paying for a finite number of leaves to take the waters.

By 1932, the frequency of spa-breaks in the colonies was managed by a special commission, the "consultative commission of hydromineral and altitudinal spas in the colonies."[71] During the two world wars, the Ministry of the Colonies paid especially close attention to the matter of local spas in the colonies, given that functionaries were generally prevented from returning home during these times of crisis (because of naval blockades, submarine threats, cost, and so on). In a circular to colonial governors issued in 1941, Pétainist authorities instructed, "The numerous difficulties caused by current circumstances do not permit us to ensure the regular leaves and replacements for military and civilian functionaries. We therefore urge you to use *stations climatiques* to the maximum. There, Europeans and their families will find better conditions to repair their health, while awaiting the possibility of returning for a furlough in France."[72] This circular went on to guarantee funding for these cures and even mandated the search for new highland sanatoria. The governor of Réunion Island replied, "Our . . . *stations climatiques* and *thermales* of Hell-Bourg and Cilaos especially, are perfect substitutes for sick leaves to the metropole."[73] Colonial spas, it seemed, were capable of replacing the very need to return to the motherland.

Related Therapies and Prophylaxes

To be sure, French hydromineral spas and hill stations were part of a much larger medical and paramedical response to the tropics—a response that was quite simply believed to make empire possible. In its loosest definition, any product, article, or practice that could reimmerse colonials in the homeland could be considered a cure of sorts. Such cures operated as a buffer against both the tropics themselves and the proverbial *cafard*, or homesickness, that was considered one of the banes of the colonizer.[74] Appropriate colonial conduct could also provide a preventative cure from diseases still largely associated with degeneration.[75]

Colonial guidebooks advocated pell-mell the use of hydrotherapy, climatology, a strict code of colonial conduct, quinine, liver pills, a rationalized diet, a regimented habitat and wardrobe, temperance, sexual moderation, and a host of other rules. Interestingly, as William Cohen has noted, French medicine resisted the regular prescribing of quinine as a prophylactic until 1945 (in spite of the fact that it had been French chemists, Pierre Pelletier and Joseph Caventou, who had been the first to isolate the drug from the chinchona tree, also known as the quinquina tree, in 1820).[76] If anything, mineral baths and other rituals held a higher place in the canon of French colonial behavior than the preventative use of quinine, whose efficacy has since been demonstrated. According to Cohen, "The medical guide for military posts in Indochina in 1885 did not mention quinine as a preventative against the fevers of the area, but rather recommended that: 'In all cases regardless of the heat, the men must fall asleep without having their stomachs covered with their [flannel] belts. They must further cover their eyes if they pass the nights in open air.' "[77] Philip Curtin has remarked that such prescriptions shared a set of formulaic features. After tracing the premodern humor-based origin of these recommendations, Curtin notes, "One way to deal with the special perils of the tropical world was to elaborate a set of hygiene rules for self-protection. Most of them stressed the importance of careful attention to perspiration, diet, liquid intake, hot and cold, with an emphasis on moderation and regularity."[78] Thus, if hydrotherapy itself constituted a highly regimented bourgeois practice, it was easily matched in its amazing degree of regularization by colonial practices of these sorts. For if the bourgeois needed structure to establish his or her social rank, the colonial required it more ominously to maintain racial and national identity and good health.

Sometimes, French doctors acknowledged, the colonial lifestyle itself adversely impacted the health of colonizers. Besides the important question of alcohol, which I will discuss in chapter 7, diet also preoccupied French colonial hydrotherapists. Erica Peters has shown how attached French colonials were to eating French in the colonies, as a way of constantly reasserting Frenchness.

Eating French sometimes posed a major challenge in remote Laos or Niger, for instance. In such cases, after 1890, colonials often resorted to canned goods.[79] According to G. F. Bonnet, writing in 1945, this compensatory diet ironically ended up contributing to the need for a cure at Vichy: "Food is often deficient in the colonies, especially in remote areas. The use of canned goods, the rarity of fresh vegetables, often lead to symptoms of under-vitiminization. And the abuse of meats . . . encourages gastric secretion, as does the excess of violent condiments (peppers, gingers, curries, peppers)."[80] Here, colonizers were caught in a catch-22. Their health would deteriorate one way or another, regardless of whether they "ate native" or whether they "ate French" out of cans. A Vichy cure, of course, promised to relieve all such "gastrointestinal" ills, be they "due to lifestyle or climate in the colonies."[81] When it was not the climate or the "exotic other" that threatened to harm the fragile health of the colonizers, it was the behavior and lifestyle of colonials themselves.

Comforts and comportments were only part of the picture. The tropics were also believed to literally sap and poison the French organism. Soon, an entire sector emerged around treating the colonial body with pills, lotions, drinks, and potions (see figure 1). Some strike us today as paramedical at best, quackery at worst, while others seem entirely legitimate. Quinine, for instance, had been utilized by the French to treat malaria since the 1830s, although the French, unlike the British, very rarely used it as a prophylactic, and the reasons for its efficacy remained largely mysterious.[82] Interestingly, quinine was employed in conjunction with a host of other treatments. It was combined with bleedings and leechings until 1870.[83] It was likewise used in conjunction with hydrotherapy — and this combination endured well into the twentieth century. In the words of one doctor, writing in 1927, "Quinine . . . is the necessary auxiliary of a thermal cure."[84] Revealingly, quinine was relegated to the role of auxiliary. Even a medical manual for colonial doctors from 1945 — clearly won over to the use of quinine as both a cure and a prophylaxis and even advocating the use of DDT to keep mosquitoes at bay — still counseled washing down quinine with Vichy water.[85] Both quinine and mineral waters were believed to act upon the proverbial colonial liver — as were the countless miracle pills advocated in both hydrotherapy and colonial guides.

Thermalisme for colonials was thus often practiced in tandem with other therapies.[86] The most distressing, in hindsight, is certainly the dual use of

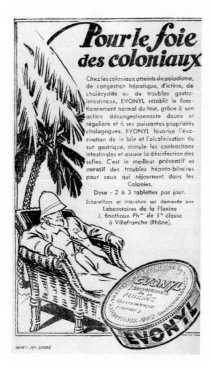

FIGURE 1. Advertisement for liver pills, promising a "gentle and regularizing decongestion" of the liver: "the best . . . preventative and curative for hepato-bile related troubles for those who live in the colonies." *Annuaire médical des stations Hydrominérales, climatiques et balnéaires de France* (1933), 8.

hydrotherapy and arsenic ingestion. Writing in 1931, Vichy's Max Vauthey expressed some reservations about the number of fatal accidents among patients following such a treatment. But he fell short of condemning the method outright, insisting that positive results could still be obtained, so long as "the arsenic treatment be moderate at first, progressive and periodically controlled by biochemical tests." [87]

The Question of Efficacy

Did any of this actually work? Given that this book is a cultural and social history of medical and paramedical practices, and given that I am not trained in medicine, I would not presume to answer the question thoroughly. Nevertheless, several points seem clear. As we will see in the next chapter, European scientists gradually recognized the largely chimerical nature of the "scramble for altitude" in the colonies. Altitude proved no panacea for Europeans. Whereas in 1823 French doctors in Guadeloupe imagined that a height of 400 feet (121.0 meters) above sea level could guard against most colonial ills (malaria and yellow fever in particular), a century later British doctors in India deemed that even 5,000 feet (2,743 meters) might not be sufficient for immunity from malaria (see chapter 3). In the climato-miasmatic paradigm of 1823, altitude provided salutary coolness; in the mosquito-vector logic of a century later, it might at best weaken the ardor or dull the senses of the anophele mosquito. But even this proved largely illusory. Two recent studies (2002–3) have suggested that altitude constitutes at best a minor factor in malarial distribution.[88]

As for hydrotherapy, it seems clear that if mineral springs had any effect whatsoever on malaria, one of the world's top killers, responsible for over a million deaths a year, the World Health Organization and countless other bodies would have jumped at such an affordable treatment of a lethal disease. There remains, of course, no effective malaria vaccine to this day, and treating the disease, once contracted, still poses a major challenge. A recent development, however, underscores the irony of French colonial doctors' scoffing at the indigenous folk practices they opposed to their rational hydrotherapy. Artemisinin, the active ingredient in sweet wormwood, an ancient Chinese herbal remedy, has recently proven the most efficient drug in combating malaria, as it overcomes previously drug-resistant strains.[89]

The amazingly elaborate systems deployed or endorsed by French colonial medicine to combat colonial ills can, of course, be studied without allowing efficacy to enter into play. Their most revealing aspects involve the construction and elaboration of countermeasures and prophylaxes, their application and implementation both in the colonies and at home.

Conclusion

Liver pills, rules of return, furloughs home, and spa accreditations were all directly shaped by the acclimatization debates. The belief that spas could serve as surrogates for home was rooted in the legacies of climatic determinism and in the transformative logic of spa science. At its zenith, this determinism had led to fears that prolonged stays in alien lands would trigger alterations of culture, behavior, race, and physiognomy, on the basis of *mésologie*. Hygienists enrolled hydrotherapy and climatology to control and soften the effects of the tropics on whites. In the arsenal of tropical medicine, only they seemed capable of "reminding the body of temperate climes." [90] Long after the Kochian, Pasteurian, and Rossian turns, French colonial doctors continued to mandate *thermalisme* and *climatisme* as guarantors of healthfulness, Frenchness, and whiteness. Legitimation bred success. Throughout the colonial empire and in France proper, colonizers, be they functionaries, missionaries, soldiers, or private citizens, thronged to spas and resorts, transforming them into nexuses and symbols of imperial power.

CHAPTER 3

Highland Hydrotherapy in Guadeloupe

A FRENCH NAVAL PHARMACIST STUDYING THE THER-
mal springs of the Caribbean island of Guadeloupe in 1864
observed, "The light strikes the water here . . . obliquely,
so that the bodies of the bathers take on a corpse-like,
pale appearance. The effect is so pronounced as to make a
Negro seem white in this basin."[1] This vignette illustrates
some of the tropes and complexities of colonial hydrotherapy. Of course, springs in French colonies were ascribed almost miraculous curing qualities, as in Europe.
But in a colonial setting, they were seen as operating other
miracles as well. They re-created France overseas, offering homesick colonizers smaller replicas of the bourgeois
leisure settings of Vichy, Royat, Aix-les-Bains, Dax, and
Bagnères-de-Bigorre. These waters, in other words, by
acting as agents of Frenchness and whiteness, reflected
the motherland overseas. Thus a pharmacist could fancy
that by immersing a black Guadeloupean into local spring
waters — then the imagined preserve of whites — one could
seemingly blur racial boundaries. So potent were the supposed qualities of these local waters that, at least under a
certain angle, they could give the appearance of erasing
the line between colonized and colonizer. Spring water was
indeed a powerful agent.

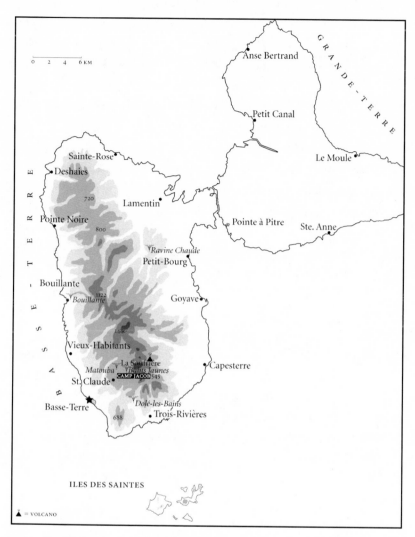

MAP 2. Guadeloupe circa 1930, showing major spas.

Spas, of course, were only one expression of power on the island, an oft-ignored one at that. As in Réunion, slavery constituted the main form of labor in Guadeloupe until 1848. Sources registered the presence of African slaves on Guadeloupe in the 1640s; by the 1660s they outnumbered the European population. Whites themselves were far from homogeneous, some of them being of foreign extraction (Dutch, Irish), others indentured servants themselves. The French Revolution in Guadeloupe, so richly studied by Frédéric Régent, Laurent Dubois, and Jacques Adélaïde-Merlande, marked a first liberation for slaves. Yet its dénouement proved tragic: Napoleon dispatched a metropolitan force to reintroduce slavery and quell the rebellion led by Louis Delgrès against its reintroduction. The rebels chose Matouba as their final redoubt. There, in May 1802, rather than return to bondage, they tore the white from the French tricolor flag and mounted a fierce last-ditch gun battle before taking their own lives in a massive explosion. It is not without irony, then, that this site was subsequently reinvented from a siege of resistance into a seat of colonial leisure and power around the Matouba spring. The very slopes that Dubois describes as laboratories of liberty would also serve as bastions of privilege, leisure, and power, places where colonial authorities sought health and home. Indeed, the same troops sent to enforce the reestablishment of slavery and quell Delgrès's resistance ended up staying and recuperating at Matouba, on doctors' orders, in the face of an outbreak of yellow fever.[2]

Old Waters in the New World

In one sense, Guadeloupe's spas show how Europeans surrounded by the exotic Other sought out the slightest trace of the familiar in their new environments. Far from being universally seduced by the exotic, they favored banal replicas of home. The quintessentially French spa model served as one such reminder of home. But spas obviously fulfilled much more than an affective function: from the very beginning of their presence in the Caribbean, the French had sought out both spring waters and the highlands — a tandem that was already believed to provide a prophylactic refuge from the nefarious effects of the tropics.

Guadeloupe's thermal springs are described by some of the earliest French accounts, around the time of the French annexation of the island in 1674. The island's springs captured the imagination of early European visitors, no doubt appearing as familiar waters in a foreign world. Early French sources recognize that indigenous peoples had long utilized the island's hot waters and had in fact guided Europeans to them in the seventeenth century.[3] What is less clear is how the Carib peoples and the Arawaks before them had viewed these springs. The Arawaks certainly attributed significance to them, as evidenced by the name they gave Guadeloupe, Karukera, the island of beautiful waters. No doubt they had ascribed different meanings to the springs than would French colonizers, who by the late seventeenth century began to employ them to treat "a host of diseases." Father Jean-Baptiste Labat recalled that in this period a swampy sulfuric pool (likely Ravine-Chaude) had already gained a reputation among the French for curing cold sweats and nervous contractions.[4] A French traveler returning from Guyana had specifically sought out Guadeloupe's waters to treat what Labat termed an acute case of oedema. Another account, Father du Tertre's *Histoire générale des Antilles*, dated 1667, portrayed Guadeloupe's hot springs as "most salutary." Despite their "stench and murkiness," du Tertre contended, the island's springs had proven their efficiency in curing diseases.[5] Nevertheless, one case he presented casts doubts on actual results. He cited the example of a certain Monsieur de Poincy, who died shortly after taking the waters to heal his spleen.[6] At a site that corresponds to the description of Ravine-Chaude, du Tertre described a more successful treatment of "several people afflicted by different ailments."[7] Here, immersion in a naturally warm pool for some eight days produced quasi-miraculous recoveries. Du Tertre indirectly ascribed this cure to the strong sulfur content of Guadeloupe's waters, which he discovered by boiling spring water and studying the residue after evaporation.[8] One is tempted to suggest, however, that the author's quest for water cures stemmed largely from the perceived toxicity of the tropics. This was allegedly reflected in their very soil, which was thought to exude "venomous vapors" or miasmas.[9]

Within this system of knowledge, Guadeloupe's waters came to signify a healthful and natural Europeanized antidote to an environment described as inherently putrid and fetid. But colonizing nations clearly elaborated different countermeasures against the tropics. To combat mysterious pathologies, the French in Guadeloupe resorted to the ancient elements of water, air, and fire (du Tertre had already established some rapport between the sulfuric content of Guadeloupe's springs and the island's volcano).[10] This would bring them to concentrate on the slopes of the active Soufrière volcano, much like their unfortunate counterparts in Martinique who perished on the flanks of Mount Pelée after it erupted in 1902.[11]

Early-nineteenth-century French medical guides to the Antilles reveal the multiple problems facing prospective colonizers, who were incapable of identifying a root cause of tropical morbidity beyond climate—a ubiquitous concern from which there appeared to be no escape in the so-called torrid zone. Indeed, in this pre–germ theory era, climate was blamed for everything from jaundice to chronic fatigue. Michel-Etienne Descourtilz, former head doctor in Saint-Domingue, wrote a sanitary guide for the French Caribbean in 1816.[12] He presented a series of hygienic aphorisms intended to regulate and dictate the everyday actions and conduct of the colonizers. First of all: "Because one of the main causes of yellow fever is the torrid heat, newly arrived travelers should avoid the rays of the sun and should only go out in the street . . . morning and evenings." Next: "One should seek out pure and temperate air within the torrid zone, where opposite and strong winds crisscross, so as to refresh the atmosphere which is so saturated with humidity, as is proven by the abundance of rain, the many insects, the rapid oxidation of metals, and the sudden putrefaction of living bodies." Further on, Descourtilz writes, "You should prescribe warm baths for people who are experiencing poor perspiration; to workers. . . . These baths should have maximum effect when they are accompanied by vigorous massage."[13]

M. G. Levacher's health guide of 1840 for the French Caribbean also listed a number of practical ways in which to wage the uphill battle against climate: First, French authorities must insist that arriving Europeans be dispersed around the islands and that their laundry be changed regularly. Second, the utmost cleanliness need be achieved, and care should be taken to avoid the overcrowding of hospitals. Third, lazarets, or quarantine stations, should be established on nearby islets, as a sort of decompression zone for incoming Europeans. These islets on the east of the Antilles presented the additional "advantage of being well ventilated and containing no swamp whatsoever." Fourth, "warm baths are of invaluable utility for the arriving European. He should adopt this habit and continue it thereafter, though in moderation." Fifth, "clothes should be light, and frequently changed." Finally, great care should be taken to follow a rational diet in the tropics: this included taking two regular meals, "as one would in Europe; they should be varied, moderate yet generous. One should avoid excesses of spices, local peppers and salt . . . ; the very best drinks with which to accompany meals are Bordeaux wines."[14] These cardinal principles centered on three overriding considerations: hygiene, the rejection of the Other (the fear of creolization through cuisine), and the reproduction of the comforts of home (epitomized here by Bordeaux wine). Highland spas would speak to all three of these colonial concerns. This cautionary list shows how balneology came to be considered an element of the colonial lifestyle —

one of many commandments which guidebooks dispensed to would-be colonizers of the French Caribbean. Soon, full-fledged hydromineral spas came to
occupy a central place as a staple of the colonial landscape and regimen.

Dolé and Camp Jacob: From Sanatoria to Sites of Power

By the early nineteenth century, Guadeloupe's naval and civil administrators
were beginning to see the potential of the lush, mountainous, and breezy southwestern corner of the so-called Basse-Terre (*basse* cardinally, not topographi-
cally). The island's governor, Admiral Louis Léon, Comte de Jacob, set about
determining an appropriate location for a military hospital and rest station near
the island's capital of Basse-Terre. On 13 December 1823, Jacob convoked his
health council to advise him on the altitude needed to achieve immunity from
yellow fever.[15] Six days later, the council reported that an altitude of greater
than four hundred feet could suffice, so long as soldiers remained there permanently and the chosen site was well removed from swamps.[16] Three years after
these initial deliberations, a certain Dr. Vatalle produced a memorandum outlining conditions and locales for a possible health station. Vatalle concurred that
freshly arrived troops needed to be sheltered from the devastating effects of
yellow fever, but he pointed out that many of the highland areas, which seemed
largely free of yellow fever, were unfortunately rife with dysentery. The optimal emplacement, he found, lay near Matouba (a hydromineral spa in its own
right), the site that would indeed be chosen for Camp Jacob. On the matter of
living conditions and diet, Vatalle, like Levacher, urged the administration to
substitute the current regimen of rum for one of wine.[17]

    Vatalle, Jacob, and their colleagues considered disease avoidance an abso-
lute priority. They had every reason to do so. In years of yellow fever epidemic,
on average one-ninth of all hospitalized patients in Guadeloupe perished.[18]
Heat, swamps, rum, lowlands, whatever the culprit might be, it needed to be
stemmed rapidly in order for a French colonial presence to be sustained under
such conditions. In April 1829, plans began in earnest for a military encampment on the highlands around Saint-Claude and Matouba, near Basse-Terre.
That same year, the head of the French royal navy's fortifications branch added
an important variation to Camp Jacob's original function. Rather than serve as
a permanent encampment, it would be used as a kind of tropical decompres-

sion chamber for troops. This period of seasoning would last for some twenty months after their arrival from France.[19] The term used to describe the future Camp Jacob is significant: *camp d'acclimatement*, or "acclimation camp."[20] The most critical phase, this official contended, was the first winter (*hivernage*), after which most Europeans could be considered acclimated. Camp Jacob was thus conceived as a sort of antechamber to the tropics for incoming white troops. It would be used, in other words, to facilitate and accelerate acclimation. But what would become of ailing Europeans living or serving in the colony whose chronic afflictions and high mortality rates seemed to belie the reliability of acclimation theories?

During the deliberations over Camp Jacob, proponents of the original permanent encampment project turned to a second site for a military convalescence establishment reserved for troops already stationed on the island. Governor Jacob was easily convinced, since this scheme, planned for Dolé-les-Bains, promised to save government funds by diminishing the number of sick days and, better yet, "by saving on transporting convalescents back to France."[21] But Dolé-les-Bains, as its name suggests, was chosen above all for its spring waters. The document of 1832 calling for this sanitary encampment presented Dolé's waters as "favorable to men afflicted with dysentery or intermittent fevers."[22] "Intermittent fevers" usually encompassed both yellow fever and malaria—a testimony to the curative qualities then ascribed to Dolé's springs. The advocates of this project were adamant on separating the treatments for new recruits on the one hand and for seasoned men on the other: "Newly arrived soldiers must be sent to Matouba, and it seems to us that the sanitary camp of Dolé should be reserved to convalescents and to men diagnosed with diseases requiring a mineral water cure."[23] Here hydrotherapy's action was broadly defined as curative, and climatology's as prophylactic.

In 1831, Guadeloupe's privy council embraced this vision, concurring that "the Dolé military station could serve as a convalescing center for soldiers who need a change of air, and who could no doubt recover here in the colony, rather than costing the administration large sums for repatriating them to Europe. The establishment would be of evident use for sick soldiers for whom the waters of Dolé will henceforth be prescribed as a curing agent by the Health Council."[24] This passage again dwells upon the savings inherent in curing European troops on location. A key concept had been coined: the administration could cut costs by creating in Guadeloupe the kind of rest and reinvigoration facilities that were becoming immensely popular in metropolitan France. Dolé would for some sixty years hold a virtual monopoly in the ranks of colonial administrators, since a simple decision from the colony's health council could send an official there for a lengthy stay free of charge and complete with a per diem (this state of affairs changed by 1900, with the increasing subsidization of cures in the metropole).[25]

Irrespective of motivations, one can conclude that by the early to mid-nineteenth century, the twin measures of mineral water and high altitude cures were becoming enshrined by the navy and civilian administration as rational, European countermeasures meant to combat yellow fever, malaria, and dysentery. At the time, they were dispensed in Guadeloupe primarily by two military and government establishments at Camp Jacob/Matouba and Dolé-les-Bains, founded with an eye to saving the administration from sending bureaucrats and soldiers back to France on health leave. In this way, pragmatic financial concerns dovetailed with the recognized need for white troops to find *ressourcement*. Mineral springs could literally act as surrogates for home. Over the next several decades, private businessmen and enterprising local doctors would begin to establish climatic and hydrotherapeutic services for the public at large, developing the spring at Ravine-Chaude, erecting an admittedly rudimentary civilian establishment next to the military one at Dolé-les-Bains (the grand hotel of Dolé, and the modernization of Dolé's basins would have to wait until 1917–20). The trend mirrored on a much smaller scale the increasing privatization and profitability of the spa industry in metropolitan France during the mid-nineteenth century.[26]

A Colonial Space for the Elite

Camp Jacob could, according to the French colonial doctor Alexandre Kermorgant, boast of being the very first colonial highland health station anywhere. Writing in 1899, Kermorgant commented on the evolution of the Saint-Claude/Matouba region since Camp Jacob's inception: "[Today,] the highlands of the isle are becoming a refuge for the wealthier classes as well as for the ill."[27] He added that the great advantage of Camp Jacob stemmed precisely from this growing, close-knit community of decision makers, functionaries, convalescents, and health seekers. In his words, "Miniature sanatoria have sprung up around Petit-Bourg, Sainte-Rose, at Trois-Rivières, at Gourbeyre, and finally at Matouba, situated some 100 meters over Camp-Jacob, itself part of the community of Saint-Claude. Every day, new houses are erected in this area. The scenic beauty of the site has led to its name of 'the Switzerland of the Tropics.' . . . As for Camp-Jacob, its principal advantage is that troops, bureaucrats, and the governor all reside there. The camp's hospital holds 120 beds. It is thus much more than a camp; it is a veritable health city [*ville de santé*]."[28] Hardly dissimulated beneath these remarks was the fact that by the turn of the century, this particular region, and indeed the high slopes of the Souffrière volcano, had emerged as a "white settlement," bringing together colonial officials at the very pinnacle of the pyramid of colonial command, luxurious planters' residences, colonial hospitals, and spas in a single region. Already in the mid-nineteenth century, Matouba served as the meeting place for the local aristocracy, and Saint-Claude had earned the reputation of Guadeloupe's "most metropolitan" town.[29] In fact, to this day, the residence of Paris's representative, the highest ranking French official on the island, the prefect, is located at Camp Jacob.[30] The mushrooming of elite estates around these centers of authority in the nineteenth century betrays the nexus of power formed around the spas and sanatoria in the highlands of Saint-Claude/Camp Jacob/Matouba. The area had not merely become posh (although paradoxically, as we shall see, some of the spas themselves were often rather dilapidated); it had also established itself as a place to "network." The fact that this twinning of ruling, elite, and bourgeois settlement occurred at and around spas was, of course, no coincidence. Douglas Mackaman has shown how the spa in nineteenth-century France became a playground for a growing bourgeois clientele seeking both a medical regimen and a highly structured, normalized leisure activity.[31] Although there are no statistics or social data to establish a reliable profile on spa-goers in nineteenth-century Guadeloupe, one could certainly speculate that the nineteenth century in Guadeloupe saw a similar rise in the social stock of spas. It also mirrored another early-nineteenth-century French phenomenon: the emergence of the spa as a bourgeois enclave from which the poor were increasingly excluded.[32] But in a colonial context, race must be grafted onto considerations of power and class.

Throughout the nineteenth century, black Guadeloupeans, like their counterparts across the Caribbean, tended not to benefit from the "optimal conditions" of the Saint-Claude/Matouba/Camp Jacob area, especially access to fresh, clean water. The historian Dominique Taffin has shown how a cholera epidemic in Guadeloupe in 1865 was largely covered up by the French administration in an effort to hide "the miserable living and demographic conditions of the black majority on the island."[33] Meanwhile, as we have seen, the freshly arrived metropolitan French population concentrated in the mountainous, breezy western half of Guadeloupe, known as Basse-Terre region. It showed a predilection for the region around Gourbeyre, Dolé, and Matouba. In other words, much more was at stake than the availability or proximity of health care: Europeans had carved out for themselves what they perceived to be the only healthful corner of Guadeloupe. And they had big plans for the region. In 1917, Dr. Pichon, the head of Guadeloupe's health services and a former professor at the Ecole de Médecine coloniale de Marseille who would become the staunchest promoter of hydrotherapy, gymnastics, modern hygiene, and tourism in Guadeloupe, expressed the hope that "the area between Matouba and Dolé, encompassing Saint-Claude and Gourbeyre, should one day become a vast health station and villégiature for the entire Antilles, and, why not, the Americas."[34] This mountainous, volcanic half of Guadeloupe, new home of the white administrative classes, was constantly contrasted with the island's flat, sugar-cane producing eastern half, known as Grande-Terre. Grande-Terre, in almost every respect, stood as the antithesis, the sanitary foil, to Basse-Terre.[35]

Here, geology rivaled topography as an underlying determinant of healthfulness. In his treatise on yellow fever, *Memoirs of West Indian Fever* (1827), the English doctor John Wilson had already arrived at the following diagnosis for Guadeloupe:

> Guadeloupe, judging from a cursory view of its exterior, is generally a calcereous formation. In many places there is exposure of naked lime surface; and while the island is generally unhealthy, those places are peculiarly so. Pointe-à-Pitre is especially worthy of attention. The District is generally marshy and unhealthy, but the dry and more elevated positions are productive of West Indian Fever, and deadly in a very high degree. About a mile east of the town is ... Fort Louis and a mile further east Fleur de Pays; they occupy points of a calcereous ridge, which extends some distance along the sea coast, and which, from its com-

parative elevation, absolute dryness and contiguity to the sea, might have been deemed a situation favorable to health. These forts have been distinguished by the mortality of the fevers which have assailed the troops, a mortality scarcely equaled in other ports of the West Indies.[36]

Grande-Terre had thus emerged by 1827 as a lethal place, not least, experts thought, because of what lay beneath it. For this doctor, geology outweighed altitude. Pointe-à-Pitre, the island's largest city, appeared unhealthy indeed compared to the small capital of Basse-Terre. Meanwhile, on the hills over-looking Basse-Terre, in Saint-Claude, Matouba, and at Camp Jacob, the white administrative classes would continue to cling to the formula of altitude, com-bined with volcanic soil, the healthful waters that derived from it, and winds, to stave off disease.

By the nineteenth century, Guadeloupe's spas were thus emerging as multi-functional sites of white authority. In this sense, the Saint-Claude/Matouba/Camp Jacob triangle can be seen as a forerunner of the summer capitals of the British Raj, although admittedly a smaller seat of colonial power.[37] The parallel did not escape the attention of the Belgian colonial doctor Georges Dryepont, who noted in 1900, "In the East and West Indies, English and French alike have gained advantage from highland areas as sites for . . . dwelling and refuge in the hot season; they have also both established medical posts, sanatoria, hos-pitals, Hill Convalescents Depots (sic), whose effects have proven beneficial to patients." [38] This passage reminds us of the original rationales for hill spas. In the colonies, the need for highland encampments, the quest for mineral water spas, debates over clothes and diet, and the development of typologies of accli-mation were all derived from an obsession with tropical heat. Like the British in India, the French believed that they "[kept] better in the hills." [39]

As the ideal of acclimation came under attack, the search began for micro-climatic bastions permitting the survival of the "French race" in the tropics. Between 1870 and 1900, French scientists conducted batteries of tests to deter-mine which areas of Guadeloupe were most salubrious for Europeans. These studies were framed as part of a renewed fear that whites might degenerate even in milder tropical settings like Guadeloupe. Indeed, in 1899 Georges Treille argued, "We know that, even in our oldest European colonies [that is, Guade-loupe, Martinique, and Réunion], the number of whites is constantly dropping, either because of economic factors, which trigger return voyages to Europe, or because of an absence of new blood, as a result of which white people have progressively lost their resistance to the climate, or ended up assimilated into the other ethnic elements which surround them." [40] Revealed here is nothing short of a fear of submersion, degeneration, and loss of identity through miscegenation—and this from a scientist who, unlike many of his colleagues, actually believed in the possibility of acclimation. For Treille's school, highland spas seemed to counter the pernicious influences of climate on multiple levels: first by creating a segregated European community, second by enhancing resistance to the climate within a microclimate akin to Europe's, and third by lowering the morbidity that ravaged newly arrived Europeans. In this last instance, yellow fever or malaria could be substituted for a more general anguish about degeneration. In this perspective, physical *and* moral regeneration and hygiene could be achieved in Guadeloupe's highland resorts.

Altitude Therapy in Guadeloupe

We saw in chapter 1 how Europeans turned to highland areas in an effort to escape disease. This was not just a construct. There was some degree of hard science behind highland health stations, although we know today that their foundational logic was flawed: Europeans believed they were fleeing miasmas, when in fact they were to some extent managing to flee mosquitoes. By the 1890s, the British in India concluded that neither cholera nor malaria could strike above an altitude of 1,500 to 2,000 meters (though some cautioned that only elevations of 2,500 meters had proven absolutely safe).[41] By 1924, British scientists in the Raj cautioned that even 5,000 feet (2,743 meters) did not provide absolute malarial immunity.[42] This of course represented a significant shift when compared with the 400 feet (121.9 meters) once recommended by Guadeloupe's health council earlier in 1823. Meanwhile, Alfred Jousset's study of 1883 noted that while an altitude of 1,000 to 1,200 meters was considered optimal for a hill station, Camp Jacob in Guadeloupe had shown that even a 545-meter-high sanatorium could prove invaluable. Interestingly, its usefulness was not merely physiological, but also psychological, for Camp Jacob "reminded the European of the homeland." [43]

Throughout the nineteenth century, altitude constituted the prime yardstick of tropical healthfulness. Kermorgant notes that Camp Jacob enjoyed a temperature average some five degrees centigrade cooler than the island's capital Basse-Terre, even though it was only five kilometers away. Camp Jacob owed its reputation to its elevation of 545 meters above sea level—an altitude still insufficient by any contemporaneous account to prevent malaria.[44] Nevertheless, according to Kermorgant, this high-altitude refuge was especially beneficial from July to October, when malaria ravaged the eastern lowlands of the island. French doctors never ceased to wonder at the supposed natural immunity of Camp Jacob. A report from 1897 noted that of all the gendarmerie brigades on the islands, Camp Jacob's seemed to report the fewest sick. It was consequently recommended that the brigade in question be enlarged and that the camp be made a "vacation residence" for French gendarmes.[45]

Among the many studies of Guadeloupe's highlands, those relating to immunity from yellow fever seemed to yield the most convincing results. Dryepont observed that in both Jamaica and Guadeloupe, the highlands had been spared the worst of yellow fever epidemics. In Jamaica, Dryepont noted, the rate of mortality dropped from 130 per thousand to 35 per thousand ever since troops had been moved from the lowlands to the mountains.[46] Similarly, in Guadeloupe, Camp Jacob had sheltered soldiers from the worst of a yellow fever outbreak in 1869, as demonstrated in the following table.[47] Little wonder, then, that Guadeloupe's administrators, bourgeoisie, and planter classes thronged to the hills. In Liliane Chauleau's words, "The most common way of preventing yellow fever [in the nineteenth century] was to take refuge in a hill station: the Camp-Jacob in Guadeloupe, or the Camp des Pitons in Martinique."[48] While the Camp Jacob area's relative protection from yellow fever seemeds indisputable, results were much less convincing with respect to malaria, which was fast becoming the number one killer on the island, accounting for a quarter of all hospitalizations by the turn of the twentieth century.[49]

In 1907, René Pichevin, an expert on colonial sanatoria, turned his attention to malaria rates in Saint-Claude/Matouba/Camp Jacob. Pichevin observed that troops stationed in the area were somewhat less vulnerable to malaria than their compatriots posted in the lowlands of Martinique.[50] But figures remained startlingly high. In lowland Martinique, 292 out of 1,000 soldiers had contracted malaria by 1904, as opposed to 286 out of 1,000 in highland Guadeloupe. A later study undertaken in 1932 by a certain Marcel Léger concluded that Guadeloupe in general had emerged as more malarial than Martinique.

TABLE. Yellow Fever Outbreak in Guadeloupe, 1869

Location	Average rate of yellow fever contraction (per thousand)
Les Saintes	660
Marie-Galante	570
Pointe à Pitre	230
Basse-Terre	210
Camp Jacob	140

Moreover, Léger noted, the entire island of Guadeloupe seemed contaminated, though he very curiously admitted to not having tested the highlands of Saint-Claude/Matouba.[51] This unwillingness to disprove Saint-Claude/Matouba/Camp Jacob's claims of malarial resistance is no doubt telling in itself. If Pichevin's figures are at all reliable, Guadeloupe's highland spas actually offered very little by way of respite from malaria. Fantasies of small oases of France, perceptions of temperateness, and illusions of salubrity proved more important than medical realities.

Nonetheless, Pichevin's preliminary findings, especially when added to Dryepont's more convincing conclusions concerning yellow fever, contributed to the growth of highland sanatoria and spas. The best way to avoid disease, they advocated matter-of-factly, was to avoid infected zones. Of course, implicit in these conclusions was the idea that whites, while appropriating the coolest, most comfortable areas of the island, would also avoid the inhabitants of so-called infected zones.

To be sure, skeptics began to make their voices heard in the early twentieth century. In 1904, military doctor Cassagnou bravely set his sights on Camp Jacob's, Matouba's, and Saint-Claude's putative immunity from yellow fever. He pointed to several outbreaks of the disease at Camp Jacob in 1852, 1853, 1854 and 1869, then assessed the likelihood that each of these had been imported from the lowlands. Cassagnou based his revisionism on insect-vector hypotheses. Interestingly, he reexamined the same data his predecessors had used to show precisely the reverse: "The traditional belief in Matouba's total immunity from yellow fever," he insisted, "rests on very flimsy foundations." Even Cassagnou, however, acknowledged that Matouba in particular seemed to offer some protection from disease, when compared to coastal areas. He refrained from imputing this partial protection to climate alone, invoking a mix of factors, including temperature, moral, and hygienic conditions.[52] Cassagnou's revelations could have undercut the legitimacy of Guadeloupean altitude therapy; in the event, they barely dented what proved a deeply entrenched belief and practice. Armed with the longstanding endorsement of several medical branches as effective antidotes to tropical ills, both water and altitude therapies continued to thrive in the twentieth century.

Hybrid Water Cures?

Camp Jacob and Dolé-les-Bains were intended to complement, not rival, each other. The decision in 1832 to create two distinct sanatoria, one for seasoned men (hydrotherapy at Dolé), the other for new arrivals (climatology at Camp Jacob) does, however, suggest that hydrotherapy was conceived as a long-term project, involving continual reimmersion into healthful spas. *Thermalisme* was thus imagined as a permanent, highly rationalized, and highly ritualized practice for Europeans in the tropics.

But in reality, no matter how much French scientists might try to recast it as a modern, specialized, intrinsically French treatment, hydrotherapy was an ancient and richly diverse practice. In Guadeloupe, as elsewhere, the thermal establishment did not by any means hold a monopoly on balneological modes. Interestingly, several local, nonwhite Caribbean influences may have at least indirectly shaped modern colonial Guadeloupe's version of hydrotherapy. In his history of yellow fever dated 1929, a certain Dr. Cazanove described an ancient and nonscientific treatment for yellow fever known as the "mulatress' treatment." Sometimes attributed to mulatoes, other times to slaves, the method called for "frequent baths . . . and purging drinks."[53]

A much older text, from 1816, defines this same treatment as follows:

Curative method of the Creoles and Mulatresses:
This method, undertaken without principles or calculations on the part of the ordinary people who utilize it (often by experience or precedent, by comparing the sick) consists of:
Frictions to the body with fresh lemons, cut in half.
Ingesting this same substance. . . .

Washings using this same bitter substance.

Ordering, depending on the cases, hot or cold baths, aromatized with large quantities of lemons or bitter oranges.

Practicing, after the onset [of fevers], a bleeding of the foot, followed by rubs.[54]

Ironically, then, this popular Antillais folk cure appears to have influenced or at the very least preceded the modern therapy that white Frenchmen were by the nineteenth century seeking to establish as inherently European. Indeed, this local folk cure, rejected by Dr. Cazanove as a "medical curiosity," nonetheless bears some parallels with the supposedly legitimate hydrotherapy practiced by the colonizers, at least in its ritual bathing.

This unacknowledged medical hybridity underscores the ambiguities and *métissage* of what was by definition a Creole society in Guadeloupe as much as it illuminates the gray areas around European medical practices in the colonial sphere.[55] In reality, people of color played an important role in Guadeloupean hydrotherapy — as practitioners most notably — even before the abolition of slavery. The French medical claim of a hydrotherapeutic monopoly is put to the lie in other ways. Gérard Lafleur has recently documented slave uses of Dolé's springs, circa 1841. In a remarkable example of limited entrepreneurship, slaves on the Dolé estate had somehow managed to rent out some twenty-two cabins for bathers, thereby gaining a small measure of financial autonomy. Only after slavery was abolished in 1848 did the spa become the property of the colony.[56] While it is thus readily apparent that the white colonial French claim of holding a monopoly on hydrotherapeutic practices and even management or control in Guadeloupe was flawed, the insistence on defining water cures as agents for and reflections of civilization is of course telling in itself. Dismissing both clinical and colonial *métissage*, French colonial doctors prescribed hydrotherapy as a distinctly French cure in a decidedly non-French tropical environment.

Another, more sinister purpose lurked behind the colonial spa's medical veneer. In 1932, a regular patron of the poshest Guadeloupean spa, Dolé-les-Bains, asserted in a Guadeloupean newspaper, "My villa was sheltered from the malevolence of the race by a series of hedges."[57] It would seem that certain spas were de facto racially segregated. Thus the sulfuric spring at the Sources du Galion appears to have drawn a predominantly black clientele,[58] while Dolé and Saint-Claude seem to have attracted primarily European functionaries. Though black servants and, occasionally, black children could be seen by the side of spa pools, they were not the regular patrons of Dolé-les-Bains prior to 1946. Seeking out spring waters in the highlands was, for many whites, a means of escaping not just the tropics, but their inhabitants as well.[59]

Proliferation and Specificities

Perhaps the most surprising dimension of Guadeloupean hydrotherapy resides in the very number of spas involved. By the 1930s, no fewer than ten mineral water spas had been developed, for a population of 267,407 in 1931 (up from 182,112 in 1901, 145,417 in 1876, and 102,986 in 1817).[60] Each Guadeloupean spa gradually carved a clinical niche for itself, relying upon legend and word of mouth to advertise its curative qualities. Rumor had it that the spring at Ravine-Chaude was discovered by a mangy dog, healed by the spring's waters.[61] After falling in, the animal was miraculously cured of his rheumatism, mange, ulcers, and sadness from having lost its master. In short, the waters of Ravine-Chaude were said to accomplish "veritable miracles."[62] In another case, this one involving a human subject, its spring waters supposedly cured a patient who had been totally paralyzed by rheumatism.[63] Accordingly, Ravine-Chaude is known to this day as a treatment center for rheumatism and for reinvigoration, its waters being used primarily for immersion — it is recommended that clients bathe in them a minimum of two hours a day (see figure 2).[64]

Until the full-blown commercial development of Dolé-les-Bains, Ravine-Chaude/Lamentin was the only spa in Guadeloupe that seemed to live up to metropolitan standards. Kermorgant commented in 1901, "This is the only spa [on the island] where steps have been taken to attract bathers; the price of the therapy is one franc per bath."[65] Ravine-Chaude's waters, at thirty-five degrees centigrade, heavily sodium bicarbonated, and calcium rich, were also purported to heal kidney ailments, liver afflictions, and gout.[66] In addition, its alkaline mud was utilized for the external treatment of rheumatism and dermatological conditions.[67] Finally, this cure-all spring was believed to relieve the symptoms of malaria, making it, like Vichy and Encausse-les-Thermes in metropolitan France, the quintessential specialist in colonial diseases.[68] Then, around 1984, a new use was found for Ravine-Chaude's waters when psychiatric ailments began to be treated at the spa.[69]

From the late nineteenth century onward, teams of French scientists had

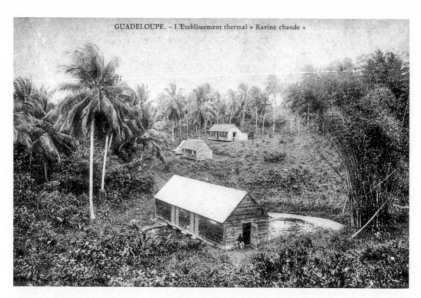

GUADELOUPE. - L'Etablissement thermal « Ravine chaude »

FIGURE 2. Ravine-Chaude du Lamentin, circa 1900. Courtesy of the Archives départementales de la Guadeloupe. All rights reserved.

analyzed, classified, and developed each of Guadeloupe's major medicinal springs. In keeping with their function as little pieces of Europe, each spa was equated to a metropolitan site. The waters at Ravine-Chaude were compared to those of Saint-Gaudens in the Pyrenees.[70] For its part, Saint-Claude's setting earned it the epithet "the Switzerland of the Tropics."[71] A Guadeloupean-born scientist elaborated in 1926: "The temperateness of its climate, the beauty of its site, the luxuriance of its vegetation, the beauty of its flowers . . . enchant the European uprooted from the old continent, and submitted for so long to the natural rigors of the tropics."[72] That luxuriant Saint-Claude in no way resembles any part of Switzerland was inconsequential to homesick European colonizers seeking reinvigoration. At Saint-Claude, colonizers were drawn to both the cool atmosphere and hot waters of the island's highlands. Such practices illustrate to what extent the colonizers sought to counterbalance and in fact neutralize their new surroundings. Where the air was hot and the waters temperate, they sought out the alleged purification of boiling waters and the cool breezes of the highlands. Saint-Claude/Matouba typified the merging of altitude and mineral water therapies in colonial Guadeloupe. In the words of Edouard Chartol, at Saint-Claude/Matouba "Hydrotherapy and Climatology complement one another."[73]

Most scientists divided Guadeloupe's ten exploited mineral springs into four categories:[74]

A) Sulfuric properties: 1. Bains chauds du Matouba, 2. Sources du Galion, 3. Source Saint-Charles, 4. Sofaïa. B) Salinated waters: 5. Eau du Pigeon, 6. Dolé-les-Bains (Bain Cappé, Bain d'Amour), 7. Ravine-Chaude du Lamentin. C) Heavily salinated waters: 8. Eau de la Fontaine bouillante. D) Heavily salinated and ferric waters: 9. Bains jaunes, 10. Bains Beauvallon.[75]

Sulfuric content seems to have been directly related to the spa's location vis-à-vis Guadeloupe's volcano, the aptly named Soufrière.[76] The closer a spring was located to the dome, the more its waters were defined as "sulfuric, chlorinated, rich in calcium and magnesium, heavily mineralized in general, and containing very heavy quantities of iron and magnesium."[77] Thus, Matouba, on the slopes of the volcano, featured high sulfur content, while Dolé-les-Bains' three springs, as well as Ravine-Chaude, fell under the saline category.

Each was, and still is, purported to treat vastly different afflictions. By the twentieth century, Dolé-les-Bains claimed an impressive array of functions, curing arthritis, kidney and liver ailments, chronic malaria, and constipation.[78] The waters emerging from Dolé's main spring, La Digue, were thirty-three degrees Celsius, only slightly cooler than Ravine-Chaude's.[79] Dolé also benefited from its reputation as the island's only luxury resort, thanks to the efforts of the retired colonial doctor Pichon, who installed a grand hotel and villas near the hot and cold springs around 1920. Dolé-les-Bains, though not on especially high terrain, represents, thanks to its gentle breeze, the quintessential example of a resort considered at once a *station thermale* and a *station climatique*. In other words, both its waters and its climate were markedly different from the ambient setting.[80] Pichon described Dolé's climate as a "perpetual spring" — no doubt a cure-all in itself for colonials bemoaning the temperature extremes of the tropics.[81] Dolé's main attraction, however, resided in its "elegant and comfortable hotel."[82] The colonial spa specialists Matignon and Abbatucci marveled at the fact that Dolé, like the great spa at Vichy, was operated by an exploitation company, or Société fermière.[83] An advertisement in a local Guadeloupean newspaper promised guests a "truly modern cadre . . . , irreproachable service, perfect cuisine . . . ," and, almost as an aside, "thermal springs . . . especially efficient in treating many diseases."[84] Dolé-les-Bains thus proved salutary for colonial administrators seeking not merely a cure from ailments ascribed to the tropics, but also an escape from the tropics themselves. Dolé-les-Bains seemed as close as one could come to France in Guadeloupe. Etiologically, the roots of both *dépaysement* (homesickness) and tropical ailments were woven together at Dolé-les-Bains and soon became interchangeable.

For their part, Matouba's waters were deemed miraculous on another score. Perched a thousand meters above sea level, these springs were located in a cool, wooded area offering an "enchanting cadre" for the *excursionniste* — a term which at once combined the notions of tourist and patient.[85] Matouba's waters emerge at a temperature of fifty-four degrees Celsius. They were considered providential as a drink, to the point that Matouba waters were served in all of the island's hospitals.[86] Clinically speaking, a certain overlap with Dolé can be discerned, as Matouba specialized in liver, stomach, and rheumatic treatment. For unlike Ravine-Chaude and Dolé, access to Matouba's springs was difficult, especially after an earthquake destroyed the main path to the spa in 1897.[87] Taking full advantage of the enchanting and isolated cadre, Matouba's exploiters explicitly targeted honeymooners, a strategy that clearly set them apart from competitors. Marketing, it seems, had become crucial to turning a profit in the competitive world of the Guadeloupean spa. By 1979, when a brand new thermal establishment was inaugurated at Matouba-Papaye (rebaptized Centre Harry Hamousin), an entirely different set of diseases was targeted: ear, throat, and nose ailments as well as joint and dermatological disorders.[88]

Furloughs and Competition

Because the colonizer's identity was perceived as being permanently under siege in the tropics, resorts and spas came to serve in part as agents for reaffirming Frenchness overseas. Naturally, for patrician functionaries, *ressourcement*, or reinvigoration, could be sought directly in the metropole. By 1920, even low-ranking colonial officials were allowed regular leaves of absence for cures in the metropole. As we have seen, however, a remarkably complex post–World War One scale of furloughs ranked the French Caribbean as much more salubrious than French West Africa, South America, or Indochina, for instance. Consequently, a functionary in Guadeloupe was allowed to return to the metropole only every five years, as opposed to every two years for those stationed in French Guyana and French Somalia.[89] This meant that the average colonial administrator posted in Guadeloupe would have to seek reinvigoration on location.

The system of furloughs was itself intimately connected to other normalizing tropical prophylaxes—which included immersion in and drinking of mineral waters, the avoidance of lowlands, and the quest for *ressourcement*. Although some elements of this prescriptive canon may have been uniquely French, much of the canon itself mirrored that of France's colonial rival, England. Harish Naraindas has identified the following mainstays, born of the intersection of colonial social practice and tropical medicine in late-nineteenth-century British colonialism: "The sanatorium, the hill station, the voyage, and the furlough (back to good old England!)." [90] As we have seen, the very same set of concerns—to which we should add hydrotherapy and perhaps the countless cure-all tablets for liver ailments advertised in Guadeloupe's newspapers—constituted the mantra of French colonizers in the Caribbean.

Much evidence suggests that a tension resulted from return rules and furlough tables, a tension opposing the ideal of the posh, bourgeois metropolitan spa on the one hand, and its Guadeloupean counterpart on the other. Guadeloupean spas, in other words, were constantly attempting to shake off the label of "poor settler's resort." Paul Carnot, a professor of medicine at the University of Paris, while conceding the "useful virtues" of spas in the colonies, nonetheless concluded that "it is still the spas of metropolitan France proper . . . that best suit our colonials, for they offer not just the virtues of their waters, but also the charms of the French climate, [and] a gaiety and luxury surrounding their cures. [These] are crucial considerations for tired colonials." [91] For colonials frequenting the small, ramshackle basins of Ravine-Chaude (see figure 2, above), Vichy and Royat must indeed have seemed something of an El Dorado. The ultimate result of these constant comparisons with metropolitan resorts was a pronounced inferiority complex on the part of Guadeloupean spa advocates. In his study of Guadeloupe's springs in 1926, Edouard Leroux noted, "Our functionaries and inhabitants can draw many medical benefits from the island's springs. One must not forget that colonial diseases like hepatitis, anemia, etc. . . . can spread quickly. In such cases, one cannot recommend European spas in the Pyrénées, Auvergne or the Vosges, which require a long trip and are moreover only open from May to October. We should be grateful that our remarkable spas are open all year round."[92] Even while underscoring the competition between local and metropolitan spas, Leroux betrayed a sense of clinical inferiority to French spring waters. The advantage of taking Guadeloupean waters, he contended, resided in proximity and availability rather than inherent merit.

Elsewhere, the struggle to keep colonial administrators on location was made more explicit. During a heated debate in 1927 at Guadeloupe's Conseil Général, the island's main elected body, a politician argued that the colony would gain from "rheumatic officials staying here in Guadeloupe for treatment, rather than going to France."[93] Some even suspected that the French colonial governor of Guadeloupe had systematically refused to accredit the island's thermal spas, for fear that he and his colleagues would be "prevented from being sent to Vichy or . . . Vittel," on the grounds that a suitable local alternative existed.[94] The colonial economy, whose main hallmark involved dependency on the motherland, thus extended to the medical realm, much to the regret of Guadeloupean promoters.

Of all metropolitan spas, Vichy especially represented a threat to Guadeloupe's hydrotherapy sector. An article in Guadeloupe's main newspaper in 1937 stated plainly, "Everyone knows that Vichy is the place for liver and nutritional treatment, and that a colonial official or an inhabitant of warm climes concerned for his health should imperatively take its waters regularly. It is a scientific fact that Vichy's waters combat the nefarious influence of [our] climate, which diminishes vitality and provokes a series of liver and intestinal afflictions. . . . It is therefore only right that Vichy should have earned the title of 'port of call for colonials everywhere' . . . it is an oasis to which all those who live in the tropics head."[95] By suggesting that the tropics were inherently toxic and that whites stationed there would find a detoxification at Vichy, the latter's promoters struck gold. Within this paradigm, Vichy dwarfed Guadeloupean spas on many registers: through its alleged clinical superiority, its social function as a center of colonial *vie mondaine*, and its cultural construction as an oasis for homesick and alienated colonizers.

In this peculiar context, the Great Depression signaled something of an unexpected boom for Guadeloupean spas, for it rendered seasonal repatriation too expensive a proposition for most colonizers. While metropolitan spa magnates grappled with the sudden drop in foreign attendance, Guadeloupean spa operators, and the colony's governors, began to hatch grand development schemes to transform Guadeloupe into the thermal resort of the Caribbean.

Before 1929, Guadeloupean springs had attracted a loyal but limited foreign or outside clientele. For instance, the Québecois poet, journalist, and politician Rémi Tremblay seasoned at Dolé-les-Bains. On a much more consistent basis, the island had drawn French colonial officials from Guyana, whom the furlough grid already pampered by allowing for health leaves for the metropole every two years. French Guyana, deemed especially inclement by the French to this day, had represented a major source of clients for Guadeloupean resorts.[96] Local Guyanese legislation had recognized the Guadeloupean spa at Dolé-les-Bains as a full-fledged *établissement thermal*, no different from Vichy. An article from 1924 discussing the question of Guyanese officials at Dolé observed, "The difficulty of life in the colonies, the excessive cost of travel, the abnormally high cost of living in France for most incomes have driven those who wish to relax in cooler and less debilitating climates than those of Guiana to seek out a quiet spot in the Antilles, one within easy access and possessing a modern hotel. Dolé-les-Bains will continue to draw more and more of our compatriots from Guiana."[97] This solid base of outside customers certainly contributed to some of the delusions and ambitions of Guadeloupean developers around this period.

A Guadeloupean *conseiller général* had exclaimed in 1927, "Who knows if the development of the spa at Ravine-Chaude will not usher in a new era of prosperity for all of Guadeloupe?" To this, a more skeptical colleague had retorted, "The dreams of building a palatial hotel at Ravine-Chaude to receive American millionaires . . . are inspired by sheer fantasy."[98] By 1935, with Guadeloupe's resorts undergoing a renaissance, another scheme was hatched to attract foreign clientele — principally American — to a new luxury spa at the Bains Jaunes, atop Guadeloupe's volcano.[99] This dream of attracting American spa-goers remains illusory to this day.

Behind the debates of the Conseil Général in 1927 lay unmistakable sympathies for some spas over others. In this way, local rivalries also contributed to the development of many of Guadeloupe's spas. The net result was that in Guadeloupe between the wars, some ten different resorts competed in a relatively limited and certainly exhaustible market. Aficionados of one spa regularly attacked rival resorts in the local press, through tortured, pompous, but

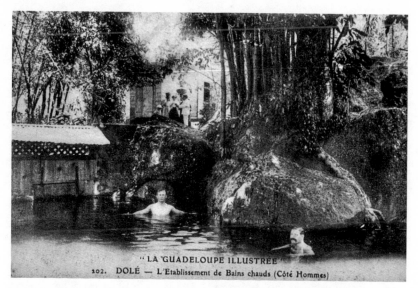

FIGURE 3. Gender segregation at colonial-era Dolé-les-Bains (caption reads "Dolé, men's side"). Courtesy of the Archives départementales de la Guadeloupe.

telling metaphors: "The resort of St. Claude . . . is one of the beautiful daughters of our colony; she can and must take on airs. But if her beautiful contours render her physically attractive, what more gracious a set of qualities than modesty and submission for a young lady. St. Claude, my dear, you should limit your desires and accept that mother has passed on different qualities to each of you: to you St. Claude the blonde it has reserved the color blue, but for your brunette sister Dolé-les-Bains, it has chosen scarlet."[100] If Guadeloupe's spas were racialized as "islands of white,"[101] to borrow Dane Kennedy's expression again, they were also manifestly gendered in the eyes of the colonizers.

In addition to being feminized themselves, as in the above passage, Guadeloupean spas were strictly segregated by gender. Such separation had been a hallmark of spas in metropolitan France since the 1830s and was in no sense unique to either Guadeloupe or the colonial realm.[102] If anything, French spa owners in Guadeloupe were reproached by their customers for being behind the times on this score as on many others. Thus, in 1924, a male representative of the Guyanese lobby complained in a Guadeloupean newspaper of the absence of any real privacy at Dolé-les-Bains, citing both hygienic and prudish considerations. Not content with the rather low barrier separating male and female baths (see figure 3), he requested the installation of private baths, given that "not all men are Adonises, and not all women are Phryneas — many people, for obvious reasons, prefer not to show themselves in tight bathing outfits."[103]

Reinventing Guadeloupe's Spas

In Guadeloupe today, thermal spas have ceased to be used exclusively by the onetime colonizers, and with the advent of departmentalization in France in 1946 and of a social security system covering thermal treatment, they have in fact seen their client base change drastically.[104] My admittedly unsystematic personal observations at Ravine-Chaude and Saint-Claude suggest that far from attracting American tourists, as had initially been dreamed, or even of serving the metropolitan administrative classes, these spas now cater primarily to the local nonwhite female bourgeoisie. These same baths had once been practically reserved for whites and had featured a gender barrier. Metropolitan French tourists, for their part, now congregate on Guadeloupe's relatively few beaches, lined by large hotel complexes on the southern coast of the Grande-Terre — once deemed the least healthy part of the island. By the same token, the former colonial establishment once devoted to treating the white and principally male body has now reinvented itself as a beautifying agent for the black female body. One can hardly miss the irony in Ravine-Chaude — the site once believed to cure diseases induced by Guadeloupe's perceived toxicity — now being either redefined as a wholesome indigenous site or promoted as an exotic destination.

Indeed, the very spas that once served as reminders of France for homesick colonials are now being fancifully reinvented by some into exotic and tropical places in their own right. When the leading French scientific thermal association met for its annual convention in Guadeloupe in 1990, a representative of Toulouse's tourist office advised Guadeloupeans to market their spas to metropolitan (white) vacationers seeking *dépaysement*. This visiting expert urged Guadeloupe's officials to "develop leisure-related infrastructures in Guadeloupe, to reinforce in the face of Caribbean competition, the attractiveness of Guadeloupe as a tourist destination, by underscoring its originality, and satisfying the growing desire for *dépaysement* of [metropolitan] clienteles."[105] In short, this outsider recommended the creation of a modern thermal chain in Guadeloupe, "one capable of offering in a tropical and Caribbean setting, an original and diversified panoply of baths and basins."[106] Such arguments encapsulate at once the continuities and changes in Guadeloupe's spa sector: a now indigenized spa industry has been advised to look back to metropolitan France for prospective clients seeking exoticism in the very venue where Europeans had once found the comfort of home.

In a similar vein, a recent edition of *Fodor's Guide to the Caribbean*, the bible of cruise travelers, describes Ravine-Chaude in terms that still evoke both metropolitan-colonial comparisons and the resort's continuing but largely fruitless effort to attract foreigners (mainly Americans): "It's not Vichy, but this modest spa is a good place to soak after tackling the trails. It draws upon the area's healthful geothermal waters and caters almost entirely to locals, though efforts are being made to upgrade it for an international clientele."[107] Ravine-Chaude continues to be compared unfavorably to Vichy but is regarded — by Fodor's at least — as an inherently local site, while for centuries it had been considered an import, a piece of France transposed to the tropics.

CHAPTER 4

The Spas of Réunion Island: Antechambers to the Tropics

IN 1923, THE POET RAPHAËL BARQUISSAU PENNED the following verse about Cilaos, the magnificent, rugged cirque sheltering one of Réunion Island's famed spas:

> C'est un champ de bataille immense que tu foules.
> Ici, noir, lapidé, farouche, hoquetant,
> Terrible, un jour Vulcain fit crouler le Titan
> Dont le sang généreux et rouge encore coule
> Aux sources où tu viens pour rajeunir ton sang.[1]

> [You tread on an immense battlefield,
> Here, black, lapidated, fierce, hiccuping,
> Menacing, one day Vucan toppled the Titan
> Whose generous crimson blood still flows
> To the springs where you come to rejuvenate your blood.]

Beyond the tortured references to volcanic activity and to mythological combat, this poem speaks to several of Cilaos's striking features. It stresses Cilaos's impressive natural setting, of course, but more important for our purposes it suggests its role as a distant battleground between maroon slaves and Creole settlers (the Titans being primitive pre-Greek deities defeated by the Greek gods). And, critically, it evokes springs. The latter are depicted as re-

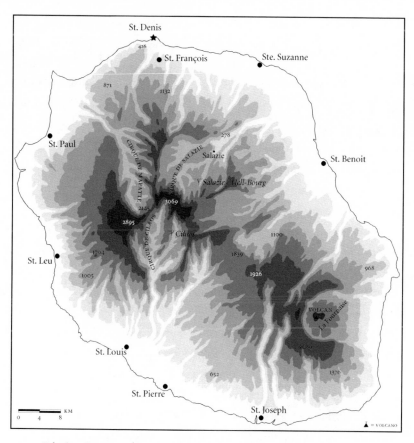

MAP 3. Réunion circa 1930, showing major spas.

juvenating the blood—a fairly accurate rendition of the curative qualities as-cribed to Réunion's spas. Since the nineteenth century, Réunion's spring waters have been believed to cure a wide range of ailments, to assuage homesickness, and perform racial revivification. Located in the heart of the island's mountain-ous interior, they seemed to provide ideal *stations climatiques* and *thermales.* Their situation rendered them vital gateways to the tropics—sites to which one would travel to find health after visiting nearby Madagascar, for example. Reaching their apogee in the heart of the romantic era, they exerted powerful attraction over *curistes*, travelers, tourists, and poets alike.

The oft-renamed 2,500-square-kilometer (1,553-square-mile) Indian Ocean island of Réunion—first known as Santa Appolinia (1506), then Mascarin, then Bourbon (1649), later Réunion (1793), then Ile Bonaparte (1806), before Réunion finally stuck in 1848 — had been uninhabited prior to European settlement in the seventeenth century and the subsequent introduction of Malagasy and African slaves. It became an important stopover and base of operations for the Compagnie française des Indes orientales, which ran the island as a private fiefdom. Only in 1766 did the French crown take over direct rule of the island from the *compagnie*. Bourbon, then Réunion, would long retain its role as a staging base. The French colonization of Mauritius, Seychelles, and Madagascar was undertaken from and largely staged in Bourbon/Réunion. In the eighteenth century especially, Bourbon was considered a breadbasket in the Indian Ocean, exporting many of its crops (coffee, wheat, corn, rice, nutmeg, vanilla) to the nearby Ile de France (modern-day Mauritius). Although slavery was certainly the main form of labor, unlike other islands, Bourbon did not emerge as a "sugar colony" until roughly 1815, after which the sugar sector experienced "prodigious" growth.[2]

On Bourbon, one historian has written, nobility mattered little: for Europeans, success was measured by the number of one's slaves.[3] Debates continue to surround the precise breakdown of slave origins on Bourbon, but Pier Larson is certainly correct in suggesting that the percentage and influence of Malagasy slaves have been consistently underestimated.[4] The overall number of slaves on the island doubled practically every twenty years until 1778. Emancipation, proclaimed in 1794, was not applied in Réunion (unlike the Antilles) during the first French Revolution, and by the time of the definitive abolition of French slavery in 1848, the island counted some sixty-two thousand slaves, hailing predominantly from Madagascar and East Africa. This said, Réunion's remarkable cultural mosaic reflects a host of other influences, including important waves of immigration from South Asia and from East Asia after 1848.

The island's cleavages were not limited to the binary of slave/nonslave. Maroons, or runaway slaves, emerged as a sizable category, establishing a parallel society in the rugged interior of Bourbon's highlands. Authorities estimated their numbers at 4,403 in 1829.[5] Nor did free people constitute a homogenous unit: a large number of poor whites, or *petits créoles*, found themselves on the margins of society. Politically, the island was torn along partisan lines. The Revolution of 1789 divided Bourbon, as did the era of British occupation between 1810 and 1814. So too did the question of abolition, resolved only in 1848. Later crises would shake Réunion, including the opening of the Suez Canal, which isolated an island previously at the crossroads of global shipping lanes. Nevertheless, throughout the nineteenth century the island retained a certain cachet in European imaginations, not only as a healthful oasis in the tropics, as we shall see, but also as a site of romantic mise-en-scène, as in George Sand's novel *Indiana*.

Réunion's Interior: From Maroon Haven to Romanticized Alpine Spa

The earliest written evidence attesting to human use of the island's hot springs dates from 1689. A Huguenot text from that year, aiming to establish a place of exile for persecuted Protestants on the isle, contains two notable observations for our purposes.[6] The first reads, "The air is good here, and one remarks a prompt recovery amongst the ill who disembark on the island." Already, Réunion was presented as a healthful island in a sea of disease — a leitmotif for centuries to come. A second passage reveals that "the island is rich in rivers and fountains . . . whose water is both admirably good and healthful. Some even say that there are purgative waters."[7] Here the curative potential of Réunion's hydromineral springs is already suggested. Both passages would prove prescient.

Réunion's highlands soon provided a different kind of haven, this time for maroons. Here, the mountains seemed either a space beyond civilization or a site of freedom, depending on one's vantage point. Both images lent themselves to the nineteenth century's romantic imagination. This was, to use Edward Alpers's phrase, "a history of massive flight, relentless pursuit and brutal punishment."[8] Various testimonies suggest that by the early nineteenth century maroons occupied the region of Tsilaos by the thousands, taking refuge in its virtually impassable peaks. The French, mindful of the dangerous precedent set by a parallel maroon society, had launched successive attacks on them in the mid-eighteenth century, with mixed results, for the maroons became masters at guerilla tactics. These manhunts attracted Creole scouts hired to track down maroons (rewards were issued for each severed maroon hand). Many of these Creole auxiliaries subsequently settled the area.[9] *Tsilaos*, meaning "place one doesn't leave" in Malagasy, would later become Réunion's largest spa, under the Frenchified name of Cilaos.[10] Most French historical narratives describing the arduous colonization of the island's rugged interior systematically efface the maroon legacy. They distinguish between the maroon era and the "discovery of Cilaos by civilized men."[11] The maroon trackers, in other words, wrote this history at the expense of the maroons themselves.

Standard accounts of Réunion's other major spa, Hell-Bourg (named after Rear Admiral Anne Chrétien Louis de Hell, the island's governor between 1838 and 1841), in the region of Salazie (derived from the Malagasy term *Soalazy*, signifying large cooking pot), should be read just as critically.[12] Most claim that the waters were used only after the arrival of the first French settlers in the area circa 1831.[13] Shortly thereafter, most narratives agree, the region of Salazie was settled by Francs-Créoles, another utopian society, constituted of indebted and disenfranchised poor whites squeezed out of the coastlands by the sugar magnates.[14] Closer scrutiny reveals Salazie's nonwhite past to be just as notable as Cilaos's. A poet provides a romanticized corrective. In a tome entitled "Les Salaziennes" (1839), a Réunionnais admirer of Victor Hugo, Auguste Lacaussade, lauded maroon resourcefulness and endurance, stressing the maroons' "useful labor" in tilling the soil and marking the landscape of Salazie.[15]

Archival records show that in 1834, only three years after Salazie's supposed discovery by Europeans, droves of slaves were using the springs. The French official responsible for the spa wrote with distress of the welfare and health of these "sick and especially leper slaves." A year later, his sympathy turned to disgust. He asked the director of the interior how he was expected to transform the site into a bona fide (read bourgeois and French) spa, when visitors wanting to admire the scenery had their gaze averted to "individuals covered in revolting ulcers." In subsequent correspondence, the same official asked, "Where shall we place sick slaves, especially lepers? And where should we bury them when they die?" This soon occurred. In 1835 a slave named Pierre-Louis perished at the spring, where he had "come to take the waters for some time now." The *conservateur des sources* berated the slave's owner, a certain Mademoiselle Prévert Brunac, for failing to provide food or shelter for him and letting him die in miserable conditions. That same year, the same official wrote to his superiors, "There are currently a few free people at the springs, but many more slaves." By 1835, he wrote of Indian lepers taking the waters. Clearly, black slaves, Indians, and free blacks were all using the springs for medical purposes and subsequently congregated at Salazie in large numbers. One can speculate

that the springs not only stirred medical hope, but also offered spiritual meaning to some of these pilgrims. For his part, the *conservateur des sources* saw his
main challenge as "bringing order to the spring." His two principal activities in
the 1830s involved preliminary engineering work to tap the spring and create
basins and the relocating of the many slaves away from the springs' immediate
proximity.[16]

The process of laying white claim to the island's springs had begun. By 1839,
the colonial administration was ordering the construction of a hotel in Hell-
Bourg to attract French patients and tourists (the two categories merge and
overlap) to the springs. The man responsible for overseeing the spa was already
speaking of its "delicious and salubrious climate" and its waters' "effectiveness
as an applicable remedy to diseases so common in tropical lands."[17] In 1852,
a group of promoters went further still, asserting that at Salazie "Providence
decided to place the cure near the disease."[18] The disease was the tropics. The
cure was not just Salazie, but also Cilaos, and indeed, to some degree, the very
island of Réunion itself—constructed as a tropical exception.

A Healthful Island

Long before the 1830s the entire island of Réunion had earned a reputation for
healthfulness. Richard Grove suggests looking to islands like Mauritius, considered paradises in European imaginations thanks to influential writings like
Bernardin de Saint-Pierre's *Paul et Virginie* (1788), to find the "seeds of modern
conservationism."[19] Closely related, I would suggest, is the idea of Réunion as
a kind of thermal panacea.

Armand d'Avezac's *Iles de l'Afrique* (1848) painted a portrait of an island that
was not merely paradisiacal, but actually healing: "[On Bourbon] chronic diseases are unknown, as are obstinate ills . . . , passed down through heredity."
D'Avezac rhapsodized: "If one were to erect a temple to physical health somewhere, it would have to be located [in Réunion]. The isle has not changed. As
in the olden days ships disgorge the sick in its ports, and they are cured without any medication or treatment, without any other attention than their simple
stay on this hospitable isle, which is more efficacious than all of medicine's
resources."[20]

Paul Gaffarel's description of Réunion in 1888 reveals this same favorable bias, even recycling some of d'Avezac's vignettes. The island's hydromineral spas, he insisted, represented merely one manifestation of a more generalized and profound healthfulness:

> By a fortunate combination of conditions rare in hot climes, this picturesque island was at the same time one of the world's most salubrious. Pure air, beautiful skies, abundant waters, fresh breezes, all is made to make this island an enchanted one. One would not think oneself in the tropics. . . . The first explorers noted . . . that wounds healed quickly here, that fevers and endemic disease were unknown. . . . Bourbon emerged as a promised land. It is still today one of the most healthful sanatoria one can recommend. One finds thermal waters whose restorative qualities are rare indeed. Thus navigators from other nationalities often drop off patients here. It is an incomparable sanitarium.[21]

Nowhere is the concept of Réunion as sanatorium more clearly laid out than in J. Auber's pamphlet *Bourbon Sanatorium* (1903). Armed with legions of statistics, Auber demonstrated how much lower Réunion's morbidity was than that of its Indian Ocean neighbors Mauritius and especially Madagascar. He described Mauritians as follows: "Less favored on their island, they come every year seeking the health and reconstructive climes of Bourbon."[22] Madagascar's toxicity had supposedly been demonstrated during the French conquest of the island in 1895. Sainte-Marie, off the east coast of Madagascar, was deemed a "veritable necropolis." In sharp contrast, Auber posited Réunion's unconditional salubriousness: "How many fever victims died in wait and in fear of being able to return to France for winter, when they had our altitudes there to rescue them nearby? Salazie's 919 meters, whose average . . . temperature is 18.38, and minimum 6 degrees centigrade. Or Cilaos's 1214 meter elevation, where seasonal temperature averages run from 12.26 to 18.01 degrees?"[23] For this doctor, Réunion's potential resided in its remarkable healthfulness (tropics as paradise in the Bernardin de Saint-Pierre mold), in contrast to neighboring isles, considered positively lethal (tropics as necropolis).

How did contemporaries account for this putative Réunion exception? Geography, insularity, and altitude are part of the answer. But Auber added another revealing ingredient, identity:

> The mere sight of our mountains and the beauty of this colony, as well as the contact with locals, are enough on their own to transform one's opinion. They

produce, at first contact, a vitally important and valuable moral reaction. . . .
First, it is the sight of well-designed towns, well-kempt, well policed. . . . Shops
remind us of France . . . The hustle and bustle is that of a European town . . .
One finds mores from a bygone time, but they are pleasing for they seem very
provincial, very French. Réunion is like a remote little piece of France, and just
as Europeans are now used to thinking of Algeria as a second France, they are
starting to conceive of Réunion as an isolated little département. . . . Is this not
the very definition of sanatoria, of sea resorts, of spa towns, of changing air . . . :
leaving behind difficulties, pains, sorrows, by immersing oneself in leisure and
tranquility, where one feels well? The analogy between Réunion and French
resort towns is striking.[24]

Here, all of Réunion is described as a health station. Location and topography
are invoked, to be sure, but the main explanation for the Réunion exception
involves identity and culture: the Frenchness of Réunion's Creoles, the appearance of their towns, the goods in their boutiques. Remarkably, in 1903 this
doctor associated the notion of "changing air," or summering at a spa town,
with Réunion's cultural Frenchness. Changing air and *ressourcement* shed their
premodern or miasmic tones and instead became laden with mesological and
almost eugenic meanings. Réunion thereby emerged as both a laboratory and a
strategic French clone in the heart of the Indian Ocean. Nostalgia, homesickness, and race intertwine in this medical analysis of Réunion's sanitary assets.

Créolité and *Francité*

Auber's discourse reflected the racialization of the anti-acclimation turn. He
was not alone in focusing on the Frenchifying impact of Réunion's microclimates upon the local Creoles. Jean-Marie Mac-Auliffe evoked the remarkable
fertility and hardiness of Cilaos's highland Creole women: "The women are
robust and very fertile. They marry young, and have large families early. For
instance, a forty-five-year-old woman, who came to me to treat her adoptive
son's fractured forearm, had eleven children and fifteen grandchildren, which
had not prevented her from adopting two orphans. . . . Creole women are
brave creatures. Their children are white and pink, fed by their mothers. They
proliferate everywhere and are a pleasure to see."[25] Cilaos's elevation and its
temperateness were accredited with ensuring fertility, healthfulness, and in-

creased whiteness. Cilaos was quite simply capable of influencing and even conditioning race.

The Mauritian journalist Charles Leal has left a useful firsthand testimony of Réunion's resorts, dated 1878. Leal observed of Hell-Bourg,

> Everything conspires to lend the thermal station of Salazie great importance. One can reach it easily in all seasons, especially during the *hivernage* [known as the least healthful season], when, in spite of rains that are moreover no more abundant than on other parts of the isle, the temperature rarely rises above 27 degrees at noon. It drops to 14 degrees in the morning and evening, and energizes and revitalizes one's organs. All, even the vegetation, speaks to the beneficial aspect of the climate. Children have a pinkish hue, unknown on much of the island. They play among the ubiquitous flowers, . . . while their mothers, fortified, fresh, and just as pink, forget their rustic environment, and shed their Creole nonchalance.[26]

Leal saw in the whiteness of the town's Creoles a sign of the healthful influence of the local microclimate. But he was doing more than simply choosing his travel destination based upon the healthful appearance of its inhabitants. He was quite plainly construing Salazie as a tonic potion. Even the Creoles' purportedly innate torpor was thus dissipated by contact with Hell-Bourg's salutary climate — salutary, of course, because of its Europeanness. In short, Hell-Bourg was capable of re-Europeanizing Indian Ocean Creoles.

Such was the dominant view of highland Creoles as mesologically conditioned by their microclimates. The view had significant repercussions on everything from social relations to high politics and even war. On his favorite topic, the stationing of troops in Réunion rather than Madagascar, Auber insisted, "I speak out strongly against sending Creole soldiers to Madagascar, where current generations are growing sickly, where the race is being subjected to a weakening, and anemic influence. Not only our troops should stay here, but soldiers from the metropole should be stationed in the highlands of Réunion, where they would be kept in a much fresher condition in the event of a war in Madagascar."[27] To Auber, mesology dictated that Réunion's Creoles would become racially unstable when transferred to Madagascar.[28] Worse yet, miscegenation would further dilute their race.

Here, we are taken back to Virchow's and Navarre's debate about Réunion's *Créoles des hauts* (highland Creoles, in local Creole dialect). Were these Creoles still Europeans, asked in essence Navarre and Virchow? Had they really acclimatized? And, if so, had this acclimation eclipsed their Frenchness? To Virchow, Réunion's Créoles des hauts stood as an exception to the rule of racial rootedness and fixity, an exception no doubt enabled by topography and climate. To Navarre, however, the Créoles were anything but a vibrant example of Frenchness: "[Are they] truly acclimatized?" he asked. "No, they simply survive." What is more, Navarre added, "the little whites of Réunion island . . . are . . . more racially mixed than is acknowledged, and can moreover, only cultivate lands between 600 and 1600 meters, in other words in microclimates, whose conditions are much closer to those [of Europe]."[29] In short, the Creole was tributary to his or her microclimate, to living in the rugged crests of the Cirques of Salazie, Mafate, and Cilaos. Each of these cirques, not coincidentally, possessed mineral water springs.

These regions, in sum, were believed to keep the Creoles French. They had, after all, permitted a similar acclimation of European fruits and vegetables. Jacob de Cordemoy, a native of Réunion and head thermal doctor at Hell-Bourg,[30] wrote with wonder about the European crops in his island's highlands, "Thanks to its highland climate, Réunion . . . produces vegetables from temperate lands. They are most readily produced in the plateaus, in valleys and canyons, where land is very fertile . . . (Cilaos, Salazie). There grow . . . outstanding lentils . . . red, white and black beans . . . peas, cabbage, cauliflower, artichokes, etc, and finally potatoes. Potatoes thrived on the island's highlands . . . Until 1906 (when *Phytophtora infestans* destroyed this crop), Réunion was able to export up to 20,000 kilos of potatoes to Madagascar and Mauritius."[31] The connection between produce, Frenchness, and healthfulness was anything but tenuous to French colonial science. Jean Lémure conflated his analysis of Salazie's waters with that of its comestibles:

> There exists a hydromineral spring near the town of Salazie. Water springs from a volcanic fissure at a temperature of 32 Celsius. It is clear, limpid, gaseous, bicarbonated, but four times less than Vichy's. The proportion of free carbonic acid is about equal to that of Vichy, its content in iron higher. It is a pleasant drink, very efficient in the cachexies of warm countries. There . . . one finds a varied sustenance: sheep, poultry, game, river fish, fresh milk and butter, excellent vegetables: peas, green beans all year round: potatoes, sweet potatoes, artichokes, salsify, even asparagus and all manner of salads.[32]

To this day, Cilaos produces two crops that seem to certify its Frenchness: wine grapes and green lentils. The latter are reminiscent of the massif central—the area of France with the second highest concentration of mineral spas after the Pyrenees. The wines available in white, rosé, and red in many ways define Frenchness in a setting where rum would otherwise be the dominant spirit.

Cilaos and Salazie were conceived as infinitely precious in multiple and interconnected ways: as breadbaskets, as convalescence centers, as sites of refuge,[33] as guarantors of Frenchness, and as solid shields against disease. In this particular respect, however, the Creoles themselves seem to have resisted aspects of modern French medicine. In 1864, de Cordemoy railed against the superstitious nature of Créoles des hauts. He wrote with disdain of their preference for folk cures like holly (*houx*) over quinine in the treatment of malaria. He noted with scorn that know-it-all Créoles des hauts women thought themselves wiser than all the "grand masters of science."[34] Grand masters of science like himself advocated "rationalized," "European" cures like quinine and hydrotherapy. In 1865, they could not account for the precise functioning of either medicine but were persuaded of their respective efficacies.

Malaria

In the realm of disease in particular, the so-called Réunion exception defied reality. Malaria had appeared on the island around 1865. Most chroniclers blamed outsiders, primarily Indian migrants, for having introduced it (Mac-Auliffe was so specific as to name the ship on which the Indian "culprits" had allegedly introduced the disease in 1864).[35] Malaria was the bane of colonials. The deadly disease was in fact at the root of Madagascar's and Mauritius's unhealthy reputations. In Mauritius, the malaria epidemic of 1866–67 killed some 40,000 people out of a total population of 360,000.[36] Malaria had so terrified nineteenth-century doctors that a medical thesis from 1861 had recommended that soldiers on sick leave in Réunion avoid the island's western coast, closest to Madagascar (some six hundred kilometers away), for fear that oceanic trade winds from the great island might carry malaria.[37]

Auber's and Mac-Auliffe's cheery eugenic picture in the 1890s and early twentieth century flew in the face of medical evidence. In 1899, wrote a certain Dr. Merveilleux, infant mortality on Réunion (accounting for 24.3 percent of deaths on the island that year) ran higher than mortality in those over sixty, whereas it should stand at roughly half. Malaria alone accounted for 377 of those 1,306 infant (under two) deaths and for 737 of the 2,064 deaths in those under twenty. Total deaths in all ages that year stood at 5,369, of which 1,761 were imputable to malaria (out of a total population of 173,192).[38]

And yet, few medical experts seemed fully to grasp the meaning of malaria's presence in Réunion after 1865. Even fewer recognized that this new state of affairs destroyed Réunion's illusion of immunity. In 1902, Mac-Auliffe, an indefatigable promoter of Cilaos, refused to acknowledge any blow to either Réunion or his spa: "Even in these new conditions [malaria having become endemic to Réunion], Cilaos remains an excellent sanatorium for malarial patients from Madagascar and Réunion's lowlands. The number of daily triumphs here over malarial cachexie constitutes the best proof of it."[39] Similarly, the *Annales d'hygiène coloniales* stubbornly clung to pre-1865 clichés. It wrote in 1899, "Ever since malaria made its appearance on the coastline, the island has admittedly lost its reputation for healthfulness. Nevertheless, Réunion remains an unrivaled sanatorium. . . . Our neighbors in Mauritius appreciate the comforting and reinvigorating effects of Réunion's highlands. They migrate every year in droves to Réunion's highlands, to strengthen their fragile health."[40] Even tainted with malaria, the island retained its reputation as an "unrivaled sanatorium." The island's Frenchness, it seems, blinded its promoters to the stark reality that tropical disease had indeed reached its shores.

Like any other mineral water spa in this era, Cilaos and Hell-Bourg were believed to treat specific diseases. By some uncanny coincidence, in the midst of the intensely malarial South Indian Ocean zone, the waters of the two spas were found to possess curative virtues against malaria. De Cordemoy noted, "The [spring] waters of Salazie work very effectively against tropical afflictions, most notably malaria. They are efficient against tropical anemia, often of malarial origin."[41] Very early on—indeed, long before malaria became endemic to Réunion itself—Cilaos and Hell-Bourg had specialized in the treatment of malarial patients. Many came from Madagascar. Already in 1861, in his medical thesis, the naval surgeon stationed in Réunion, C. Gaudin, lobbied for a military reform: "There would be great advantages to order the immediate transfer to Réunion of men [on campaign in Madagascar, Nosy-Be, Mayotte] stricken with serious intermittent fevers."[42] According to Gaudin, Réunion offered far more than a return to some miniature France. He was persuaded, like many of his colleagues, of the efficacy of the island's waters in treating malaria. He submitted a case study into evidence:

> Sir N. a noncommissioned officer in the *infanterie de marine*, 25 years of age, arrived from Madagascar. He reached the Saint-Denis hospital on September 28, 1853, in a state of complete anemia. He experienced two bouts of intermittent fevers. . . . The fever was broken, after the second bout, by a large dose of quinine. After the patient had recovered some strength, we judged it appropriate to move the patient from debilitating heat, and transfer him to Salazie. I have had many an occasion to see patients, arriving moribund in Réunion, be literally reborn, through the influence of climate alone. Then, once in convalescence, they are sent to the mountains to gain strength, robustness and even the pink hue they had brought from Europe. . . . In this young man, the fever did not recur, the anemia dissipated, and the spleen . . . returned to its normal volume. The waters were administered to the patient with great care. It is only gradually, and over the space of one month, that he managed to drink five glasses morning and evening. Whole baths were only administered for the last twenty days, three times a week. We began with sprays and showers, as well as lotions of mineral water on the patient's limbs; then these techniques were alternated with baths.[43]

Gaudin thus attributed the patient's rapid recovery to the influence of climate, to quinine, and to the waters (both external and internal cures). Salazie and Cilaos were soon presented as veritable antidotes to tropical diseases. The commercial vein was a rich one, if one considers the devastation wrought by tropical disease—and the fears it instilled—in the nineteenth century.

A Military Role

Gaudin's and Auber's case studies, and their concerns, largely focused on Salazie's role as a military sanatorium. Gaudin raved about Salazie: "Before we had this resource, we had only one recourse to save extreme cases, repatriation."[44] Repatriation, he acknowledged, was both costly and delicate, making Salazie all the more precious a sociomedical tool. In a guide to Salazie's waters, copublished in 1857 with L. A. Petit, the lead doctor on the island, Gaudin further refined this argument: "We have a military convalescence center on Mont Saint-François [overlooking the capital of Réunion, Saint-Denis]. . . . We have obtained some good results there on men exhausted by tropical heat, and by previous diseases. But experience has proven that Saint-François is insufficient for chronic, persistent afflictions, where the human economy needs to be more profoundly transformed, and in those where one must enrich the blood in essential minerals it is lacking. In those cases, we must urgently submit our patient to hydrotherapy."[45] Salazie/Hell-Bourg was thus considered the ultimate weapon, to be used after lighter means—Saint-François (a *station climatique*, but not *thermale*)—had failed.

Gaudin's and Petit's numerous examples suggest intense military use of this ultimate recourse. Patient B, a sergeant in the *infanterie de marine*, twenty-eight years old, arrived in Réunion in 1854 suffering from malaria and hepatitis. He was hospitalized three times for recurring, nagging relapses. After a third outbreak of "Madagascar fever," the sergeant was finally evacuated to Salazie. He remained there for three months, drinking five glasses of mineral water morning and evening. The results were miraculous: "He has completely recovered and is in fine health. . . . His liver has returned to a normal size. The Sergeant has returned to military service, and his health has been strong since then."[46]

An officer in the naval artillery corps arrived at Réunion from Madagascar in 1855 suffering from fevers and a "very pronounced malarial cachexie." He entered the hospital a rake: weak, thin, and battling liver ulcers. He was sent to Salazie for two months, where he was treated by Doctors Herland and Doré. They reported that "his condition improved daily thanks to the climate and to the waters taken carefully and scientifically through both baths and drinks."[47] The fevers soon recurred, however, and he was dispatched for a second cure to Hell-Bourg. Toward the end of this second stay, the patient wrote to Gaudin and Petit, "Gratitude dictates that I thank you before even leaving Salazie. . . . Ever since my stay at the spring, my health has improved day by day, my strength is returning. Now, without imprudence, I can take long . . . walks in the mountains. My appetite and sleep are both excellent. My only regret is not to be able to stay longer under the repairing climes of Salazie."[48] Not all patients were so lucky, of course. Obituaries occasionally recorded the demise of military personnel in Salazie. In August 1895, for instance, the local press reported the death of a naval doctor named Moutard, who had been stationed in Tamatave, on the east coast of Madagascar. He had come to Hell-Bourg, in the words of the press, "to recover from the fevers he had contracted in Madagascar."[49] He was not saved by Salazie or by its waters.

Popularity

Such tragedies notwithstanding, Salazie and Hell-Bourg saw their reputations rise substantially throughout the nineteenth century. In 1839, entrepreneurs seeking to develop the spa, noted that "in the last two seasons, the fourteen pavilions erected to serve as lodgings, comprising some thirty rooms in all, have proven insufficient. At present, demand is higher than ever. As a result, many people having come expressly from Mauritius to take the waters, cannot profit from the current spa season. This shortage of housing demonstrates that the importance of the infrastructures is out of step with the spa's real needs."[50]

Although Hell-Bourg's population was admittedly not composed exclusively of bathers, its explosion was nevertheless a direct consequence of the spa's popularity. By 1852, what had been a hamlet of fewer than fifty permanent inhabitants only two decades earlier had become a thriving town some 4,000 strong[51] (by way of comparison, the town of Vichy itself counted 6,428 inhabitants in 1866, only half of whom seem to have been permanent residents).[52]

Soon Hell-Bourg's prestige and desirability would rise to such an extent that, like Camp Jacob/Matouba in Guadeloupe, it would be chosen as the site for the governor's villa. Salazie held a special place in the heart of Henry Hubert de Lisle, the island's first locally born governor (in office 1852–58). He confided to his wife at the height of the Southern Hemisphere's summer in 1857, "Never is the sweetness of Salazie's climate better understood than at these times. It is February 20, the heat at Saint-Denis is intense . . . Here [in contrast,] we enjoy a delicious, fresh atmosphere. Balsamic air invades us, and one can stand a fire in the evenings."[53] That same month, Hubert de Lisle noted that "the square in front of my Salazie villa is perpetually busy. One sees all the beauties of the spa pass by." He entertained Saint-Denis' high society: magistrates, naval commanders, the director of the interior, the island's treasurer, and a certain Madame Desmolière. He took the precaution of mentioning to his wife, "This last invitation should not irk you, for there is no higher virtue on the island than her."[54] Hubert de Lisle subsequently invited "several local bigwigs" for a lunch near the springs. The governor concluded, "I am enchanted by this habit of coming to the spring during the *hivernage*, while one suffocates in the low-lands."[55] Emulation did the rest. The island's plutocracy soon vied for summer cottages near the springs, and by 1861, Gaudin was writing of Salazie's "elegant villas, in the shadow of a charming hospital."[56] The legacy of this golden age of Salazie remains palpable to this day. Its lavish villas and cottages have made Hell-Bourg the only overseas French town to be officially recognized as a "plus beau village de France."

In season, the spa's success was considerable; less so out of season.[57] A letter to the editor appearing in 1885 found Hell-Bourg "sadder and sadder" in the off-season. Porters, guides, and hotel owners were described as entering a kind of hibernation—a slumber from which the town would emerge only with the next spa season.[58] All the more proof, perhaps, that the town's very existence was intimately associated with the success of the spa.

Cilaos, the island's other main spa, soon experienced a similar boom, in spite of its remoteness. The mayor of Saint-Louis (to whose district Cilaos was initially assigned) wrote to the director of the interior in May 1851, "You will understand, as I do, Monsieur . . . the urgency of passing a law, when you consider that in Cilaos at present there are 60 to 80 bathers coming from all over the island, and from Mauritius, and that I receive daily scores of more requests for bathing permits."[59] The mayor hoped to legislate shorter baths or at least a bathing timetable. Hydrotherapy was unmistakably *en vogue*. Indeed, its popularity was such that it was causing trouble. The mayor of Saint-Louis explained, "The incidents and disorders I have mentioned to you [arguments over baths] are increasing, and demand prompt resolution."[60]

Order and Disorder

The science and practice of hydrotherapy by their very nature required tranquility, routine, rationality, regimentation, and discipline. At Vichy in 1895, *curistes* found the presence of prostitutes around the springs an abomination, not so much because of prostitution itself, but because of its proximity to the springs—site of bourgeois tranquility, probity, and order par excellence.[61] Disorder threatened Salazie ever since the 1830s, when slaves were seen as standing in the way of the site's transformation into a site of bourgeois leisure and medicine.

In 1854, thirty-two petitioners wrote to the island's governor about an unruliness of another sort. The "cantine" they wrote, illegally installed near Salazie's springs, "created a hotbed of disorder." Indeed, they argued, "not only do these cantines afford domestics with the opportunity of continuous debauchery, but . . . sailors and soldiers, sent to convalesce at Salazie's hospital, are thereby provided an easy access to alcohol, thereby prolonging their disease, and increasing your spending."[62] Upon receiving this missive, the governor sprang into action, asking his director of the interior to close "these establishments that are dangerous for the health of our soldiers and sailors."[63] The petitioners' emphasis on the corruption of sailors and soldiers and the threat of additional expense because of relapses during a cure seem to have hit a nerve.

Contagion and disease posed an even greater threat to the reputation of health spas. Yet the very popularity of Réunion's spas paradoxically increased the threat of epidemics.[64] The British traveler William Dudley Oliver wrote of Hell-Bourg in 1896, "This popularity is by no means an unmixed blessing. The large influx of people and the consequent overcrowding have affected the healthfulness of the place. I have known instances of fourteen and sixteen persons being crammed into a house, which according to English ideas, would contain six; sanitary precautions are entirely neglected, and the result can hardly be wondered at."[65] Similar trends can be discerned at Cilaos. In 1912, the governor wrote to the consul of Mauritius, reassuring him that only four cases of tuberculosis had been proven at Cilaos.[66] His compatriots should continue to visit Cilaos without fear, he concluded. That same year, the plague made its appearance at Cilaos. The colony's register of laws contains a decree from 1912 mandating the disinfection of all houses in Cilaos between the departure of one occupant and the arrival of another.[67]

Attracting Foreign Tourists

Were the spa-goers patients or tourists? The two notions went hand in hand at Cilaos and Hell-Bourg, as at any other hydromineral spa. Certainly, considerable hopes were pinned on parlaying Réunion's healthfulness—and hence its highland hydromineral resorts—into tourist destinations. In an age when Mauritius, the present-day postcard destination, was considered unhealthy precisely because of its lowlands and beaches, the idea was to capitalize on Réunion's exceptionally temperate highland microclimates. In a word, Mauritius's Creoles, it was hoped, would come to Salazie and Cilaos to reimmerse themselves in Europe (even though many had lived in the Indian Ocean for generations, making the notion of return problematic). And they did, in large numbers. Already in 1839, the director of the interior received the following letter from the "former curator of thermal waters":

> When you honored us with a visit to the thermal springs of Salazie, it did not escape your sage attention that if we succeed in attracting foreigners to this site, it will prove beneficial to the prosperity, not only of Salazie, but of the entire colony. Because here one finds comfort, the gentle, salubrious and delicious climate, and an efficient remedy for the diseases so common in the tropics, we are sure to see ill Mauritians, and Indian notables, coming to find health here. No doubt, things augur well for Salazie's future, when one considers that Vichy — whose waters are analogous to ours — was but a tiny town, no further along than Salazie, only twenty years ago. Whereas today, it is a site of great luxury, boasting magnificent buildings, walks and roads.[68]

Thus, in the very early years of Salazie's development, one finds bold promotional campaigns for attracting foreign tourists and patients. The parallel with Vichy is equally striking. No doubt authorities in Réunion hoped to reproduce the success of the new *reine des villes eaux*, as Vichy was becoming known: a cosmopolitan, elite destination, and by the same token an economic motor for a previously depressed region.

In 1852, the director of the interior received a long letter from entrepreneurs seeking to exploit Salazie's waters. The group suggested that major improvements would need to be undertaken in order to attract "wealthy inhabitants of British India especially, so subjected to liver and spleen diseases, so admirably treated by Salazie's waters." To incite them to come, one would have to "ensure that they found in our establishment the luxury and comfort to which they are accustomed."[69] Another document, from 1839, elucidates this marketing campaign: "Patients coming from India would certainly prefer Salazie to Cape, where there are no mineral springs, and to Europe, whose distance is so great as to constitute an obstacle to travel."[70] Before the digging of the Suez Canal (1859 to 1869), many in Réunion held out the hope that they could make their island at least a stopover, if not a destination in its own right, for Britons seeking temperate oases, conjointly with hydromineral cures, in the tropics.

Mauritians, however, remained the main target. According to de Cordemoy, "The most assiduous visitors of our Réunionnais hydromineral spas are the inhabitants of the neighboring island of Mauritius."[71] Special care was taken to court Mauritian elites.[72] The group seeking to exploit Hell-Bourg in 1852 made the following case: "A survey undertaken in 1839 . . . showed that fifty-two visitors from Mauritius had spent some 85,000 Francs. This sum, of course, was spent only partly in Saint-Denis hotels, and in transport to Salazie. The majority was spent on shopping and jewelry, fashion and those thousand articles of French industry that our neighbors so greatly appreciate."[73] This mid-nineteenth-century advertising campaign was thoughtfully sketched out. Salazie and Cilaos, it was hoped, could contribute to making all of Réunion a tourist destination and trading booth for French luxury goods.

Cilaos's popularity reached its zenith around 1900, with Mac-Auliffe's nomination to the post of hydromineral doctor in residence. Up until then, the dizzyingly dangerous journey from Saint-Louis to Cilaos, along sheer cliffs on the back of porters, seems to have dissuaded all but the most intrepid *curistes*. In spite of these difficulties, Mauritians had come to appreciate this site by the late nineteenth century. Again, isolation rendered Cilaos's situation tenuous. Until the construction of a one-way road in 1932 (specific times were set for cars to go up and to descend), its remoteness meant that fewer amenities and commodities were available there than at Hell-Bourg.[74]

An archival document, a petition dated 1917 and signed by sixty-four Mauritian notables, shows mounting dissatisfaction with Cilaos's backwardness, imputed once again to its isolation:

> Cilaos, as you know, has been the favorite site of *villégiature* for many Mauritians, who seek calm, health and rest from its waters. Unfortunately, from year to year, the bathers frequenting this *station thermale* and *climatique* observe with some pain that it is stagnating, and indeed on a downward trend. . . . Mauritian families who travel to Cilaos generally seek calm and tranquility. For this reason, they tend to avoid hotels, and prefer renting villas for the season. There are many such villas on the plateau. But these villas are in a greater and greater state of disrepair. Many are filthy and lack upkeep. . . . The *établissement thermal* itself, which should be Cilaos's very raison d'être . . . offers a pitiful spectacle to bathers. The cabins are in complete disrepair. . . . The bathing tubs are . . . barely ever cleaned. In fact, bathers only deign sit in them with disgust. The cabins often smell terribly.[75]

Réunion's tourist office, or Syndicat d'Initiative, wasted no time in responding. It was reacting to the petition, of course, but also to fresh competition. Indeed, an answer needed to be found to the governor-general of Madagascar's intensive investment in Madagascar's large spa, Antsirabe. The latter was threatening to lure both Mauritian and even Réunionnais clients away.[76]

At the beginning of the twentieth century, this same tourist office had formulated grand pretensions, looking to South Africa for possible spa-goers. In a brief to the governor-general entitled "Our thermal stations and the question of tourism on Réunion," the Syndicat d'Initiative outlined a plan:

> Already, Mauritians are assiduously frequenting our thermal spas, especially Cilaos and Salazie. However, the number of vacationers from our sister island remains too low to serve as the basis for a grand tourism scheme requiring massive public works and spending. A few days away from Réunion, a new economic motor is growing, destined to a brilliant future. That is South Africa, whence we can hope for an important influx of tourists. . . . Indeed, South Africa's own climate is rugged . . . and all the families of rich financiers . . . from these regions head to the coast in the winter in search of a gentler climate, as well as entertainment. But the entire coast along the Mozambique Canal presents no charm whatsoever, nor any tourist sites. . . . People knowing these areas well declare that there is a large and wealthy potential tourist base there, indeed a virtually bottomless well of wealth, which would be all too happy to find a wonderful tourist site only five days from Durban, a site boasting fine thermal and altitudinal stations for the sick and the convalescent.[77]

To be sure, Réunion was not alone in seeking new tourists from South Africa: Madagascar and more recently the Seychelles have likewise sought to tap into this pool of potential tourists.

In any event, the South African lead raised considerable hope in Réunion. In 1914, the newspaper *La Patrie créole* reported the alleged intention of an "English engineer, charged by a large Transvaal financial institution . . . to investigate whether it would be possible to acquire and manage our different spas, such as Cilaos, Hell-Bourg and the Plaine des Palmistes." The archives do indeed contain the business card of a certain Jules Paillotte, an Englishman of French origin residing in Johannesburg. He had apparently sought to acquire a kind of exclusive monopoly over a casino and a *cercle des étrangers* — comparable to a similar club at Aix-les-Bains. His ambitions went further still. He claimed to want to operate all of the spas as well as the hotels in those spa towns, which he would help erect, and to install electrical lighting and tramways in Saint-Denis.[78] None of this materialized, and South Africans proved largely chimerical. Attracting tourists from a rival colonial empire, especially from a vast colony like South Africa, proved more challenging than expected. One could also surmise that big game hunting, safaris, hikes, seaside resorts, and so on held greater attraction for Afrikaner and British tourists than French-style highland colonial spas.

Hydrotherapy's Heavy Lifters

Attracting tourists implies the presence of basic infrastructures and transportation routes. This was achieved at Hell-Bourg after Governor Hubert de Lisle decided in the late nineteenth century to order the construction of a road to Hell-Bourg, in part at least to facilitate access to his personal villa.[79] As early as 1864, various firms competed for coach service to Salazie.[80] Matters were different at Cilaos. Until 1932, Cilaos's rugged terrain had precluded all but the most rudimentary means of transportation. As de Cordemoy attests, *curistes* traveled all but seven kilometers of the path from the coastal town of Saint-Louis to Cilaos (a distance of some thirty-six lateral kilometers and over one vertical kilometer) on the backs of human porters: "This rather painful ascension on foot is much more comfortable in a porters' chair. It is the best-suited means of locomotion at present. Imagine a simple chair, laterally fixed by ropes to two long stretchers. This is the mechanism, too pompously referred to as a *fauteuil*. . . . Depending on the weight of the traveler, the number of porters varies from four to eight. Two by two, they carry the *fauteuil*, and switch over to another team of two every two kilometers or so."[81] Charles Leal recounts seeing one of his Mauritian friends arrive in Cilaos on one of these chairs: "We had been in Cilaos for twenty days. Mr. Souchon arrived last week, escorted by twenty porters, twelve for his person and eight for his luggage. I was sitting at a lookout plateau when his *fauteuil* arrived. . . . Frankly, our dignified friend inspired pity. He regretted having undertaken the trip. His nerves were frayed and he was still shaking, telling me that he was considering returning that very day so as to get over these impossible paths once and for all."[82] Leal's light-

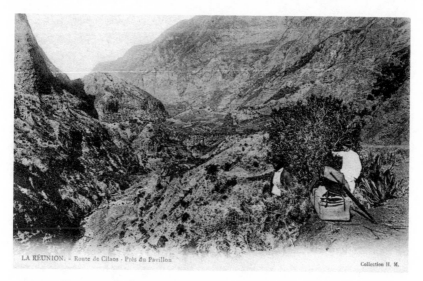

LA RÉUNION. - Route de Cilaos - Près du Pavillon   Collection H. M.

FIGURE 4. Two porters by their stretcher en route to Cilaos. Postcard, author's collection, date unknown.

hearted account sheds some light on porters, a profession entirely dependent on the economic spin-off of the spas.[83]

In 1902, fifteen of Cilaos's porters, several of them Créoles des hauts, signed a petition arguing that this tributary status made them in effect slaves to one Maximin Hoarau, the supervisor of the thermal establishment. Hoarau apparently managed their finances, taking a large percentage of their meager profits, and insisted that they purchase supplies from his private store.[84] In the nineteenth century, porters had played a central role in spa life at Salazie as well. In 1857, the porters at Salazie seem to have been predominantly Malagasy ex-slaves, formally liberated after the general abolition of slavery in all French colonies in 1848.[85] Gaudin and Petit recommended the use of *fauteuils* on the grounds that they were "less tiring and faster" than walking—clearly thinking of the carried rather than the carriers.[86] Although none of the passengers seemed to recognize it, portering was grueling and risky work. A porter's song on the Cilaos path attests to these risks, but also to the different origins of the porters themselves, some former Malagasy slaves, others Creoles: "Ah, Oh, ombé tsi manday là. Chemin Cilaos va tuer nous."[87]

The British traveler William Dudley Oliver spent considerable time around 1895 taking the waters at Cilaos and Hell-Bourg. His description of Cilaos's natural beauty and settings is cast in superlatives. He was persuaded that it would soon become the main spa on the island—which it would in fact become after Hell-Bourg's waters began cooling in 1920. A hurricane three years later would seal the Salazie spring's fate, and today Hell-Bourg is only a *station climatique*, no longer a *station thermale*.[88] Oliver wrote of the necessity of connecting Cilaos to the coast by a decent road. But in the meantime, like all tourists seeking authenticity and uniqueness, he found the Cilaos Cirque's very isolation—and the uncanny means of locomotion employed to reach the spa—to be one of its main curiosities.[89]

Oliver provides other interesting details. Three of his porters stopped unexpectedly in Cilaos, claiming to be homesick and demanding to be paid for having to wait for their customer in Cilaos. Oliver, it seems, wanted to keep porters around while taking his cure, so that they might take him on shorter hikes around Cilaos (hikes, once again, whose cardiovascular benefits would be largely lost on the "hiker"). His porters threatened to leave if they were not paid in advance for this unusual service. To mollify them, Oliver tossed five francs to the head porter, a certain Monduc.[90] Oliver suspected him of having immediately drunk the profit on rum.

In the nineteenth century, portering occupied a surprisingly central place in both empire and hydrotherapy. Little wonder, then, that we should encounter it at their confluence. Douglas Mackaman has analyzed the symbolic and practical functions of the sedan chair in nineteenth-century metropolitan spas. According to him, "The bath or sedan chair was little more than a boxed-in seat mounted on two carrying poles. This simple mode of conveyance . . . brought . . . many bathers from their hotels to a spa and then back again."[91] Although the chair bore similarities with Cilaos's, the differences traveled were incommensurate: a few hundred yards at Vichy or Dax and a grueling trek at Cilaos. Portering of this sort—over long distances and difficult terrain—constituted a striking feature of European imperialism. Indeed, the image of porters, some of them former slaves, carrying bathers was of course laden with colonial power signals. Réunion, as an *ancienne colonie* (like Guadeloupe), was reputed to be less unabashedly exploitative in its social relations than new colonies like Madagascar or Equatorial Africa. But here was a practice directly mirroring the infamous palanquin, the means of locomotion adopted by the French in Madagascar, most notably. Even at the time, the palanquin was perceived as an instrument and a symbol of colonial domination. The imperative of hydrotherapy and the sedan chair phenomenon at metropolitan spas seem to have justified the utilizing of palanquin-like practices in the old colony of Réunion.[92]

Practicing Temperateness, Experiencing Réunion's Spas

A testimony offered by the reporter L. Simonin in 1862 gives a sense of the fairly rudimentary state of Cilaos's facilities at that point. Simonin wrote in a popular travel magazine, "Imagine a large natural pool. . . . The ground is covered in gravel, the edges sealed off by flat stones, and near the entrance lies a large underwater stone on which one is seated. The basin is vast: entire families come and move about at will. Each basin is covered by a roof and hemmed off by a straw curtain."[93] Still, observed Simonin, "the primitive" nature of the establishment did not detract from its promise; if anything it enhanced it. Several settlers had boasted that Cilaos represented nothing less than the fountain of youth.

On one of his many rambles around Cilaos, Oliver traveled to Saint-Pierre for an overnight stay. There, on the coast, he spent an infernal evening, devoured by mosquitoes and tormented by the heat. This reminded Oliver of Cilaos's raison d'être. Mosquitoes, he noted, were virtually unknown at the health station. In fact, to assuage the itch from his numerous bites, Oliver found no better remedy than a hydrotherapeutic cure at Cilaos.[94] Oliver's remarks were typical of travelers at the time. The Réunionnais deputy François de Mahy was likewise struck by the thermal shock between Cilaos and coastal towns: "After Cilaos, here we are in Saint-Paul. What a contrast! In Cilaos, a European climate. Here a tropical one par excellence."[95]

The date of Oliver's account, 1895, is significant, for it coincides with the French conquest of Madagascar. Many seriously ill patients were taken from Madagascar to Saint-François and Hell-Bourg for treatment that year and the next—although not nearly enough to satisfy the likes of Auber. Oliver met several of them, mostly in Hell-Bourg. He observed of Hell-Bourg's military hospital, "While I was there, [it] was generally full of soldiers invalided from Madagascar. They at any rate had had enough of that ill-managed business. Some of that noble band of volunteers, which Réunion sent to the Madagascar

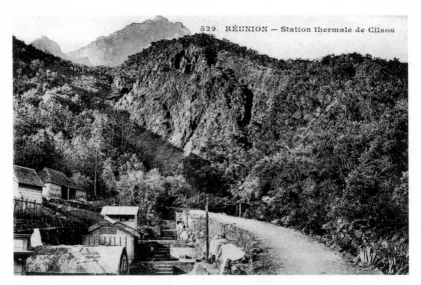

FIGURE 5. Cilaos, *bains de la commune* (communal baths). Postcard, author's collection, date unknown.

expedition, also appeared at Hell-Bourg."[96] In other words, both metropolitan French soldiers and Réunionnais Creole volunteers were seeking treatment — or rather "French air and waters" in Hell-Bourg.

Oliver also met many Mauritian tourists, with whom he was able to converse in English. He faithfully transcribed the rationales for their lengthy stays in Réunion's highlands: "When I speak of Réunion as a health resort, I do not wish to be misunderstood. It is not merely a question of passing a few weeks among pleasant surroundings, or of escaping disagreeable weather. It is an absolute necessity for Europeans dwelling in tropical climate to have some place to which they can go to recruit their exhausted energies. And in this, to my mind, consists the great value of Réunion to the people of Mauritius."[97] Leisure, argued Oliver, never entered into the picture. At stake were health and whiteness, in short, survival.

Oliver, like Leal, had a sharp eye for detail. He found the actual hydrotherapeutic installations at Hell-Bourg to be rather lacking: "The bath houses, known locally as the Douche, are two melancholy-looking wooden buildings, which by no means add to the beauty of the scene."[98] Oliver was just as attentive to balneological practices. At Cilaos, he catalogued the two hydrotherapeutic options presented to would-be bathers: one in a romantic, albeit

no-frills natural surrounding, the other in a formal, though equally rudimentary hydrotherapeutic establishment: "A small cascade in a ravine higher up
had been made into a douche by turning part of the stream through a stem of
bamboo. This arrangement, though somewhat primitive, answered its purpose
admirably. A screen of aloe leaves sheltered one from the public gaze, and a
kind of sentry-box served as a dressing room . . . The bath houses were small
wooden sheds, and the presiding genius was an old and long-bearded Creole. A good many people also drink the waters. When I was there a saucepan
was provided for that purpose."[99] Oliver's account is all the more illuminating
because it was published a year before Cilaos's bathhouses were refurbished.
Thereafter, new bath buildings were founded, relegating the structure Oliver
had known to the title of *bains de la commune* — six "mere" pools covered by
simple wooden cabins, remarked Kermorgant with some disdain.[100]

Drinking Cures

Patients who came to drink, rather than soak in, the waters made up a distinct
and important category. For one thing, by the turn of the twentieth century,
Salazie seems to have been used, in the words of Kermorgant, "almost entirely
for internal use, whereas at Cilaos balneology play[ed] a more important role
in treatments."[101] Cilaos, in other words, attracted both *buveurs* and *baigneurs*,
drinkers and bathers. Doctors certified the potency of Cilaos's drinking waters
in the same way they did those of Perrier, Evian, Vichy, and Thonon. But they
added a critical caveat. For the waters to be most effective, they would have
to be consumed at the source. Much the same was being said in the metropole to promote drinking at the springs themselves. This conclusion was tied
to the amounts of sediment in suspension as well as to the amount of gas at the
spring. More pragmatically, it delighted Cilaos's promoters. Scientists had in
essence mandated a lengthy stay in a spa town, over the alternative — already
quite prevalent — of consuming bottled mineral water. Such was the opinion
expressed by the pharmacist M. Réland in 1904: "On the left bank, and higher
up than the warm waters, there exists a cold spring, which the inhabitants of
Cilaos drink as mineral water. These waters are less mineralized than the hot
ones. . . . Neither keeps long, for a few days after my return, the waters that I
had taken as samples featured deposits of their earthy carbonates. If one wants

to achieve positive results in consuming these waters, they, like Salazie's, must therefore be drunk on location, or shortly after bottling."[102] Cilaos was thereby able to attract an entirely new clientele. Whereas its baths were reputed to cure malaria, rheumatism, bout, spinal diseases, phlebitis, and diabetes, the waters consumed orally were believed to act upon the liver, the intestine, and the stomach.[103]

This begs a broader remark about the most tangible carryover of colonial hydrotherapy. Many of the springs examined in this book — Dolé-les-Bains, Rano-Visy (see chapter 5), and Cilaos most notably — are tapped to this day for bottled mineral water. In fact, this has proven the most lucrative legacy of colonial hydrotherapy. Cilaos bottled water, fast-tracked for official mineral water status in 1972,[104] and now sold everywhere on the island, features a label vaunting pristine nature and altitude. The link with the logic of colonial *thermalisme* and *climatisme* is manifest. It nevertheless runs contrary to Réland's stance in 1904. No longer is it paramount today to ensure that active mineral elements be in suspension, by drinking the water directly at the source. The notion of pure, alpine spring waters, clones of Vichy or Evian, suffices.

Epilogue

Questions of distance, authenticity, and efficacy would haunt the new, cutting-edge hydrotherapy center at Cilaos from its very inception in 1985. The previous establishment's location in a shallow ravine had made it vulnerable to flash floods in hurricane season. The new plan was to continue tapping the springs in the ravine (sources Irénée and Véronique), but to bring the waters up to a higher plateau (named Matarum) via a conduit. Yet this short pipeline contravened the decree of December 11, 1972, on hydrotherapy and spring waters, which held — in keeping with Réland and others — that waters lost some of their efficacy in traveling. The law was modified with the help of a prominent left-wing French minister in 1983, and in 1987, the new *établissement thermal* Irénée Accot was inaugurated.[105] Today, the spa offers Jacuzzis, aqua-massage, shiatsu, and algae therapy, a far cry from the intrusive techniques practiced some sixty years ago — and from the more rudimentary pre-1897 installations for that matter.[106] One senses, moreover, that spa culture has been profoundly transformed. The spa that had once attracted settlers from around the Indian

Ocean and beyond now caters essentially to locals. Extrainsular tourists seem to prefer the beach.[107] The more intrepid, who do cross Cilaos, usually do so as the starting point of a mountain trek rather than as an end destination for hydrotherapy.

As Pascal Duret and Muriel Augustini have noted, today the vast majority of outside tourism to Réunion comes from metropolitan France. By and large these metropolitan French tourists crave three things: beaches, exoticism, and difference, when, of course, Réunion's status as a French *département* — since 1946 — might make them ponder some degree of sameness. As a result, argue Duret and Augustini, exoticized identities are being manufactured specifically for the tourism industry.[108] Where does this leave sites like Cilaos? As in Guadeloupe, the mineral spas that once brought more visitors to the island than any of its other attractions have now been eclipsed by seaside resorts — on the very coast once identified as unhealthy by Gaudin and others. Cilaos is visibly playing catch-up to the seaside resort of Saint-Gilles: recently Cilaos's mayor promised to build a casino to try to rival that of Saint-Gilles's.[109] Cilaos's claims to Frenchness have become more of a tourist liability than an asset, although efforts are certainly under way to exoticize everything from Cilaos's wine to its Creoles. Visiting scenic Cilaos or Hell-Bourg today, one easily forgets that these sites were once considered critical for settlement and empire. They were seen as nothing short of tonic agents, capable of protecting and revivifying colonials and of extracting Creoles from their "torpor" while simultaneously "re-Frenchifying" them.

CHAPTER 5

Leisure and Power at the Spa of Antsirabe, Madagascar

THE HIGH-ALTITUDE MINERAL WATER SPA OF ANT-sirabe in central Madagascar encapsulates the nexus of power, medicine, tourism, and leisure that makes colonial spas and hill stations a rich source of investigation. For here, once again, was a particular form of colonial tourism — distinct from the pillaging of Angkor by Orientalist adventurers, from exotic tours of the South Pacific, and from automobile rallies in North Africa, about which much more has been written.[1] Instead of looking for the exotic, at Antsirabe colonials actually went to remarkable lengths in their quest for the familiar. Antsirabe thus involved lateral colonial tourism within the island colony of Madagascar, with the goal of achieving *ressourcement*. Such reimmersion in the motherland was to be achieved by soaking in Antsirabe's temperate climate and bathing in its familiar waters — waters that, as we shall see, colonial doctors legitimized in purely metropolitan terms by stressing their similarities with Vichy's. Colonial settlers, soldiers, and administrators alike came to, or seasoned at Antsirabe, in their own words *pour se refaire une santé* (to rebuild their health), with the multiple connotations that this entails: reproducing bourgeois leisure practices, operating within a rigid climatic mold, and asserting the restorative qualities

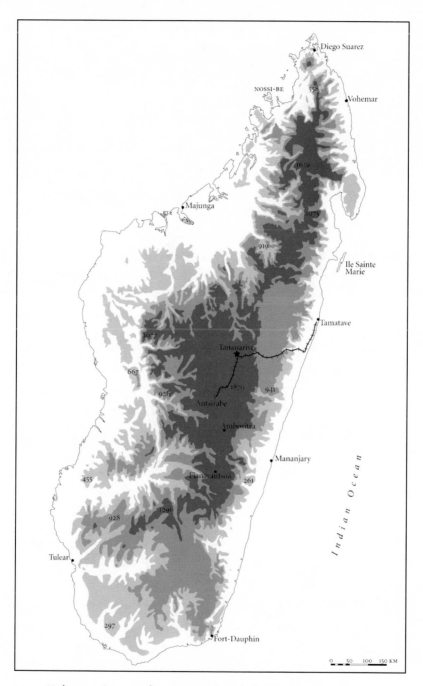

MAP 4. Madagascar circa 1930, showing Antsirabe and other principal cities.

of reimmersion into France, or at least what they considered a piece of France ten thousand kilometers away. In this chapter, I will examine how a preexisting Malagasy site was appropriated and reinvented as a space of colonial villégiature and power.

Spring Waters in Malagasy Cultures

Even triumphalist colonial narratives recognize that the Merina and Betsileo people of highland Madagascar had, long before the French invasion of the island in 1895–96, used the waters of Antsirabe, meaning "place where there is much salt" in Malagasy.[2] But such accounts are also careful to argue that prior to the invasion, the Merina had supposedly "not developed or properly exploited" the waters.[3] This piece of colonial mythmaking sought to establish a French monopoly over the "proper," "scientific," and "medicinal" uses of springs. An interesting British account written by J. T. Last in 1894 held that

> the natives cannot account for the water being hot, so conclude that the place must be the seat of some supernatural power, and therefore deem it the proper place whereat to make their prayers and offer their sacrifice. But although they cannot understand the reason for the water being hot, yet they quite appreciate the springs as a healing source. The natives of the district, and also many from a distance, when afflicted with rheumatism and kindred diseases, resort to the spring, when they both bathe in and drink the water. The medicine-men also recommend it strongly, thoroughly believing in its healing powers.[4]

As we shall see, the belief that Antsirabe's waters cured rheumatism became widespread after the Malagasy prime minister's son recovered from this affliction following a hydrotherapeutic treatment at Antsirabe in 1879. But the originality of this testimony is to show how supposed European cures and Malagasy beliefs surrounding early inhabitants known as Vazimbas (see below) were cross-fertilized in the late nineteenth century.

Sifting through these layers of colonial writings, one is hard put to reestablish the many precolonial practices surrounding the hot springs of highland Madagascar. The work of the anthropologist Maurice Bloch lends us a sense of the significance of water in a host of Merina rituals — the Merina being the highland ethnicity that had come to dominate most of Madagascar under the reign of Radama I (1810–28). Indeed, Bloch argues that water was literally equated with *mahery*, or power, in Merina culture.⁵ Water played a crucial function in a host of rituals, ranging from circumcision rites to the elaborate royal bath ceremony.⁶ Bloch's interpretation of the royal bath provides helpful context:

> For the royal bath, youths whose father and mother are still living . . . went to fetch water from certain special streams and lakes. These streams and lakes are associated with creatures called Vazimbas. Vazimbas are represented as rather vague indigenous inhabitants of Imerina who were defeated by the Merina and especially by ancestors of the royal line. . . . However, because of their original ownership of the land, their spirits still control certain aspects of its fertility and have thus to be worshipped rather as nature spirits. This non-human fertility is symbolized in most Merina rituals by water. . . . Once this water had been obtained, it was brought back to the palace and warmed. The monarch, at the very moment of the turn of the year, took off the old clothes in which he had been dressed, and stepped into and then out of the bath . . . [After the bath, he/she] then sprinkled the people with water. . . . Receiving this water was a sign of filiation, either political or kinship . . . , and so if any slave received the blessing of the water of the bath he was automatically freed.⁷

Although mineral or naturally warm waters were not necessarily part of this ritual, the conflation of waters from the royal bath with power and privilege would have profound repercussions for the spa of Antsirabe. Moreover, French hydrotherapy would graft new medical meanings onto the waters' already sacred association with the Vazimbas. Thus, at Antsirabe some Malagasy bathers were careful to perform a series of Vazimba-related rites, including throwing coins into the baths, braiding grass near the spring, or presenting animals in sacrifice, before taking the waters.⁸ In fact, one of Antsirabe's springs was known even to French doctors as the "Vazimba hole."⁹

Alfred Grandidier, the famed colonial cataloguer and ethnologist of Madagascar, provides another illustration of the importance of mineral waters and springs in Malagasy societies. He too notes the abundance of "sacred springs and ponds and fords (*rano masina, ampitsaha masina*)" across the island. He then cites a secondhand account: "Mr. Mondain recounts having seen in 1902 inhabitants of Ambohimanga gathering around a small pond to the south of the town, and danc[ing] frenetically around a patient drinking some six liters of water. The said water was considered *masina* (holy) and was attributed the virtue of predicting the outcome of diseases."[10] In 1893, an Englishman, James Mackay, described the following Malagasy water treatments for malaria, involving both cold showers and vapor baths: "The native treatment of malarial fever consists in sending the patient out early in the cold morning dews and mist to take exercise. Then he is made to bathe, by having a cold douche all over him. After that a form of vapour bath is improvised with some steaming decoction, the materials being various herbs. Lastly he is not allowed to lie down."[11] Clearly, the spiritual and the medical were fused in these Malagasy water rites — rites that would rapidly enter into contact with the equally ritualized culture of colonial hydrotherapy.

Precolonial Antsirabe

Antsirabe's post-1800 history can be broadly divided into four eras: the precolonial era; the missionary period in the late nineteenth century when Norwegian Lutheran missionaries attempted to infuse European medical meanings into the springs; the colonial era itself, begun in 1895–96 with the brutal French conquest of Madagascar and ending with Malagasy independence in 1960; and post-1960 independent Madagascar. The Norwegian presence at Antsirabe might at first seem surprising. Prior to the French protectorate over Madagascar, established in 1885, and the French invasion and subsequent annexation of the island a decade later, various Protestant and Catholic missionaries as well as several imperial powers, most notably Britain and France, had jockeyed for position and influence on the great island. When Queen Ranavalona II acceded to the throne of Madagascar in 1868 and reversed her predecessor's hard line on Christianity and foreign missions, the Norwegian Missionary Society (founded in 1842) joined in the scramble for Madagascar.[12] They carved out several zones of influence on the island, chiefly in the capital Antananarivo and the region of Vakinankaratra, where Antsirabe is located.

Several sources show how prior to the French conquest, the Norwegian Lutheran Mission, especially Doctor Borchgrevink and Pastor Rosaas, set about converting Malagasy elites to specific therapeutic virtues of Antsirabe's waters. In particular, these Norwegians were convinced early on that Antsirabe's waters were "closely allied to [those] of Vichy"[13] — hence their ascribing to Antsirabe the Malagasy name of *Rano-Visy* (Vichy water), which has stuck to this day. Rosaas's diaries suggest that it was in 1879, the very year he claims to have discovered the main spring where the queen's bathhouse would later be erected, that a Professor Waage in Oslo (then Kristiania) established the parallel between the mineral content of Antsirabe's and Vichy's water.[14] Interestingly, Rosaas again coded Antsirabe as a site of European medicine, by first treating a Norwegian named Mrs. Petersen with the waters and then utilizing its growing reputation to gain leverage and ascendancy in elite Malagasy circles.

Rosaas's rising influence is perhaps best reflected in the saga of the Malagasy prime minister's son Panoelina (known more formally as Rapanoelina), who had fallen ill upon returning from England in 1879. Rosaas and Borchgrevink prescribed repeated immersion in Antsirabe's sulfuric springs over several years, a treatment that allegedly cured the young man entirely of his state of virtual paralysis.[15] Word of Panoelina's recovery spurred a rush to take the waters. Numerous Andriana (Merina "nobles," loosely translated) scrambled to reserve private baths at the spa. Prime Minister Rainilaiarivony and Rosaas exchanged copious correspondence over which Andriana could be lent the keys to the queen's bath.[16] In 1880, Madagascar's minister of foreign affairs, Rainimaharavo, in turn asked to take the waters of Antsirabe to treat his gout. He wrote effusively to his uncle the prime minister about his subsequent recovery.[17] That same year, other Merina notables took the same waters to treat a gamut of afflictions ranging from kidney ailments to lung disease, rheumatism, and gout.[18] In 1882, unable to keep up with demand and eager to maintain control over an establishment that had become synonymous with privilege and favor, the prime minister instructed Rosaas as follows: "From now on, unless you receive a letter from me, do not let anyone bathe in the Queen's house or in mine."[19] Antsirabe's sudden popularity cannot be imputed entirely to Andriana emulation or to the word of Panoelina's recovery. The prestige associated with the Merina tradition of the royal bath, and indeed the Merina equation of power and water, had undoubtedly spilled over onto new hydrotherapeutic practices.[20]

Many other Antananarivo notables, unable to make the 169-kilometer trip to Antsirabe, asked to have the waters brought to them. Thus, an Andriana by the name of Rainizanoa wrote to Rosaas, "If you have sparkling water with

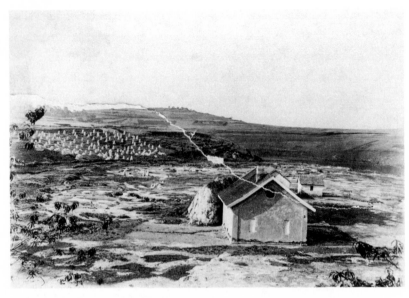

FIGURE 6. This earliest known photo of the queen's bathhouse, circa 1882, also shows surrounding Andriana structures and, in the background on the left, probable calcite formations. (The identical picture at the FTM geographical institute in Antananarivo is listed as dating from 1898.) FTM, Album 10, 107. Courtesy NMS. All rights reserved.

you, I would like to have some because it is difficult to find it here." Ratsi-manohatra, for his part, asked, "I would like to get some Vichy water from you because I finished mine." And Rakoto requested, "I ask you again if you can do me the favor of getting me some Vichy water."[21] Borchgrevink seems to have been happy to oblige, at least for these influential Andriana. As early as 1879, the doctor noted that he "sealed [the bottles] so that they keep their efficacy."[22]

Rosaas and Borchgrevink were keenly aware of the power they had derived from the celebrated cure of Panoelina. First of all, the Norwegian Lutherans were able to gain an edge over their competitors. Rosaas observed in his diary, "There were rumors about, according to which Jesuits were trying to get a hold of the springs here, and our friends advised us to apply to the Queen and ask permission to construct a bathhouse for her." Further on, Rosaas acknowl-edged other fringe benefits: "A rather large sign-up for our school can also be viewed as a fruit of the baths." Finally, he noted, "Luckily, the spa brought our mission great services. We gained a better relationship to the [Malagasy] Gov-ernment, all the resistance from the people ended, and many have now gained better health at this bath. In 1884 the bath was solemnly given to the Queen [Ranavalona III], and the keys handed over to the delegate Isak-andriana; but these were returned to us again on the Queen's behalf, and we were allowed to use the three departments to the East. All this was a great honor in the eyes of the people."[23] Antsirabe's missionary era thus saw the springs become associated with European medicine and, most important, saw them parlayed into an instrument of considerable power.

The Norwegian missionaries remained active at Antsirabe throughout the colonial era. Tensions between French and Norwegians flared up repeatedly. In 1911, for instance, secular French medical authorities protested that the Lutherans were duping "credulous" Malagasy by combining standard European medicine (at their private mission hospital) with liturgical chants so as to "speed recovery." This made it all the harder to convert Malagasy patients to rational French medicine, argued the report.[24] Still, in times of crisis, Norwegians and French came together to repel the threat of indigenous resistance.

Of all the conflicts that erupted in the wake of the French conquest, none marked Antsirabe, and indeed all of Madagascar, more profoundly than the *menalamba* insurrection, begun in November 1895. The rebellion's targets included the French invaders but also the Merina rulers, accused of accommodating the French, as well as the missions, tokens of the Christianization of the Merina crown.[25] The rebels claimed to defend both the authentic values of the Merina monarchy — against what the monarchy had become — and traditional religious practices, like talismans, now threatened by evangelization. Stephen Ellis, the leading expert on the insurrection, deems it at once a civil war, a struggle for national liberation, and a war of religion. Antsirabe played an important role in the rebellion, for it was there the rebels launched their first direct attack on a European center. Under the local leadership of Rainibetsimisaraka, some fifteen hundred Malagasy rebels, wielding their signature red flags (symbols of the royal line, not of Marxist revolution), descended on Antsirabe in May 1896. There, a French witness recounts, two European men, sixteen women, and nine children withstood a siege for several days in Pastor Rosaas's house, chosen as a redoubt for its nonflammable roof. They watched as the sanatorium was razed and churches burned in the distance. French and Norwegians had banded together to repel the attacks, purportedly killing, with considerable help from their Malagasy rescuers, five hundred rebels in the process. In Ellis's words, this account gained notoriety, in no small part because it "struck a chord in the colonial siege mentality" with its "best wild west" ending. French Antsirabe had been christened in blood.[26]

For all of these conflicts, however, the transition to French domination in 1895–96 had little effect on Antsirabe's curative reputation, on its fame as a site of health. It did, however, significantly alter the balance of power among Europeans, as we have just seen. At the moment of transition, Rosaas bemoaned that the queen's bathhouse had been ransacked by local Malagasy, after the French *résident* had forgotten to return the key (Rosaas observed indignantly, "This is how French civilization behaves").[27] In one area, however, the Lutheran missionaries had quite unwittingly laid a foundation for French colonial myth-making: their equation of Antsirabe and Vichy would become the keystone to Antsirabe's very raison d'être. As French doctors began to lay claim to Antsirabe, they sought to establish their own knowledge in *thermalisme* over both the colonized and, to a lesser extent, the missionaries.

The Question of Authenticity

One of Borchgrevink's practices — that of sending sealed bottles of Antsirabe spring water to notables in Antananarivo — fell headlong into an intense and ongoing French debate over whether the mineral potency of spring waters is diluted by bottling or transportation from its place of origin. Did it matter that these waters had been transported overland, over several days, before being consumed? A Dr. Farinaud, an Antsirabe expert, maintained in 1939 that even an hour's exposure to air rendered *Rano-Visy*'s otherwise healthful water too acidic. Drinking at the source was medically mandated.[28]

For that matter, one could ask, was it problematic that this was not actual Vichy water so much as a local equivalent, *Rano-Visy*? This question of authenticity is, of course, at the crux of Antsirabe's colonial position: colonials soon congregated there on the basis of purportedly scientific claims of its being the Vichy of the Indian Ocean. If the mineral and chemical could trump the cultural, then colonials could fancy themselves back home in Antsirabe. But if absolute authenticity was required, then colonials would be left only the costly option of returning to France regularly. French colonizers, convinced that landscape, geology, and science somehow preordained the creation of a

French enclave in highland Madagascar, set about, like their counterparts in British India, "replicat[ing] the domestic, educational and social institutions of their homeland with startling exactitude." [29] In this case, the premise of Vichy water similitude provided the foundations for such an experiment in colonial cloning.

Medical Rationales

Long before invading Madagascar, French observers had vaunted the salubrity of the high-altitude plateau around Antsirabe. In a document from 1843, Nantes' chamber of commerce offered a key for reading the island's climatic variations: "Once established in the district of Imerina (central highlands), we would be able to radiate from the center of the island to the periphery. All the plateaus of the interior offer a climate as healthful as that of France. Authentic documents leave no doubt on this matter: the principle even stands at the basis for Hova [read Merina] successes. They [the Merina] fall sick just like us in the coastal areas; upon contracting fevers, they return to their high Imerina plateaus and reimmerse themselves into a European-like clime." [30] This environmental-racial view of Merina (whom French ethnographers mislabeled Hova) fragility endured into the twentieth century. [31] A colonial medical report from 1904 reads, "Light skinned, and hence vulnerable to mosquitoes, ignoring the rules of hygiene . . . the Hova [or Merina] can live . . . only in his homeland. It is well known how vulnerable this organism [*sic*] is to malaria, and how he is decimated every time he enters a climate warmer than Imerina (the central highlands). We have seen this on the coast. Merina cannot live there, nor can they develop or found families." [32] Once again, the anophele mosquito paradigm was simply engulfed in the earlier tide of racio-climatic determinism.

Precisely because of their purported climatic fragility, the Merina were likened to the French (that both groups claimed to rule the island only reinforced this parallel) and deemed mesologically predisposed to thrive only on the salubrious central highlands. This only confirmed long-standing French medical bias in favor of the highlands, at the expense of the coastal zones. Macé Descamps' *Histoire et Géographie de Madagascar* (1846) reported even that some travelers "had declared the [plateau's] climate to be superior to that of France."[33] Similar judgments were passed in the period immediately following the French conquest of Madagascar. The French tropical doctor Georges Treille marveled at the immigration and settlement opportunities offered by Madagascar's high central plateaus: "Madagascar must be ranked as a settlement colony, and it should be possible, in fact, to encourage not only the immigration of healthy men, but also that of women and children."[34] As we saw in chapter 1, the theory that idealized temperate microclimates, whether located in higher altitudes like Antsirabe or cooled by currents or breezes, held such areas to be the only colonizable regions of the tropics. In this perspective, the ultimate measure of a settler colony was the possibility of bringing European women and children to it. Thus, the high plateaus around Antsirabe were explicitly contrasted to the island's supposedly nefarious coastal areas. In fact, Jean Lémure pointed to the lengthy Norwegian missionary presence around Antsirabe as a sign of its colonization potential.[35] Treille, for his part, explained, "The entire chain of the high plateaus compensates by the excellence of its altitude, for the current vice of its coastline. There can be no doubt that Europeans will be able to settle durably in the Imerina and the Betsileo areas" (Antsirabe lay near the juncture of the two).[36]

As Philip Curtin has observed, "French medical opinion . . . was convinced that the highlands [of Madagascar] had always been malaria-free."[37] Specialists differ on whether or to what degree Madagascar's high plateaus had ever been exempt from malaria. Yvan Paillard's findings suggest a massive increase of malaria in the island's central highlands — including the district of Vakinankaratra, where Antsirabe is located — between 1895 and 1908. Gwyn Campbell provides a convincing answer to the mystery of malaria's rapid spread, one that shifts the chronology earlier. Campbell asserts that the *fanampoana*, or requisitions, used by the Merina monarchy in the nineteenth century were largely responsible for malaria's increasing occurrence in Madagascar's highlands.[38]

One thing is certain: colonial doctors were at a loss to explain what they considered to be a mysterious increase in malaria in the central highlands around the turn of the twentieth century. A medical report of 1904, while grudgingly recognizing that a malaria outbreak had occurred in Imerina and Betsileo in 1878 (in other words, prior to the French invasion), nevertheless theorized that the rise of malaria in the highlands around 1900 could be attributed to population movements from the coasts to the highlands and improved transportation routes between the two areas in the wake of the war in 1895.[39] Better to have induced the rise of malaria, it seemed, than to have been wrong about the healthfulness of Madagascar's highlands.

The French conquest of 1895 proved the most important test to the vision of Madagascar as a colonizable island — an idyllic vision shared by many French settlement advocates that had elided malaria from the central highlands altogether.[40] Such visions of Madagascar as a partial paradise were shaken by the tremendous losses to malaria incurred by invading French troops in 1895–96. Interestingly, however, this medical debacle would only reinforce a French bias against the coastal regions, in favor of the highlands.

Curtin has shown that the French military conquest of Madagascar "has the worst reputation for medical failure of any military campaign in the European conquest of Africa." [41] Of the 15,000-man force, 5,980 were lost to disease, primarily malaria, over a ten-month campaign; by comparison, only 13 French soldiers perished in combat. Such cataclysmic losses led the French to seek refuge from the disease.[42] Colonial doctors recognized at the time that 72 percent of fatalities were due to malaria — a low estimate according to Guy Jacob.[43] Already, Curtin notes, precautions had been taken to put soldiers through a series of decompression chambers before subjecting them to Madagascar: many had been posted on the less malarial island of Réunion, in hopes of achieving some degree of acclimation.[44] It is in this context that one should understand one of Antsirabe's earliest colonial functions: that of a military sanitarium or convalescence center that would in a sense combine the functions fulfilled by both Camp Jacob and Dolé-les-Bains in Guadeloupe. Antsirabe was to serve as a kind of antechamber to the tropics, one that could act both as a base for freshly arrived soldiers and as a retreat for those having endured long stays in the colony.[45]

Not all colonial experts agreed on the supposed healthfulness of the high plateaus, or on their utility for that matter. General Joseph Gallieni, the "pacifier" of Madagascar, saw "little to be done" in the central plateau.[46] This sparked a brief but intense polemic. Settlers in the highlands were outraged to hear Gallieni suggest that "the entire economic future of our new possession is to be found in the coastal regions of the island." [47]

Even Antsirabe's healthful reputation was put to the test, after successive localized epidemics of smallpox in 1897,[48] and malaria in 1901.[49] In 1902, it was technically downgraded from the status of malaria epidemic, but colonial medical authorities recognized that "malaria has not ceased to occur [by any means], and in fact remains the chief cause of morbidity and mortality in the province of Antsirabe." [50] In 1906, there was little choice but to recognize the epidemic nature of the disease: 3,457 patients were hospitalized for malaria in Antsirabe proper, and 9,643 for the broader Antsirabe district that year. Given the gravity of the epidemic colonywide, local doctors searching for a silver lining actually considered the figure of 9,643 malaria cases out of a total district population of 40,406 to be relatively favorable (roughly 25 percent as opposed to the 50 percent, or 9,395, malarial patients for 19,546 in nearby Ambohimasina)! [51] Malaria would continue to prove a scourge at Antsirabe, undermining the town's claim of utter healthfulness. [52] The fact that malaria was present at Antsirabe might logically have called into question its being chosen as a health station. Far from it: it was precisely after the turn of the twentieth century that settlers, administrators, and soldiers began to flock to the highland spa.

In spite of proof that malaria and smallpox were present (and sometimes rampant) in Antsirabe, the site continued to be seen as a salubrious separator from the tropics and their diseases. A guidebook to Madagascar published in 1931 persisted in the belief that Antsirabe was "absolutely exempt from malaria." [53] Why the refusal to acknowledge the presence and persistence of malaria at Antsirabe? The answer is partly straightforward, involving the marketing and advertising of a healthful vision of the spa. More profoundly, the unwillingness to burst Antsirabe's reputed antimalarial bubble was also the result of a disjuncture between tropical science and the colonial periphery. [54]

The ultranationalist, anti-Semitic, and xenophobic French newspaper *La Libre parole* struggled to come to terms with mounting French losses during the conquest of Madagascar. In 1895, the popular newspaper speculated, against all scientific evidence, that malaria might be directly contagious from person to person, before admitting a terrible helplessness: "Quinine is proving useless, and changing air is not helping our soldiers much either." [55] A letter from an officer taking part in the Malagasy campaign lamented in much the same vein, "Ordinarily, this state of anemia ... which only gets worse and forces the European to return to his native land, only sets in after 18 months to two years in the tropics. Madagascar must be especially unhealthy for our men to be knocked out of service after only three months. They are being intoxicated." The newspaper then noted that evacuated soldiers were being sent to Salazie in Réunion. The article went on to distill for the general public the debate over what degree of altitude could offer respite from tropical disease. Drawing from the example of colonial rivals, the newspaper stated that Darjeeling's 2,668 meters or the Nilgherry Hills' 2,200 meters were far more appropriate for detoxification than Salazie's 950 meters (Réunion) or, for that matter, Camp Jacob's 545 meters (Guadeloupe). Indeed, concluded *La Libre parole*, any height over 1,000 meters might do.[56] Such knowledge of the precise altitudes of colonial sanatoria also reveals to what extent the minutiae of climatic debates filtered down to the popular press in France. Ultimately, the newspaper clung to the notion that "changing air" and altitude constituted the only salvation for French troops.

The popular press, however, was not alone in refusing to see Antsirabe's potential health shortcomings. Colonial doctors participating in the Madagascar invasion had, of course, been the first to clamor for a highland sanatorium. Jean Lémure, who witnessed the medical debacle, wrote of poor results with some of the first sanatoria attempts in coastal areas, on Sainte-Marie island, and at Vohémar, which had initially been billed "the Normandy of Madagascar." He noted that at these sites "fevers worsened instead of improving."[57] Meanwhile, G. A. Reynaud's *Considérations sanitaires sur l'expédition de Madagascar* (1898) once again drew from a comparative framework, making connections between this colonial expedition and many others, some British, some French. Reynaud found the temporary sanatorium installed by the French military on the small island of Nossi-Comba (near Diego-Suarez in northern Madagascar) to be completely lacking, in part because of its low elevations and high levels of malaria. Conversely, he wrote with great admiration of Cilaos's and Salazie's curative effects, noting that they had been underutilized during the military health crisis of 1895. He also held out hope that "new sanatoria would be installed on Madagascar's high plateaus."[58] Reynaud's optimism regarding the healthfulness of Madagascar's central highlands was unconditional, even obstinate. And once again, he drew noteworthy parallels with Salazie and Camp Jacob:

> [Madagascar's] dominant pathology is malaria.... As one climbs in altitude, one escapes its influence. As of about 500 meters, one will find few vectors of malaria, and on the Imerina plateau this affliction is altogether exceptional. Europeans who come down with malarial fever on their arrival in the highlands have

usually contracted it while staying in the lowlands. It is a fact often observed that fevers previously latent in Europeans, manifest themselves when traveling from an insalubrious hot clime to a salubrious highland. . . . Numerous such cases have been observed in patients going from Guadeloupe or Réunion's lowlands to the health camps of Camp Jacob and Salazie. . . . I will agree with the vast majority of experts, that the high plateaus of Madagascar are healthful.[59]

Pressure for Antsirabe's development came from such doctors, armed as they were with an impressive comparative arsenal of altitudinal statistics, and persuaded—in spite of much evidence to the contrary—of the unconditional healthfulness of Madagascar's central mountain chain. The ongoing French association of altitude and health proved stubbornly immutable.[60]

Antsirabe's 1,600-meter elevation and its legendary July–August frost thus came to obscure its proven (and ongoing) failure as a shelter zone from malaria. The factor that clinched the perception of Antsirabe as a panacea in colonial minds, however, was certainly its spring waters. Indeed, to one doctor in 1899, at least, a *cure* at Antsirabe was every bit the therapeutic equal to a trip home. A certain Dr. Duval asserted, "In most cases, treatment at Antsirabe would produce the same results on patients as a trip home followed by a long stay in Europe."[61] At last, a local antidote had been found to Madagascar's alleged toxicity.

The so-called French pacification of Madagascar between 1895 and 1902 occurred at the very time Ronald Ross's findings on the transmission of malaria by mosquitoes were gaining currency. It should come as no surprise, then, that the founding of the French colonial and military health station at Antsirabe was couched in two distinct logics: first in the pre-Rossian language of acclimation, fresh air, altitude, soil, and water, and soon in the post-Rossian language of mosquito avoidance. In both pre- and post-Rossian paradigms, of course, Antsirabe, with its cool nights (thirteen-degree Celsius daytime average temperature in the coldest month of July, with nighttime lows of freezing), therapeutic waters, and high altitude, seemed to fit the bill.[62] Following two different logics, Antsirabe thus promised a welcome respite from coastal malarial zones. Another pre-Rossian dimension was the French medical obsession with the liver and with the hepatic symptoms of malaria (perfectly real, as travel doctors today can attest), believed to be treatable at Antsirabe.

In short, Antsirabe was thought to operate on two levels: first, as a kind of regional prophylaxis, on the basis of its purported immunity from malaria, and, second, as a hydrotherapeutic and even climatic cure for malarial symptoms. Doctors now consider the distribution of malaria vector mosquitoes on the island to be "mainly a function of bioclimatic domains and, to a lesser extent, altitude."[63] Altitude, in other words, was certainly not the only answer, although it has some claim to medical relevance. This brief parenthesis on shifting medical rationales also shows that the climatic/environmental paradigm withstood the arrival of germ theory. As Dane Kennedy has observed, the primacy of climate and constitutions remained firmly established in the colonial hygienic discourse as a kind of shorthand, one able to withstand the late-nineteenth-century realization that disease, not climate, killed.[64]

The application of climatology and hydrotherapy raised hopes that Antsirabe could serve as more than a health resort—that it could become a panacea based upon metropolitan affinities, whether to the metropole's spring waters or to its climate. In 1899, the *Revue de Madagascar* boasted, "Nowhere in Madagascar are these two essential conditions, the high qualities unique to these waters and the beneficial climate, nowhere are they as luckily combined as in Antsirabe. . . . The alkaline mineral waters of this locale are indeed without equivalent in Madagascar, being more or less identical to the waters of Vichy."[65] *La dépêche coloniale* reported in 1901, "The action of [Antsirabe's] waters, joined to the temperateness of the climate of the island's interior, will be a precious resource for restoring the shaken health of those having spent time on the coast."[66] Another article that same year raved as follows: "Antsirabe is about 1600 meters above sea level. This elevation means that we enjoy a very cool climate and that the region is well ventilated. It is in all respects an idyllic health station."[67] As late as 1954, six years before Malagasy independence, French doctors still insisted that "favorable climatic conditions make Antsirabe certainly the most salubrious spot on the entire island."[68] The illusion of healthfulness was complete.

Tapping the Springs

The European search for Madagascar's hot springs began early on. In what is probably the earliest European description of Antsirabe (name changes and vagueness in the text make it impossible to know for certain), a French traveler to Madagascar in 1802 evoked "a village named Ranou-Mafane, which in [local] tongue, means town of the warm waters. It takes its name from a spring, emerging from the middle of a swamp, whose waters are boiling. Animals unfortunate enough to swim in it die on the spot." [69] By the late nineteenth century, Norwegian missionaries had prospected widely around Antsirabe, inventorying and tapping a number of natural springs. The queen's bathhouse, designed by Norwegian missionaries in 1880, was conceived along a highly rationalized, hierarchical design, with the queen's room, the prime minister's room, and the rooms of visiting Andriana radiating around a central basin. *Thermalisme* being a regimented and specialized practice involving equal measures of ritual and science, its colonial practitioners for their part sought to codify and classify mineral content, spring temperatures, forms of consumption, and medicinal usages.

At Vichy, one counts no fewer than six major springs: the Sources Chomel, Grande Grille, de l'Hôpital, Lucas, du Parc, and des Célestins. Each draws different crowds, queuing—depending on their diagnosis—with their distinctive drinking cups in hand or waiting to immerse themselves in warm pools for standard lengths of time. Gradually, as part of their plan to reproduce Vichy, colonial hydrotherapists established a similar gamut of springs in Antsirabe, even borrowing the actual names of Vichy's springs in some cases. As at Vichy, these were divided into two categories. Among those dedicated to bathing, because of their high temperatures of fifty-one degrees centigrade, were the Source Ranomafana I and Ranomafana II (Ranomafana signifies "hot water" in Malagasy, and there are thus numerous springs on the island known as Ranomafana). Six more were reserved for drinking cures: the Ranovisy Spring, the Source de l'Hôpital, the Source du Lac, the Source du Parc (all considered akin to Vichy's Grande Grille); the Source de la Sahatsio, used to treat malaria and anemia; and the Antsirakely spring, tapped to this day for its sparkling water, or *Visy-Gasy*. [70]

Prospecting, tapping, and developing the springs visibly elicited great pride among French colonial engineers and scientists, providing a demonstration of French know-how. Moreover, it distinguished colonial practices from indigenous ones—from merely bathing in a natural spring water basin or from simply drinking directly from a natural source. Hence, Inspector General Fillon described the engineering work on Ranomafana's bathhouses as "a way of utilizing the warm waters in rational and hygienic conditions." [71] Earlier, in 1905, a pharmacist named Réland had warned that Antsirabe's wonderful waters "only have truly salutary effects when they are taken with discernment and on the advice of a doctor." French thermal doctors and engineers, in other words, were perceived as the key to distinguishing French spring water practices from those of their indigenous predecessors.[72]

Early developments in creating hydrotherapeutic infrastructures were hampered by financial intrigues around the *compagnie fermière*—again modeled on Vichy's—that had purchased the rights to exploit Antsirabe's waters. A local administrator complained in January 1909 that "the baths for Europeans, and those for the Malagasy are both installed in rudimentary conditions. They lack hygiene, they are dilapidated, and their basins are made of wood."[73] Only between 1913 and 1916 did work begin in earnest on what would become the modern bathhouses of Ranomafana. Henri Perrier de la Bathie conducted extensive bores around the springs in 1913, seeking to channel them so as to obtain "a constant and regular flow."[74] Still, Perrier de la Bathie bemoaned that he could not pinpoint the precise *griffon* (the exact site where the spring surfaces) of Ranomafana, but had instead managed to identify a number of candidates, the most promising one located on the grounds of the Lyonnais Company pigsty.[75]

Governor-General Hubert Garbit gave new impetus to the project in 1916 (at the height of World War One, when fewer administrators were able to return to France on furlough), ordering the construction of a vast reservoir, three new pavilions, showers, a vapor bath, and pools and, in 1917, even projecting a grand new hotel, which would become the Hôtel Terminus, later renamed the Hôtel des Thermes.[76] Under Garbit's leadership, an artificial lake was created over the swamp and a second spring was tapped (Ranomafana II), solely for the purposes of leveling and regularizing the flow of Ranomafana I. World War One's impact on Antsirabe's growth was dramatic: the list of the town's European inhabitants registers strong growth in every professional category— from missionaries to merchants, industrialists, and settlers—between 1913 and 1918.[77]

Antsirabe's water conduits, installations, and baths were constantly retooled over the course of the colonial era. Experimentation sometimes proved costly, reminding all concerned, Malagasy and French alike, that potent elements were being harnessed. In 1933, as the spring of Andranomandevy was being bored, toxic gas emanations killed a Malagasy who had come to drink the waters.[78]

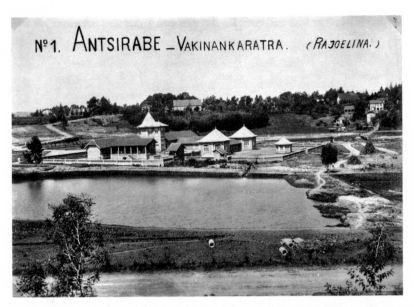

N°1. ANTSIRABE — VAKINANKARATRA. (*RAJOELINA.*)

FIGURE 7. Ranomafana under construction around 1920. Courtesy NMS. All rights reserved.

In 1945, the baths were further enlarged with the construction of another twelve cabins in a second-class bathhouse, a thinly veiled euphemism for a native bathhouse.[79] As we shall see, the baths had been segregated from the outset of the colonial era. Again, like the Great War, World War Two marked a period of sustained spa expansion. In 1941, a new decree made allowances for administrators stranded in the colonies to take regular paid holidays at local spas rather than be repatriated to the now-blockaded metropole.[80] At this time, Antsirabe grew so popular that at least one witness blamed the complete surprise of the British attack on local Pétainist forces in May 1942 on the fact that much of the French high command and officer corps was taking a collective cure at Antsirabe.[81]

Taking Antsirabe's Waters

Time and again, colonial doctors would reinforce the connection between the waters of Antsirabe's many springs and those of Vichy. The opinion was validated by the Paris-based Académie de Médecine in 1902.[82] Charles Moureu of the Collège de France conferred final legitimacy to the theory when he proclaimed in 1924 that the similarities between Vichy's Grande-Grille spring and

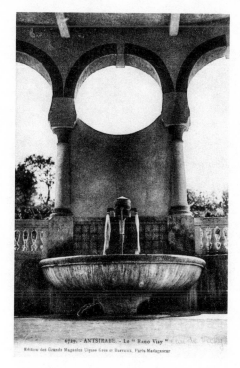

FIGURE 8. Rano-Visy source (interior view). Postcard, author's collection, date unknown.

Antsirabe's Source Ranovisy were striking. It was therefore not surprising, he noted, to see the same diseases successfully treated at the two spas.[83] Thus French doctors prescribed these local waters for exactly the same ailments as in Vichy: "congested livers, cirrhoses, malaria, and diabetes."[84] The fact that malaria's effects upon the liver were allegedly tempered by both Antsirabe's and Vichy's waters made the sites ideal meeting and resting places for colonials. Indeed, ever since 1895–96, malaria had become the bane of French colonizers in Madagascar.

Like Vichy's, then, Antsirabe's waters were thought to act favorably upon the liver, the enduring fetish of both French medicine in general and tropical medicine especially. Far from being dismissed as the twentieth century progressed, on the contrary this conviction grew more firmly established — contemporary science, of course, confirms that malaria enters the blood through a mosquito bite, before affecting the liver and infecting the bloodstream. An article of 1937 in a prestigious journal of tropical medicine concluded that Antsirabe's waters "decongested painful livers very rapidly, bringing the organ back to a normal size after the water cure." A series of examples were given,

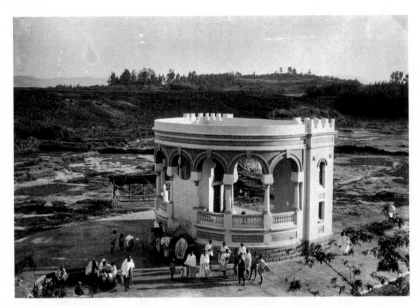

FIGURE 9. Rano-Visy source (exterior). Courtesy NMS. All rights reserved.

mostly cases of settlers in the lowlands. Upon arriving at Antsirabe, one west coast settler's malarial liver was measured at fifteen centimeters. A month later, if we are to believe this account, his liver had shrunk by four centimeters, thanks to the water cure. In the case of a malarial child who arrived at Antsirabe "in terrifying, skeletal condition," the water cure was presented as nothing short of miraculous: "At the end of her treatment, the child was transformed, she had put weight back on, and was no longer pale. Her liver was normal, and her spleen near normal."[85]

By the 1930s, Antsirabe's doctors had projected an image of a virtual Vichy-clone. The *Gazette médicale de Madagascar* summarized the waters' curative purviews as: (1) malaria and (2) "the colonial liver,"[86] a general, popular catch-all term associated with the everyday suffering brought on by the colonial condition — the condition of being a colonizer, that is.[87] In the words of *La Femme coloniale*, a magazine aimed at female settlers in Madagascar, "[Many of us] have a liver already tired by years of colonial living."[88]

To be sure, as with many spas, Antsirabe's purported curative qualities changed over time. The waters were prescribed for more than just liver ailments. Ever since 1879 its doctors claimed curative powers for rheumatism. More recently, it has been used to treat cancer and sterility (cancer because of the spring's high radioactivity).[89] Nowadays, one is struck by the range of afflictions said to be treated by the waters, including respiratory ills, gout, rheumatism, gynecological and gastric problems, diabetes, and hypertension. Some of these diseases are and were treated by immersion, others by purgative techniques, and others yet by various shower mechanisms.

Within this spectrum of balneological practices, Malagasy patients in the colonial era were likely able to maintain some precolonial rituals relating to springs and accommodate them to methods prescribed by French doctors. While European spa-going rose only 17 percent from 1928 to 1931 (from 9,398 to 11,005), Malagasy frequentation increased much more significantly — by some 70 percent (from 22,715 to 38,643).[90] Already in 1919, a Mauritian observer noted the popularity of the Ranomafana spring in particular: "The waters of the Ranomafana spring are highly appreciated by the entire Malagasy people. It is interesting to see arriving, daily, hundreds of indigenous men, women, and children, coming to seek better health from every corner of the island."[91] Antsirabe remains a site of medical pilgrimage in Madagascar. A tension can be identified here, for French thermal doctors sought to control and oversee indigenous balneological practices. When in 1941 a Malagasy teacher mysteriously died in one of Antsirabe's hydrotherapeutic tubs, a French doctor found an unexpected opportunity to advertise his services in the press: "In the interests of the Malagasy and the population in general, you should know that this native had neglected to receive medical advice prior to taking this bath, and that similar accidents could happen again. I should also mention to the indigenous public that I take patients on Monday, Wednesday and Friday afternoons."[92] This scare tactic was aimed not only at enriching the said doctor, but also at controlling Malagasy bodies and practices at the spa.

Reminders of Home

The parallels between Vichy and Antsirabe speak to other issues as well. Doctors and *curistes* alike commented on the Antsirabe region's supposed physical resemblance to the Massif Central, the volcanic center of France where Vichy is located.[93] But opinions varied. Duval, who became a staunch advocate of Antsirabe after having supposedly been cured by its waters in 1898, wrote, "The aspect of this town is that of a quaint Algerian village, lined with eucalyptus."[94] Single texts seemed torn between multiple comparisons. M. Frenée's guide (1931) to Madagascar began by likening Antsirabe's climate to that of the French south (Midi), before noting the town's physical resemblance to quaint villages from the greater Paris area (Ile-de-France).[95] Antsirabe had a remarkable capacity for reminding foreigners of home, wherever that might be. An American tourist in the 1950s at first drew parallels with Maine but was soon converted to thinking of the place as French: "Even the sky is a mild French sky, full of soft white and grey clouds."[96] Amazingly, the unique landscapes around Antsirabe (featuring massive rounded granite and calcareous formations) were consistently elided in these narratives. Instead Antsirabe was considered French largely because of its waters, sky, and other intangibles. To a French doctor, the willows around Antsirabe's main lake called to mind the grave of Jean-Jacques Rousseau at Ermenonville.[97] A recurring trope of colonial narratives involved contrasting Antsirabe to Madagascar's coastal areas and hence to the tropics: "Here the air is cool thanks to an elevation of roughly 1,500 meters. Colonial eyes tired of contemplating palms, coconut trees or . . . raffia . . . are bewildered by plane trees, poplars and pines. One is served artichokes, asparagus, 'real vegetables' from France, and in winter, potatoes, pears, peaches, grapes, chestnuts . . . in short everything that makes a colonial happy, while in Paris people will pay a fortune for a pineapple or a mango."[98] It is clearly the contrast between the coast and the highlands that triggered an effusion of nostalgia in this atypically relationally reflexive late colonial passage.[99] Such "nostalgic simulacra"[100] were omnipresent at the resort of Antsirabe: the arboretum, Vichy-inspired baths, fountains, boulevards, the grand hotel, the golf course, and, in this instance, the food,[101] all stirred powerful colonial memories of home.[102]

Settler Society at Antsirabe

In 1909, the entire province of Vakinankaratra, of which Antsirabe was the capital, counted only 210 Europeans. Fourteen more were born that year, while only two died, thereby seemingly confirming the administration's view that the area was ideal for settlement.[103] By 1955, the population of Antsirabe proper had exploded: it counted 2,070 Europeans as permanent residents (of whom 1,942 were French), 112 Chinese, 164 Indians, and 13,500 Malagasy (plus another 13,653 Malagasy in the outlying areas). One could add to these figures an important number of seasonal European visitors (*estivants*) who regularly vacationed at Antsirabe. Throughout the colonial era, and especially in its pre-boom years, Antsirabe also counted a significant population of non-French outsiders. These included Norwegians, Greeks, Britons, Italians, and a number of British subjects from the Middle East and South Asia.[104] Curiously this fact never seemed to undermine Antsirabe's putative Frenchness. If anything it appeared to reinforce the idea of a miniature Europe in Madagascar. The point seems to have been that at Antsirabe, the exogenous population appeared to be at less of a numerical disadvantage than elsewhere on the isle: whereas the overall population ratio for the entire island was of roughly 80 Malagasy for every European, the ratio in Antsirabe itself (excluding suburbs) was more on the order of 6.5 to 1. Colonial settlers had thus created an insular environment where they felt very much at home and where they perceived even the demographic balance of power to be tilted in their favor.

Antsirabe's colonial *beau monde* seemed to enjoy an idyllic lifestyle that made it the envy of settlers the island over. But if one scratches the surface, one finds no shortage of dissension among Antsirabe's whites. In 1909, the French director of the province tempered his admiration for the dynamism of the local *société* by underscoring its pettiness and vindictiveness (anything but atypical of colonial society):[105]

> I must recognize the merit of settlers who have created in Antsirabe [a host of] industries, two distilleries, one brewing company, a flour mill, a lard processing plant, lime ovens, etc. Those who did not hesitate to experiment by importing live cattle from France, those who cultivate wheat, barley, mulberry bushes, or those who create wheelwrights works, those who are mining for precious stones, those who have prospected for minerals . . . all are worthy of praise and further encouragement. They may not be millionaires, but in this healthy region, where all is inexpensive, they live very well, indeed with a certain ease. And yet, the town is impossible to administer and govern. There is amongst our compatriots, no camaraderie, no sympathy whatsoever.[106]

Still, in spite of this strife, Antsirabe's whites managed to perform and embody privilege. In its heyday (1915–48), the spa came to be seen as the *dernier cri* of colonial society, a bourgeois setting capable of rivaling a metropolitan resort.

Antsirabe as a "Pinnacle of Power"

At Antsirabe, colonial domination was not a hollow term.[107] As we have seen, the region had emerged as one of the hotbeds of the *menalamba* rebellion in 1896, and colonial repression proved particularly harsh in the area. Photos attest to the rounding up of prisoners in the heart of Antsirabe.[108] Indeed the jail was one of the first large-scale public buildings erected at the spa town. Planned in 1902 and completed the following year, it could accommodate 160 prisoners, a considerable number for what was still a village. By colonial standards, the prison could lay claim to some degree of modernity, having separate cells and even wings for women and men, for petty and major criminals, for those charged with administrative offenses such as resisting *corvées*, even for pre- and post-trial inmates.[109] According to the local director of public works, it would at once conform to the "rules of hygiene" while also featuring a Malagasy style. Like all four buildings constructed in 1903 (a girl's school, a prison, a public building, and the office of public works), it was the product of "penitentiary labor."[110]

It was around the time of World War One that colonial planners began in earnest to transform Antsirabe into a bourgeois French leisure site comparable to Dax, Vittel, or Vichy.[111] The spa produced a remarkable spin-off effect, including the construction of Madagascar's largest hotel, a symbol of French colonial *démesure*, as it could rarely (and cannot to this day) fill its hundreds of rooms with paying customers.[112] Even its fans conceded that the legendary establishment, the Hôtel Terminus, "was almost colossal on the colony's scale."[113]

Clearly, colonial Antsirabe's raison d'être was to remind colonials of a seaside or hydromineral spa back home. One source from 1934 reported, "Were it not for a few details relating to the aspect of the countryside and the customs and color of the locals, one would forget that one is so far from France. . . . As at Deauville or Vichy, the high society arrives in luxurious automobiles or by rail in a rapid *micheline*. Are we really in the colonies?"[114]

By the same token, the town became a testing ground for modernist colonial architecture inspired by one of Madagascar's conquerors, Marshal Louis-Hubert Lyautey. Indeed, ever since the first plans were laid to invade Madagascar, members of the French colonial lobby had thought of the island as an

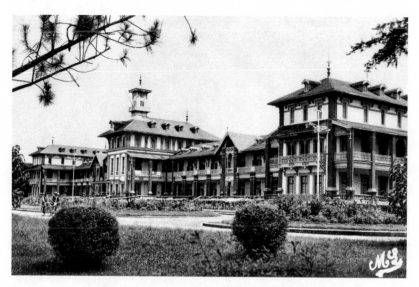

immense laboratory. In the words of one journalist, writing in 1894, "Never again will we find a laboratory like Madagascar: an inhabitable island, a climate bearable to Europeans, no Europeans neighbors, complete freedom of action." [115] Antsirabe played a central part in this French colonial tabula rasa, where social, architectural, and cultural experimentation were the order of the day. [116] Creating a Vichy replica in Madagascar, after all, was first and foremost a colonial experiment. The experiment was considered such a success that in 1931 an article ostensibly aimed at pairing Antsirabe and Cilaos in tourist pamphlets could not resist a slight of Réunion's main spa: "Cilaos deserves no less than [Antsirabe], to be ordered, conceived, and built according to the principles of the new urbanism." [117] The article's reasoning exposed a chasm between the two spas at the very time Cilaos was seeking to catch up by investing in a new hotel. At Antsirabe, the modernist *ville nouvelle* doubled as *ville d'eau*, in a marriage increasingly common in metropolitan France as well.

Colonial Antsirabe's broad avenues (figure 11) and cutting-edge architecture were intended to achieve the dual goals of defining the resort as European and of making it a symbol of French rationality and modernity with which to impress the Malagasy. Segregation was a corollary of these objectives. The place of the Malagasy in colonial Antsirabe was ambivalent: they represented a growing client or patient base for the spa, but French urban planners sought

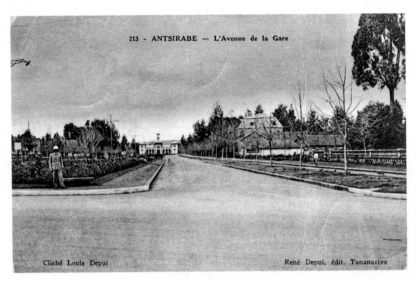

Cliché Louis Depui   René Depui, édit. Tananarive

FIGURE 11. L'Avenue de la Gare, Antsirabe. Postcard, author's collection, date unknown.

to ensure that the heart of the town remain overwhelmingly French. As Gwendolyn Wright has observed, Antsirabe was rigidly divided into sectors: cheaper
Malagasy housing was concentrated near the market to the south, while quaint
European villas ran east from the hotel through to the train station, along
grandiose avenues.[118] The Norwegian mission, the cathedral, and the artificial lake and its neighboring mineral baths lay at the crossroads of these two
worlds. Sometimes slippages occurred. Take the postcard sent home by a French
settler in 1912, on which he or she scribbled the question, "Does this not look
like a lovely French village?" over an image showing the intersection of Antsirabe's indigenous and missionary quarters (figure 12). Physical incursions,
meanwhile, proved both inevitable and intolerable to French colonial society.
A document preserved in Madagascar's National Archives betrays a scarcely
veiled attempt to restrict Malagasy access to the European quarter. In 1926,
Antsirabe's all-French municipal council voted to ban what it first termed "indigenous carts." After some discussion, the wording was eventually changed
to the more politic "animal-driven carriages," but the gist remained the same,
for Europeans rode by *pousse-pousse*, automobile, or *micheline*.[119] In another
instance, in 1946 the municipal council took on the problem of urban overcrowding. Noting the increase of "large buildings on very narrow lots, next
to other buildings in the same condition" and the harm that this was doing

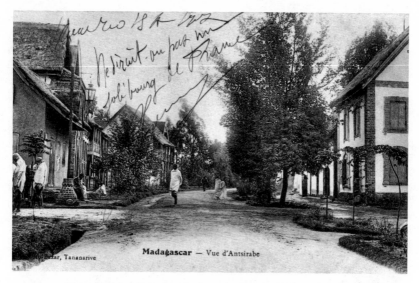

FIGURE 12. Postcard of the Missionary district at the juncture of the Malagasy and thermal quarters. The handwriting reads, "Does this not look like a lovely French village?" Dated 1912. Postcard, author's collection.

to "the beauty of the thermal station," the council endeavored to "preserve a large space around each building, comprising a garden." Legislating beauty was little more than a pretext. The council voted to enforce four zones: one commercial, another "thermal and residential," and two more suburban. This new zoning sanctioned and even reinforced Antsirabe's segregated urban grid, reifying the equation of white space and "thermal and residential quarter." [120]

Antsirabe's baths themselves were strictly segregated, a more dilapidated wing being reserved for "natives." [121] In 1919, the wealthy Mauritian traveler G. Antelme described the installations at Antsirabe's Ranomafana spring as follows: "Three of the cabins are reserved to the natives, and four others to the Europeans. Moreover, there is nearby a special cabin reserved for the Résident de la Province." [122] Within this complex hierarchy of bathing, the French résident de la province had usurped the private pavilion principle of Queen Ranavalona II and the Norwegian missionaries. Even after the modernization of the Ranomafana installations, some sought greater segregation still. A metropolitan French chemistry professor visiting the spa remarked in 1935, "The baths are somewhat small, and require, according to me, a few more renovations, in particular so as to avoid contact between white raced and indigenous bathers."[123] The addition in 1945 of a new second-class bathhouse would answer this settler demand. In this postwar scheme, scientists were careful to segregate the very waters themselves: those of Ranomafana I were reserved to Europeans, while those of Ranomafana II filled the basins of the "indigenous pools."[124] Throughout the colonial era, the practice of drinking the waters was equally embedded in local power relations: Jules Coré, who grew up in colonial Antsirabe recalls that the "boy," or better still a requisitioned indigenous prisoner, would fetch his family's *Rano-visy* or *Visy-Gasy* water every morning.[125]

Antsirabe emerged as a powerful symbol of colonial power. And at least some Malagasy were impressed. The Merina notable Rakotovao remarked in 1904, "The aligned boulevards, houses and trees; the water by the side of the road were all wonderful to watch. . . . The beauty of the housing, the hospital comprising several buildings, the purity of the water, the hot waters for bathing, the Vichy water to drink. It was truly incomparable!"[126] To this observer, medical, architectural, and sanitary forms of power and knowledge went hand in hand.

Antsirabe's importance rose steadily throughout the twentieth century, as entire infrastructures soon revolved around the spa. Making wide use of indigenous forced labor, the Gouvernement général de Madagascar ordered a railroad built in 1914 to connect Antsirabe to one of its client bases in the capital, Tananarive (today Antananarivo).[127] This supplemented the colonial road connecting Tananarive to Ambositra via Antsirabe, which had been built around 1902 with an equal reliance on forced labor.[128]

As early as 1903, the colonial administration ordered the erection of a girl's school near the spa.[129] By the 1930s, no doubt borrowing this function from British colonial hill stations of the Raj, the governor-general's office decided to transform Antsirabe into the principal site for European boarding schools on the island, offering a selection of private — largely missionary — and public education.[130] The rationale for establishing a public French boarding school in 1934 was once again couched in the language of 1896: "The salubrity of this health town justifies in itself the choice of this site for children to begin their learning process, sheltered from the terrible diseases that rage on the coast."[131]

In addition to children in boarding schools and *estivants*, who congregated there in the Southern Hemisphere's summer, December through February,

Antsirabe attracted a faithful returning clientele from around the island. As a settler, one was just as likely, if not more so, to cross an acquaintance at Antsirabe's Hôtel Terminus as at the capital. An article of 1925 trumpeting Antsirabe's popularity lists visitors from every corner of the island: Majunga, Tamatave, Tananarive, before turning its attention to closer locales, like Fiana-rantsoa, Mananjary, and Ambositra. In these towns, all within a two-hundred-kilometer radius of the spa, wrote the journalist, "inhabitants seem to have actually agreed amongst each other on a rotation scheme, so that a number of them are always present at our Vichy *malgache*."[132]

Urban Planning and Colonial Establishments

If Antsirabe was to aspire to the rank of a "quaint French town," it would require not only magnificent boulevards, public statues, flowered pots, charming public spaces, and so on, but also a set of prescribed institutions: a city hall, a social club, a market, schools, a racetrack. Some of Antsirabe's famed establishments were typical of resort towns—be they seaside resorts, high altitude resorts, or spas. In 1901 *La Quinzaine coloniale* expressed the wish that Gros-claude's *compagnie fermière* would soon build a hotel, baths, and a casino, in that order.[133]

Here again, the point was to design a French city around the springs. In 1931, as part of a beautification campaign, the mayor ordered the creation of a covered market, destined to replace Antsirabe's famous precolonial outdoor market.[134] The mayor explained: "A town like Antsirabe must have an elegant market, well laid out, capable of being washed down, where meats, vegetables and fruits would be properly ordered, and no longer exposed to dust and flies, as they are today."[135] In short, the mayor wished to see the Malagasy market replaced by a (rather wishfully) orderly French *halle*.[136] The new market was completed in 1935.[137] As part of this same Frenchification scheme, in 1941 the municipal council mandated the construction of a clubhouse between the golf course and the arboretum.[138] While these sites of socialization were for the most part de facto segregated, others, never officially sanctioned by the municipal council, appear to have tolerated or even encouraged mixity. The town's colonial brothel counted several black prostitutes and indeed a black madam.[139]

Attracting Foreign Tourists

As a health resort, Antsirabe's success depended upon attracting settlers through various marketing techniques, from word of mouth to aggressive advertising of its curative virtues. Antsirabe's most ambitious promoters attempted early on to attract outside visitors, most notably from Mauritius, South Africa, and Réunion. An optimistic 1934 directive on Antsirabe's tourism potential reads, "But a hamlet yesterday, small town today, Antsirabe will soon become the great center of tourism where, from across the Indian Ocean, all those who have only a few short weeks' vacation—too short a time to travel to Europe—can come to reinvigorate their health with our thermal springs, analogous to those of Vichy."[140] This passage contains the seeds of an ongoing debate: Antsirabe's promoters acknowledged that it could not compete with the real thing (that is, Vichy); they thus focused on attracting customers with too little time or money to travel to Europe. Already during World War One, when identifying a prospective clientele for the spa, Madagascar's Governor-General Martial Merlin concluded it would be unreasonable to expect vacationers from Réunion, Mauritius, or South Africa to throng to Antsirabe. The first two, he wrote, "will, outside of times of submarine warfare, always prefer to vacation in Europe rather than Madagascar. As for South Africans, why would they abandon the resources, comfort and variety of pleasures of the good life in South Africa, from big game hunting to music hall shows . . . to come and bury themselves in Antsirabe?"[141] In short, Merlin decided, Antsirabe should count only upon local settlers for its customer/patient base.

In this debate on Antsirabe's tourist potential, even the spa's detractors recognized that it represented the island's best hope for attracting overseas visitors at the time. In an era decades removed from the creation of mass ecotourism, colonial tourist agencies were resigned to the attitude that Madagascar supposedly presented neither the "vestiges of various ancient and disappeared civilizations so totally different from those of Europe" nor the big game hunting of continental Africa. Given that Madagascar had neither archeology nor hunting to offer, a report to the Ministry of the Colonies reasoned in 1924 that "only the town of Antsirabe, the Vichy of Madagascar, seems able to draw a regular foreign clientele. The colony has neglected nothing to make this happen: a large hotel has been built, a thermal facility has been erected, a doctor has been sent to France for training at the Institut d'Hydrologie."[142]

Antsirabe's promoters themselves seem to have been torn between grandiose pretensions, a desire to keep this piece of France to themselves, and an undeniable fear that Antsirabe fell short of international luxury standards. This tension between arrogance and shame, between seeking to market Antsirabe in South Africa and settling on local clients, came to a head in 1935 when a South African journalist printed an article on Madagascar's attractions in a Natal newspaper. The journalist, a certain Owen Letcher, was quite generous to Antsirabe, once again writing into it a set of nostalgic cues: "Antsirabe cannot fail to capture the charm of the traveler. The peach blossom and the blue of the waters suggest Japan, or, seen from another angle, the well laid-out streets and quaint pretty houses are reminiscent of some little town along the Corniche road."[143] But Letcher was much less indulgent toward Madagascar's infrastructure and indigenous people, ranting with frightful racism against Malagasy train porters, whom he described as cannibals, and against the "disgraceful" dirtiness of other cities—Antsirabe notably excepted. This tirade drew immediate reaction from Madagascar's authorities. Directives were issued for Malagasy railway agents to be hired at once in Antsirabe, Tamatave, and Tananarive and for them to be given "sober and visible uniforms." "Non-accredited natives" would be barred from handling travelers' luggage. The incident at its core implicated the ambiguous position of Antsirabe and Madagascar as a whole vis-à-vis another colonial power. Once South Africans started reading these articles and, it was hoped, ventured to Antsirabe, the supposedly lax standards of colonial segregation, etiquette, and pomp would need to be reinforced. If Antsirabe was to be truly representative of France overseas, then it would need to stand up to reproductions of Europe and standards of Britishness in South Africa—reproductions that French colonial officials in Madagascar seem to have regarded with envy.

Plans for Antsirabe to Serve as Colonial Capital

By the mid-twentieth century, Antsirabe had gained such stature that it emerged as a would-be capital for French administrators. Its purported salubriousness was proportional to the putative decay of the existing capital of Tananarive. In a letter of January 1945 to the governor-general, Emile Delmotte, a settler in Ambositra, summarized in rather crude terms the prevailing views of settlers on "Tana": "Tananarive is a pile of dung. In order to clean it, one would have to level everything down to the bedrock and the clay on which the city is built. It cannot be defended: a couple of dozen bombs would level the city completely. . . . All of its springs are polluted, proving that the rot is subterranean as well. In contrast, Antsirabe, as both a *station thermale* and *climatique* . . . is favorable to the health of Europeans. The Australians did not hesitate to abandon Melbourne—a city of some million inhabitants—to move their administrative capital to Canberra, a tiny spot in the middle of nowhere."[144] Delmotte deployed revealing tropes to associate the precolonial seat of Merina power, Tananarive, with degeneration and dirt, contrasting it to the quintessentially healthful and French Antsirabe.

The projected transfer of the capital to Antsirabe, first proposed in the 1920s and revived in 1944, was of course eminently political, for it was designed in part to undermine nationalist sentiment in the existing capital of Tananarive. In recommendations made to the minister of the colonies in 1944, Governor-General Pierre de Saint-Mart formally requested the transfer of the island's principal administrative, political, and educational facilities to Antsirabe. Tananarive, he argued, was overcrowded, its expansion was hindered by topographical obstacles, and its hygiene was lacking. Antsirabe, in contrast, being situated on a high, healthy plateau, offered endless opportunities for expansion.[145] More than this, Saint-Mart envisioned the move as the first step in a vast urban renewal for Madagascar:

> Situated on a vast healthful plateau, well served by rail-lines and roads, presenting large open areas for future constructions, Antsirabe offers the characteristics of the city we are seeking to create. . . . The program I am proposing involves transferring in the next five years all administrative services, and many educational services to Antsirabe. Individuals would buy up properties in Antsirabe very rapidly, if the town took on the rank of capital. The purchasing of lots, public works, etc., would absorb a large part of the unused capitals. Finally, the transfer would allow for public works in Tananarive that cannot be undertaken without destroying existing blocs of public housing.[146]

The governor-general was thus outlining more than a simple "summer capital" status for Antsirabe. He already counted on speculation rendering it an even more desirable location. He was, in short, himself speculating on Antsirabe. As for Tananarive, the city could be further rationalized, Frenchified, or Hausmanized if an exodus of government officials to Antsirabe could be achieved.

Two years later, Saint-Mart's successor, Marcel de Coppet (who in 1947 would brutally crush a rebellion on Madagascar's east coast, killing some seventy thousand Malagasy), fine-tuned his predecessor's rationales.[147] Yet again climate was invoked, this time metaphorically, at a time when Malagasy nationalism was making major inroads: "I do not think that Tananarive offers the proper climate of serenity and independence for a young political assembly. . . . Politically, you will surely agree that the presence of a new representative assembly in Tananarive can only reinforce the primacy of the ancient Hova capital over the rest of the island, and hence the primacy of the Merina over the coastal peoples."[148] Here, de Coppet followed to the letter Gallieni's notorious *politique des races*, which in Madagascar had basically involved pitting the highland Merina against the island's coastal peoples.[149] De Coppet continued: "Without needing to cite the examples of Washington or Canberra . . . there is obvious symbolism in the withdrawal of a federal capital from the former seat of Hova power to a *strictly European* city. Besides, it will definitely and indelibly mark the imprint of Western and French civilization on this island."[150] Here colonial disdain for a preexisting capital — derided as both dirty and hostile — was invoked as the justification for establishing a brave new distinctly European capital in Antsirabe. Antsirabe would, in turn, like ancient Roman baths, provide a lasting testimony to a powerful and influential colonial presence.

A year later, de Coppet went further still. Sensing resistance in Paris to transferring the seat of power to a spa town, on February 1, 1947, less than two months before the insurrection broke out on the east coast, he insisted, "[The idea of moving the capital to Antsirabe] is aimed at removing the young assembly from separatist influences in the former Hova capital, and avoiding the pressures that political agitators can exert, thanks to Tananarive's working masses, its large urban proletariat."[151] The proposed transfer was thus fueled as much by the perceived threat of urban proletarian nationalists as by the attractiveness of Antsirabe as a safe and healthful alternative.

Heated debates soon consumed the *Assemblée représentative*, convened in Antsirabe in January 1948. To those who remembered events in France some eight years earlier, the situation must have borne parallels with the French national assembly's emergency meeting at Vichy in July 1940. Ultimately, the

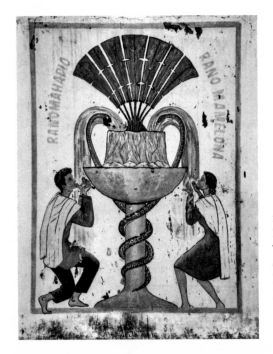

largely Malagasy-dominated assembly resolved: "Considering that the choice
of Antsirabe has proven unfortunate, as much because of the assembly space
itself . . . as for our isolation from Tananarive, we declare not wanting to meet
again in Antsirabe."[152] Only four delegates dissented.

Conclusion and Epilogue

At last, in the throes of a political crisis that augured the beginning of decolonization, settlers had hoped that the site they had long perceived as most
healthful, that to a great degree they had sought to carve out as their space,
would be made their capital. There was, in this ultimately aborted scheme
of transferring the capital to Antsirabe, a sign of both the utopianism and
combativeness of the *Zanatany*, as French settlers in Madagascar were called.
From the very beginning of the colonial period, colonials had identified Antsirabe as the antithesis of both the malarial coastal regions and the ancient
Merina capital of Tananarive. Legitimized by mutually reinforcing scientific
opinions and settler nostalgia for home, Antsirabe emerged as the focal point
of settler society in Madagascar. Here French settlers constructed a fantasy

of home and healthfulness, arguably their two greatest desiderata. Overcompensating for their avowed vulnerability to disease in Madagascar (so clearly demonstrated in 1895–96), colonials sought to transform Antsirabe into an oasis of imperial power — where *thermalisme*, a highly ritualized, regimented, and organic branch of European science, would reduce their fragility to tropical pathologies. Thus, Antsirabe's curative and therapeutic promise as a Vichy twin — constantly reasserted despite major shifts in tropical medicine between 1895 and 1960 — in due course contributed to transforming it into a symbol of imperial leisure and power. This particular kind of colonial tourism and leisure emerged as a practice for evading, negating, or neutralizing the tropics.

Ironically, while its colonial raison d'être had for so long been to remind homesick settlers of France, Antsirabe has been reinvented in recent times as an authentically indigenous cure. The spa has maintained its popularity since Madagascar's independence in 1960 — and it may well be rising today as the cost of modern mainstream medicine becomes increasingly prohibitive in this impoverished country. A present-day patient at Antsirabe's Ranomafana baths is greeted by a mural showing a young Malagasy man and woman drinking from the fountain of medicine. A recognizable national symbol, the traveler's tree, dominates the spring. The words framing the painting, "Ranomahadio" and "Rano Mamelona," can be loosely translated as "Water that cleans" and "Water that gives life." The cleansing logic of French hydrotherapy has clearly replaced any overt precolonial Vazimba references, but the entire ensemble has nevertheless been carefully indigenized, the geological goodness of the great island eliding any trace of French colonial science.

CHAPTER 6

Korbous, Tunisia: Negating the *Hammam*

IN 1930, JEAN DESPOIS DREW UP TUNISIA'S SETTLE-
ment potential index. In a didactic exercise for the broader
French public, this Tunis-based teacher proceeded to distill
knowledge that had long underpinned the logic of settlement. Europeans, he wrote, "especially those of Mediterranean origin, can acclimate very well [in Tunisia], and set
down roots." Thus, Despois reasoned, "the French can live
under Tunisian skies just as well as under French skies, so
long, of course, as they take some precautions during the
summer heat." Here geology and hydrology came to the
rescue. Despois explained: "The earth of this country provides precious remedies to its inhabitants, in the form of
thermomineral springs. . . . Those of Korbous . . . are the
only ones to have been properly developed. Well situated
in a quaint valley of Cap Bon across from Carthage, they
are accessible by a picturesque corniche road. They receive
some 5,000 patients a year." [1]

At first glance, Tunisia's premier hydromineral spa
might not seem to qualify as both a *station thermale* and
climatique, for unlike the spas examined in previous chapters it was located in the lowlands, by the sea. Such an interpretation, however, would fundamentally miss the essence
of *climatisme*. Indeed this science was predicated on cli-

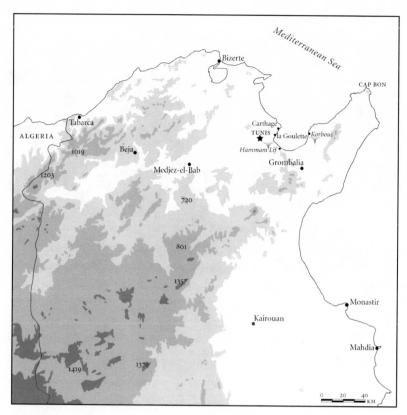

MAP 5. Northern Tunisia circa 1930, showing Korbous.

matic cures—in other words, on immersion in a microclimate or simply into a different climate from the ambient or dominant one. Whether such a change was provided by altitude, trade winds, or marine currents was irrelevant. At the international congress on hydrotherapy and climatology held during the world fair in Paris in 1937, a professor from the Ecole des Hautes études, Maurice Uzan, explained: "Korbous, a lovely hydromineral spa, also provides climatic virtues, thanks to its location on the western side of the Cap Bon peninsula, at the foot of a mountainous chain. . . . The maximum temperature in January is of 13.3 centigrade, with 15.5 maxima and 11 degree lows. There are more than 200 days of sunshine a year. . . . The dominant winds come from the northwest, and the sirocco is rare. Its thermal and barometric stability, its strong insulation, and steady ventilation give Korbous a tonic and sedative influence, proper to Mediterranean climates."[2] Albert Malinas who for some time directed the

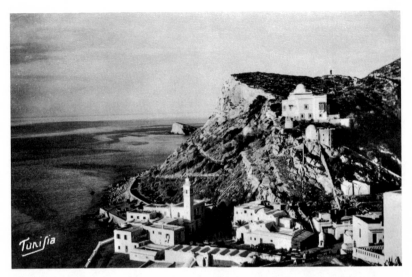

FIGURE 14. Korbous, 1950s. The minaret is the Dar-el-Bey hydrotherapy establishment.
Author's collection.

spa at Korbous, remarked, "Korbous brings together the advantages of marine
and mountain climes."[3] Here, in other words, was a site at once refreshed by
European breezes, cooled by a local mountain chain, and tempered by the sea,
mimicking Europe's purportedly mild and regulating climes.

Korbous's waters and climate rendered it such an ideal resort that its promoters tried to attract customers from faraway colonies. In the national archives of Vietnam, a document attests to this remarkable attempt to project
Korbous across the empire as a substitute for home. The document, dated 1913,
reads as follows:

> We have the honor of informing you of the precious advantages offered by the
> hydromineral spa of Korbous, since it opened to colonial officials who, thanks to
> the decree of June 19, 1913, can be sent there for treatment, in the same way as any
> other accredited spa. The climatic and hydromineral spa of Korbous presents
> distinct advantages for colonials: it operates in winter, from November 1 through
> May 31, at a time when European spas are closed; its situation on the gulf of Tunis
> ensures a temperate marine climate, exempt from humidity, providing colonials
> with an ideal transition climate, which will allow them to re-acclimate gradu-
> ally, and be able to return to France afterwards, without the sometimes serious
> effects caused by too rapid a transition from a warm back to a cold country.

Korbous presented other advantages, connected less to its situation on the route back to France than to its intrinsic hydromineral virtues and amenities:

> At Korbous . . . colonials will find appropriate and efficient treatments against afflictions contracted in warm lands. French and foreign colonials frequenting Korbous have already obtained remarkable results; the warm, chlorinated, hyperthermal and heavily radio-active waters of our spa constitute, indeed, a stunningly effective and rapid medication acting on general and organic atonies, which lie at the origin of most colonial afflictions. Our installations are every bit the rival of the most famed European ones: a personnel of professional masseurs and masseuses, employed the rest of the year in French spas; individual pools; a Roman steam bath, pulverization, gynecological and underwater apparatuses, and so on. We are able to treat successfully many diseases, amongst which I would cite: rheumatisms, laryngitis . . . chronic congestions of the liver and spleen, malarial cachexie, chronic colonial dysentery.[4]

This text speaks to many of the central tenets of French colonial hydrotherapy and climatology: the twinning of the two sciences in question, the quest for a particular niche (in this case the fact that Korbous remains open when French spas are closed), the certainty of hydrotherapy's efficacy in the treatment of colonial ills, the obsession with the Ministry of the Colonies' official recognition, the association with French spas (made explicit here through a claim on shared personnel), and the more general Frenchness of the site. The case also presents interesting particularities. Here, the spa's enterprising operator, Edmond Lecore-Carpentier, the director of the *Dépêche tunisienne* newspaper, targeted Indochina, one of the few colonies not to boast of a large hydromineral spa and a destination, moreover, on whose route Korbous was situated (via Suez). In addition, Lecore-Carpentier raised the specter of reverse thermal shock, the peril of too rapid a reentry into the climate of home. He followed the logic of *climatisme* to its natural conclusion: if the colonial needed to acclimate to the tropics, then he or she would need to take the same precautions before reentering the motherland. If spas could facilitate departure, then surely they could enable reentry. Finally, Korbous offered a treatment seldom proposed at the other spas discussed here. The Roman steam bath is noteworthy largely because of its uncanny resemblance to the Ottoman *hammam*, all the more uncanny since Korbous was used continuously since antiquity. As Alev

Lytle Croutier reminds us, "the *hammam* (Turkish bath) is an adaptation of the Byzantine bath, which itself derived from Roman thermae."[5] One would think, therefore, that the French would have found it difficult to claim any kind of monopoly over either the site or its therapeutic uses. And yet, they would stake a claim to a scientific, colonial, French, and even Roman form of hydrotherapy, contraposed to a radically other indigenous model.

Roman and Ottoman Models

France's war against Tunisia in 1881 and its subsequent designation of the country as a French protectorate marked the culmination of decades of French imperial ambitions aimed at creating a transdesert empire. As Julia Clancy-Smith has shown, the French decision to invade Tunisia was impelled in part by the need to quell resistance, which radiated in and out of Algeria.[6] Throughout their North African holdings, the French self-consciously associated their colonial enterprise with ancient Rome's—noting even that the Romans too had faced stiff opposition to their "civilizing mission." Patricia Lorcin has demonstrated how thoroughly French imperialism in Algeria was suffused with Roman connotations. Jacques Alexandropoulos reminds us that the same held true for Tunisia.[7] Throughout the French colonial Maghreb, an appropriated Roman legacy was invoked to justify not merely archeological missions, but also the basis of French colonialism. It even ended up shaping *pied-noir* identity, by conditioning the view of settler society in North Africa as a melting pot of *Latinité*, or Latinness. Most important, the Roman model enabled the relative effacing of Ottoman influence in the grand colonial narrative, in favor of a significantly older and distinctly Western Roman foundational myth.[8]

Hydrotherapy was certainly not exempt from this mythology. Indeed, the rekindling of Roman baths was central to it. At Korbous, the French lionized Decimus Laelius Balbus, the Roman "benefactor" of ancient Korbous (founded by him in 44 BCE), and emphasized the site's Latin name, Aquae Carpitanae.[9] Although French sources recognized that Korbous had been used almost continuously since antiquity, they posited that between the Romans and French development in 1904, the efforts of "local people" to improve and develop the spa were "practically nil."[10] A tourist brochure produced by Kor-

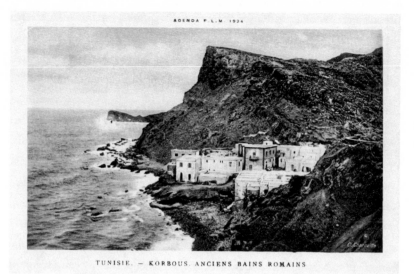

TUNISIE. — KORBOUS. ANCIENS BAINS ROMAINS

FIGURE 15. "Korbous's ancient Roman baths." Postcard, 1924. Author's collection.

bous's *syndicat d'initiative* typifies this interpretation: "Numerous Roman ruins testify to a glorious past that crumbled after the fall of Roman civilization. There remained only a lovely crique, utterly abandoned except by patients who continued to come faithfully, and a few Arab masseurs, when Mr Lecore-Carpentier . . . took the decision in 1904 to revive the spa, which he made into the lovely resort we see today."[11] Even French colonial landscaping evoked the Roman past. Lecore-Carpentier's company planted some six thousand trees in and around Korbous between 1904 and 1935, implicitly reviving Roman irrigation and agriculture after centuries of presumed Arab aridity.[12]

The history of baths and bathing should have challenged this Rome–France genealogy. In a recent study, Ahmed Saadaoui considers the hammams of Tunis "the direct descendent[s] of the Roman bath." Omar Carlier, in his analysis of North African hammams, points to Byzantium as the mediator between ancient Roman and Ottoman modes of balneology — the synthesis of which was later reexported to North Africa by the Ottomans. Carlier registers another influence, that of Iberian exiles after 1609. The hybrid result, Carlier argues, owed a great deal to both Rome and Turkey. The Roman legacy readily apparent in the North African hammam is reflected most strikingly in the fact that Tunis's forty public baths have cold, lukewarm, and hot chambers. Yet a distinctly North African hammam did emerge in the modern era, one that, interestingly, would continue to thrive in the Maghreb after the steady decline of the Middle Eastern hammam in the twentieth century.[13]

The hammam (meaning "spreader of warmth" in Arabic) defies straightforward definition. Sometimes translated as "Turkish bath," it could equally connote a steam bath, sweat bath, or public bath. It fulfilled an impressive number of roles, some religious (ablutions, purification on the eve of Friday prayers), others capitalist (its operators counted as influential members of the local bourgeoisie), others hygienic and medical, and still others social (marriages, for example, were prepared at the bath). In Jewish culture, argues Carlier, a clearer distinction was drawn between the hammam as an agent of leisure, relaxation, and sociability and the *miqveh* for religious observance.[14] In the North African hammam, gender segregation was not spatial so much as temporal: the same baths catered to men and women but at different times — typically men in the morning or evening, women and children during the afternoon. Florence Ramond Jurney's analysis of novels by Tahar Ben Jelloun and Ferid Boughedir casts the hammam as a site both of female sociability, a place of female freedom and escapism, and of ambiguous gender identity: Because of its transformation from male to female site and back, it is assigned a fluidity in novels that ascribe otherwise fixed genders to spaces.[15] We should not neglect the place of the Turkish bath in European imaginations. The hammam stirred both heterosexual and homosexual fantasies: *scènes et types* postcards intended for French male consumption showed sparsely clad Arab women in hammam settings, while Gustave Flaubert boasted in the 1850s of an amorous encounter with a bath-boy in a Cairo hammam.[16] Christelle Taraud has demonstrated how the recruitment of prostitutes often took place in the confines of the hammam at those times when it was reserved to women.[17] And Alev Lytle Croutier points to the hammam as a site of both female socialization and same-sex liaisons.[18]

Although the hammam's many roles have been studied at length, its margins and its ties to European hydrotherapy have not. For one thing, drinking cures, though prevalent at some hammams, most notably at Korbous, were not necessarily a hammam staple.[19] And fundamentally, the relationship between mineral spring and public bath appears more fluid in the hammam than in French hydrotherapy, in which *bains publics* are strictly distinguished from *stations thermales*. In the French case, the major difference between a bathhouse and a thermal spa is that the first involves the tapping of a naturally occurring, usually hot mineralized spring and the second an artificial warming of ordinary waters. One should not overstate such differences, however, for, as we shall see, similarities abound. At Vichy, as in the Maghreb, drinking establishments stand side by side with bathing ones. But at Vichy the connection with steam baths, for instance, represents a relatively late import couched in exoticism. Then again, one can easily argue that the drinker's pilgrimage to Vichy featured religious, mystical overtones. Possible distinctions with the hammam's explicitly sacred dimension are therefore once again a matter of perspective. Still, the definition of a hammam seems more elastic than that of a *station thermale*, with particular regard to the question of naturally occurring springs. Thus, Tunis's public bathhouses were, of course, termed hammams, but so too were Tunisia's other hydromineral spa of Hammam Lif and Algeria's Hammam R'Hira. Even Korbous had been known as Hammam Kourbès prior to 1881.

Demarcating French Hydrotherapy

The French stressed and distorted such differences, especially religious ones, so as to distance the supposed science of *thermalisme* from the religious and cultural uses of the hammam. French native or hammam narratives insist on three points in particular. First, they tend to mystify indigenous meanings of Korbous. The review *Tunisie revue illustrée* described in detail the post-Roman "rediscovery" of Korbous:

> Korbous is said to have been created by the marabout Sidi Amara. . . . He had come to camp in the mountains near the sea. The pious native encountered a lion with which he spent his days and nights. . . . One day, Sidi Amara descended to the sea. Touching the ground with his stick, he produced a warm water geyser, through the will of God. Soon he received the visit of his brothers who proposed a pilgrimage to the Dakhla of the Maaouines. All three mounted their horses and left, but Sidi Amara's mare stopped abruptly, as if halted by a chain. The two saints turned to Sidi Amara and told him to stay. It is not possible for a saint to accompany a saint. Stay where you are where your doctor's duties beckon . . . Sidi Amara became famous in the whole land. Patients came to seek his expertise, most notably a wealthy woman who, once cured, paid for the restoration of the Roman ruins which form a bath in the rocks. The three cabins still present today date from this era. One was sacred, and for the exclusive use of Sidi Amara." [20]

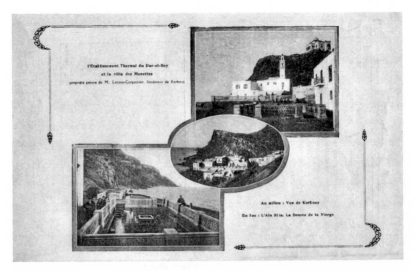

FIGURE 16. Korbous: (*bottom*) Aïn-Sbia, with pilgrims in basin; (*top*) Dar-el-Bey; (*center*) general view. Brochure *La Côte du Soleil: Korbous station thermale et climatique d'hiver.*

Although the sacred and the medical are clearly interconnected in this story, the French focused largely on the former. Henri Rajat, the director of Vichy's municipal hygiene bureau, described Korbous revealingly as "a Muslim Lourdes."[21] The equal, if not more obvious, parallel with Vichy escaped him entirely because he associated Vichy with science and Korbous with superstition. An archival document on Korbous insisted, "The Muslim, like the Jew, keeps all his faith in the waters of Korbous, because he has enshrouded them in sacrosanct legends, according to which the waters sprang up through divine intervention."[22]

One of Korbous's springs appears to have been considered especially holy by Muslim pilgrims. "For ablutions and localized baths, the Arabs have always preferred Aïn Sbia," wrote Louis Geslin in 1913. He added, "Since it has been tapped, a basin has been constructed . . . and at all hours of the day one can see Arabs lotioning their scars with the water of this miraculous spring. They dedicate large, ex voto multicolor silk flags to it."[23] This Spring of the Virgin, as the French knew it, thus elicited expressions of piety from local Muslims and equal doses of scorn from French doctors, who might well have been reminded of very similar ex voto offerings around springs in France.[24]

Second, French accounts invariably focus on a local drinking ritual known as the *medbach.* This practice should be situated in the broader context of local

Tunisian folk and prophetic medicine. The latter ascribed a prominent role to *jinn*, or evil spirits, whose effects were thought to be canceled by a host of cures, including sunlight, gunpowder, drinking potions, and pungent herbs, preferably prepared by a marabout.[25] In his thesis on Korbous, written in 1913, Geslin noted, "The mineral water, or *medbach*, is always absorbed by the Arabs in purgative doses. They divide their purgative cure in seven-day installments."[26] J. Arnaud, for his part, described the *medbach* as follows in the *Presse thermale*: "Natives practice a veritable orgy of liquids. Instead of taking the warm waters from the spring as Europeans do, they ingest it in the form of an herbal tea they name 'medbach' and which is little more than a maceration of nine species of aromatic plants from the nearby mountains. They generally alternate the absorption of natural water and this tea each week."[27] Arnaud once again distanced French hydrotherapy and its obsession with the authentic, mineralized, and telluric "source" from an Arab practice in which the potency of the spring waters themselves seemed somehow less central. Michel-Louis Bastide had noted very similarly in 1888, "The [Arab] patients who come to [Korbous] do more than take a bath in the pool, or frequent the sweat bath: they also partake in internal drinking cures. But the water they employ does not come directly from the *griffon* [spring]."[28] Here, then, resided the major difference between the *medbach* and a proper Vichy drinking cure.[29]

Third, French sources underlined the central role of the steam bath at Korbous, as at any other hammam. While they recognized its medical potential (the steam bath made its appearance at many metropolitan French spas in the nineteenth century, where it benefited from exotic cachet), they questioned its practice by Tunisians. Michael Fisher has exposed the British appropriation of the Indian entrepreneur Dean Mahomed's "Indian medicated baths and shampoos" at Brighton. Long after Mahomed built his grand bathing establishment in 1821, it was conflated with the "Turkish bath" gaining in popularity in Britain as well in the nineteenth century.[30] At Korbous, the steam bath's waters were drawn from the Aïn-Haraga spring, where it emerged at forty-three degrees centigrade. According to Geslin, this temperature "produces a very disagreeable sensation of respiratory suffocation." Geslin's opinion was, predictably, negative: "This is the Haraga so famous amongst natives: They take it at all times of the day, but preferably in the evening. They leave the Haraga congested, shriveled up, sweating buckets. Not a season goes by without a major accident. Certain Arabs take it for half an hour, even a full hour. . . . Some die. One Arab died at the Haraga a few days ago, who had stayed in the steam bath all day. Other patients came and went, nobody suspecting he was dead." [31] Far from revivifying the body, as a French "cure" did, this non-European therapy appeared to drain it, inducing a condition so near death as to make death indistinguishable. Here, then, was a practice deemed medical but irrationally practiced, at odds with European principles of balance, moderation, and regulation. Jérôme Penez has followed the nineteenth-century debates over mineral bath duration. Standard time was thirty minutes. Baths over an hour long were proscribed. [32]

Overall, a supposed Oriental Korbous of superstition, religion, and neglect was systematically opposed to a French, modern, and scientific Korbous. Before 1904, wrote Malinas, "a stay in this small and poor Arab village was a sad affair." But now, he beamed, "the *Compagnie concessionnaire* has transformed the old miserable baths into a station boasting the most modern comfort, as much in material and technical terms." [33] This was a recurring theme. Geslin observed, "Before 1904 . . . when a patient came to the Arab village, he found no decent lodging, no appropriate food for his cure, no installation allowing him to drink nor bathe in a manner in conformity with the most basic hygiene." [34] In 1902, commented one doctor, the stay of "even the most accommodating European" was "virtually impossible at Korbous" because of the extreme "dirtiness" of the site and the need to bring all belongings along. Indeed, this source specified, "the patient must bring along his bed and blankets; objects necessary for every day life are altogether absent." [35] This was not just a matter of imposing French standards. The difference between what were soon called the Oriental Korbous and the French Korbous emblematized the French colonial civilizing mission in Tunisia, by underscoring French superiority in the realm of rational hydrotherapy.

As Rajat's inability to compare Korbous with Vichy suggests, the colonizers displayed little lucidity in contrasting their balneological and hydrotherapeutic practices to those of Tunisians. A particularly striking example can be found in the archives, where an anonymous French source states, "Muslims and Jews follow a twenty-one-day cure that can be extended to forty days. The period of real activity is that of twenty-one days, divided into three seven-day chunks. The number seven is significant. It is considered a fateful number, and Arabs have a blind confidence in it." [36] Rather than remark upon the astonishing similarity in length of treatment—both hydrotherapists at Vichy and Tunisian doctors at Korbous had settled exactly on a twenty-one-day cure—this observer stressed the superstitious basis of the Arab cure's three seven-day segments.

What is more, although they characterized precolonial Korbous as something of a desert, few of these colonial texts denied the very real pre-1881 popularity of the springs among local people. Indeed, long before Korbous rivaled the popular beach of La Goulette as a favored destination for French settlers, it had attracted legions of Arab pilgrims and bathers as well as some European travelers. A pre-1881 French testimony states as follows:

> The small village of Korbous contains approximately a hundred Arab dwellings inhabited by a fraction of marabouts, the *Ouled Sidi Amram*, numbering some 50 families approximately. They come here almost only during winter—the bathing season—at which time they rent out rooms, sell milk or eggs, or fetch water at the spring. . . . This spa is frequented almost exclusively by Arabs . . . They come here in droves, and from afar, because the mineral waters have a wonderful reputation in the whole land, an amply warranted reputation confirmed by the chemical tests whose results I have just given, and by the number of cures accomplished here. [37]

Here, a French doctor recognized not only the popularity of the waters immediately prior to the French conquest (and, needless to say, well after Roman times), but also their successful pre-1881 use in treating certain afflictions (he lists scrofulose, rheumatism, gout, syphilis, and paralysis). [38] These similarities and continuities would only cause the colonizers to redouble their efforts at creating a distinct French, modern Korbous.

In reality, preprotectorate Korbous had been popular not only with Tunisians. In a book in progress, Julia Clancy-Smith demonstrates that Europeans, some visiting, others posted in Tunisia, had long taken the waters at Korbous. She cites the case of the Gaspary family, that of the French vice-consul in La Goulette, relishing the leisure, family time, and improved health they derived from Korbous in May and June 1824. She also gives the example of the English consul general in Tunis, Sir Richard Wood, who in 1858, in view of an upcoming trip to Ireland, took the waters to treat his rheumatisms (here, perhaps, the idea of reverse acclimatization, or reacclimation, was already at work).[39] All of this points to important continuities between pre- and postprotectorate Tunisia as well as to the very obvious fact that preprotectorate Korbous had been anything but repulsive to nineteenth-century elites, as colonial sources often claimed. In any event, the notion that French Korbous was created overnight was clearly as erroneous as the claim that Arabs had somehow neglected, overlooked, or abandoned the site.

"Founding" French Korbous

Lewis Pyenson reminds us that the declaration of a protectorate over Tunisia in 1881 was followed just months later by the arrival of a scientific team.[40] As in Egypt and Mexico, geologists, physicians, and botanists advanced in the traces of French troops.[41] According to Geslin, four years after the protectorate was established, the protectorate's director of mining, Aubert, studied the possibility of "properly" tapping Korbous's waters. In 1902, the springs and outlying areas were ceded to the Viscount de Méaulde and to Edmond Magnier, but neither managed to honor the conditions of their contract. The archives reveal that the process of attribution in 1901–02 scarcely took into account the dwellings and the inhabitants of Korbous, whose properties were registered on the municipal rolls but slated for either appropriation or destruction, under the rubric "expropriation for a purpose of public utility." [42]

A measure of stability was brought to the Korbus hydrotherapy venture in 1904 with the concession of the spa to Lecore-Carpentier. For inhabitants of Korbous, little had changed. Many of those who had managed to keep their homes after the initial wave of expropriations in 1902 saw them leveled by an engineering project aimed at "protecting the spring of Aïn Kebira . . . from infiltrations and imperfections from the surface." Several "Arab dwellings in the North of Korbous village" were thus destroyed because their inhabitants had purportedly compromised the purity of the nearby spring. While these efforts at maintaining complete purity proved largely vain, Malinas found some consolation: "At least we had the satisfaction of discovering the upper part of an ancient (Roman) wall." [43] Excavation served not merely to reach the *griffon*, but also to revive a Roman legacy and elide the more recent past.

Not all local influences were erased, however. The French reserved some elitist admiration for the Dar-el-Bey establishment. This structure had once served as the personal retreat of the prince Ahmed Bey, who had it constructed between 1837 and 1855. Under the French, the building was refashioned into a modern hydrotherapy establishment, boasting by 1913 an underwater shower, eight bathing rooms with individual pools, two shower massages, one "*Roman* steam bath, a gynecological cabin, a pulverization room," and so on. Geslin described the architectural ensemble as "rather singular, for the heavy architecture of the Bey palace has barely been altered." [44] The resulting architectural hybrid typified Korbous's new urban face. Very similar to Lyautey's modernist-Moorish pastiches in Morocco, it made for a singular backdrop for open-air and covered baths. How could it not have undermined the French claim to an untarnished, uncompromised French version of hydrotherapy? The explanation has to do with class. In 1888, Michel-Louis Bastide made it clear that of all Korbous's precolonial architecture, only Dar-el-Bey was "constructed in a European way." By this he meant that it offered European comforts and European hydrotherapy technology, rather than any particularly European outside appearance (Bastide contrasted the Dar-el-Bey to other Arab structures he deemed "most primitive in their installations").[45]

Such ambiguous examples of mixity notwithstanding, the ultimate goal of Lecore-Carpentier and his consorts was scarcely hidden: "To create a thermal establishment worthy of a *ville d'eau*, and to facilitate as much for Europeans as Muslims and Jews, the treatment of each by adapting to each one's customs and mores. In a word, the objective is to establish a European Korbous next to the Oriental Korbous." [46] Establishing a European Korbous started with promoting the spa to settlers, administrators, and even colonials from other empires, or other parts of the French empire, and to a lesser extent, to curistes from metropolitan France itself.

Attracting the Colonizers

Like promoters of all the other spas examined in this book, those at Korbous needed to convince multiple clienteles to frequent their resort. Having a faithful local patient-pilgrim base already in place, Lecore-Carpentier and his team turned to colonials and settlers: hence, Lecore-Carpentier's missive to Indochina in 1913 vaunting the spa's curative effects against colonial ills. Geslin's assertion that very year is in the same category. According to Geslin, Korbous would one day become "the refuge of colonials, and to patients having stayed in the new world or the tropics, who will travel here for their health, chased from London, Paris or central Europe by the rigors of winter."[47] Again, Korbous occupied a middle ground, neither tropical nor European-hibernal, a position projected as an ideal "recompression chamber" for colonials.

The task of marketing Korbous to the colonizers was complicated by a lack of mineral compatibility between Korbous and Vichy, Vals-les-Bains, Encausse-les-Thermes, La Bourboule, Châtelguyon, or any other metropolitan spa renowned for treating colonial afflictions. Whereas Antsirabe could claim a natural affinity with metropolitan antimalarial waters, Korbous's claim seemed more chemically tenuous. The *Quinzaine coloniale* in 1909 classified Korbous's waters as "hyperthermal, belonging to the chlorinated-soda family, related to the waters of Balaruc and Uriage in France. The presence of iron, phosphate, arsenic and even lithium in these waters lends them undeniable therapeutic value."[48] Unfortunately, neither Balaruc nor Uriage claimed any tropical medicine purview, the former being used to treat afflictions of the central nervous system, rheumatism, and circulatory disorders and the latter, skin disease, syphilis, and gynecological disorders.[49] Korbous's medical staff were unfazed. Malinas, while recognizing Korbous's efficacy in treating the very same diseases as Uriage, asserted their "undeniable efficacy in the treatment of . . . malarial anemia," adding for good measure, "Korbous's main action is tonic and revitalizing, for it stimulates weakened organisms, altering bodily exchanges, exciting and repairing cells."[50] In this way, Korbous was reinvented as a colonial regenerator, dissimilar chemically but not therapeutically to Vichy, Antsirabe, Dolé-les-Bains, and Cilaos.

The Stigma of Syphilis

Even so, transforming the spa into a haven for diseased colonials proved more delicate at Korbous than elsewhere because of an enduring negative association. Even Korbous's tourist agency recognized it obliquely: "Aïn Sbia," it explained, "benefits from a wide reputation in all of North Africa for its special virtues . . . which are conceived for the treatment of specific diseases so widespread among Arabs."[51]

A reading of Schoull's and Remlinger's *Les eaux thermo-minérales de la Tunisie* (1903) and Malinas's *Notice sur le groupe hydro-minéral de Korbous* (1909) can elucidate this mysterious "Arab disease." Schoull and Remlinger emphasize the effectiveness of Korbous's waters in treating syphilis.[52] This reflects in part the dominant view at the time that syphilis was best treated with arsenic. In 1909, Malinas decided to break ranks with Schoull and Remlinger because, he argued, they had contributed to stigmatizing Korbous as a syphilitic center. As Alain Corbin has shown, venereal disease evoked a dual peril — sanitary and moral — in the early twentieth century.[53] Malinas's rationale is instructive: "Schoull and Remlinger were wrong, according to me, to identify Korbous as the top treatment center for syphilis. Indeed, this reputation is mostly confined to Tunisian natives, amongst whom syphilis is extremely widespread, and is not considered a social stigma. The same cannot be said of us. We thus worry that . . . this reputation for a specific action against syphilis, while it may have decided a handful of Europeans to seek treatment here, has wrongly frightened countless others from coming."[54] Malinas identified fear of contagion more specifically as a blemish on the spa's reputation: "It is the fear of being contaminated by natives afflicted with syphilis that [drives French people away]." Here, Malinas tried to reassure the colonial public: "There is only, rest assured, a wealthy or at least comfortable native clientele at Korbous these days. The miserable wretches who were once such a burden on the town, carriers of horrid lesions, who instilled both pity and secret terror amongst bathers — they have been driven away by the proximity of Europeans, and have left for other hammams in Tunisia."[55] Here, segregation met fear of contagion in the classic colonial equation. Korbous was defined as a safe, elite, and European space, not merely because of the social class of the Tunisians who frequented it, but also because of who did not: Indigenous paupers had been driven away to other hammams.[56] The distinction between hammam and *station thermale* was thus articulated in social as well as racial and cultural terms.

Segregation

In his *Notice*, Malinas emphasized the separation of bathers: "The water of Aïn Sbia . . . is tapped into a column, and into a rectangular platform which serves as a drinking fountain. The part that is not drunk passes into a pool left to the

use of natives, who treasure it as a healing pool for wounds and skin ailments."
In this scheme, the water not consumed by Europeans descended to feed the
native bathing pool. Nearby, observed Malinas, the "Aïn Haraga functions as
a dedicated steam bath frequented exclusively by natives." [57] Such segregation
was considered sufficiently unremarkable by the French that no "Arabs Only"
sign need have been placed over the Haraga steam baths. Hammam steam baths
in Tunisia were quite simply understood to be reserved for Tunisians. Europeans, meanwhile, frequented the eerily similar "Roman steam bath" at the
Dar-el-Bey.[58]

Segregation was by no means a French invention at Korbous. Geslin suggested that to some extent French rule had actually relaxed segregation between Muslims, Jews, and foreigners. Referring neither to Aïn Sbia nor to Aïn
Haraga, but to the "second-class" old thermal establishment, largely over-
shadowed by the more luxurious Dar-el-Bey, Geslin notes, "The old thermal
establishment is frequented by men in the morning, and between 3 and 7 pm by
women, Muslims and Jews indistinguishably. Things were not always so. The
Arabs, relates Gauchery, enforced a [tighter] bath schedule. The resort func-
tioned in an odd manner: from midnight to ten in the morning, the pools were
reserved for Arabs, from ten to noon to "*roumis*" (foreigners), from noon to
one to Jews, and from one to midnight to Arab women, and often from four
until eight to Arab [men]." [59] The French thus cast the French–Arab divide at
Korbous as merely the latest ordering of the baths. Even in colonial times, at
the second-class "old" hydrotherapy establishment, class and gender seem to
have somewhat complicated the colonizer–colonized divide. Although gender
segregation was strictly enforced, it never matched the degree of colonizer–
colonized segregation, since at least men and women of the same ethnicity
were allowed to use the same waters, albeit at different times.

As early as 1901, the French civil authority in Grombalia had expressed concern that "no disposition seems to have been taken to maintain the bathing
rights of indigent natives and Europeans at Korbous." The said official, a certain Pumonti, deemed it "appropriate to oblige the exploiting company to construct two pools, one for Europeans, the other for natives, where the indigents
could be admitted for free at any time." [60] Only poor Europeans challenged
the colonizer–colonized divide in this founding logic of French Korbous, since
they were henceforth relegated to bathing in the native pool.

The Arab Korbous: Between the Picturesque
and the Modern

The colonial contribution to French modernism is now well established, thanks to the work of Gwendolyn Wright, Herman Lebovics, Paul Rabinow, and Zeynep Celik.[61] Korbous's rebuilt Arab village in many ways straddled the line between the authentic and the modern. On one hand, the French razed old indigenous dwellings and conceived a new Arab quarter that would no longer elicit disgust or fears of contagion in French bathers. On the other hand, they delighted in Korbous's exoticism and Arab distinctiveness.

In 1913, Geslin commented approvingly, "The old village has been destroyed in part, and it will progressively perish, replaced by new constructions adapted to the particular needs of a heterogeneous and cosmopolitan clientele. Europeans and Europeanized North African Jews prefer hotels. Natives, Berbers or Tunisian Jews, who come to take the waters as a family affair, prefer apartments or homes that they can rent by the month. . . . Each of these apartments features its own pool of mineral water, filled freshly every day."[62] French archival sources corroborate this view: "The Muslim, like the Jew, prefers being at home to take the waters."[63] Here, North African and European customs are distanced, Tunisian Jews constituting a marginal intermediary category. But Geslin nevertheless stresses that apartments for "natives, Berbers or Tunisian Jews" are supplied with fresh mineral water—thereby bringing "proper" European *thermalisme* even to the colonized. Geslin continues:

> New homes for native Tunisian and Algerian customers, installed a few years ago by the spa's operating company, conform to their needs and habits. They are, moreover, a model that could be imitated elsewhere at spas where the poverty and dilapidation of the native installations seem to be the rule. . . . African spas that have tried to attract patients from Europe, like Hammam-R'Hira in Algeria, or Hélouan in Egypt, have done virtually nothing to satisfy local customers. The efforts of Korbous's *compagnie des Eaux et du Domaine* are more eclectic and less exclusive. They cater to all in kind.[64]

More than any other North African spa, Korbous was seen as providing for the "unique needs" of both the colonized and the colonizers. The latter were pampered with, in Geslin's words, "two entirely new hotels . . . destined to satisfy the needs of the colonial bourgeoisie."[65] Korbous's segregation was thus sanctioned by the imperatives of cultural specificity, preservation, and authenticity.

Lecore-Carpentier and his media empire invested considerable effort in designing, shaping, and defining the new Arab Korbous. Whereas before 1904, Korbous had counted only "70 miserable rooms, . . . a rough total of some 1000 square meters," they explained, by 1935 it boasted 207 lodgings specially earmarked for Arab customers, 100 kitchens, 105 bathrooms, not to mention the 2 hotels aimed at Europeans.[66] The goal was not only to provide French hygiene to Tunisians, to establish de facto segregation between colonizer and colonized, but also to create "a convivial Muslim atmosphere." Lecore-Carpentier's team somehow presumed they could capture and embody this ambiance better than Muslims themselves. Indeed in 1939, Lecore-Carpentier's successor, his son-in-law Charles Maillet, identified this "convivial Muslim ambiance," enabled by the new (French) urbanism, as precisely the feature that attracted crowds of Algerians to Korbous, which, he stated, they preferred to "their own [Algerian] resorts."[67]

Most French accounts insist on the simultaneous modernity and authenticity of Korbous's new Arab quarter. An undated pamphlet in the archives reads, "New constructions have allowed us to receive a greater number of occupants: all of these edifices were conceived on a dial-shaped outline, in keeping with the geography of the site. Their style is Oriental, their openings numerous, with grand corridors, halls, covered galleries allowing the sun and marine air to enter."[68] French architects had simply followed prevailing colonial wisdom and the thrust of contemporaneous architectural trends by conflating elements of Oriental architecture with broad windows and open passages. They thereby hoped to preserve an exotic touch of Oriental architecture, while eliminating its purportedly unhealthier aspects — "narrow," "insalubrious," and "overcrowded" Arab urbanism. The same source observes, "One cannot insist enough on the effort accomplished by the *Compagnie des eaux thermales* in terms of these particular housing projects, which answer the needs of the Tunisian population. Korbous is the only spa in North Africa to boast such a number of rooms, independently from proper 'Hotels' which we will examine in a subsequent paragraph on 'European Korbous.' "[69] The document concludes with a nod to Korbous's purported synthesis of modernity and authenticity: "Korbous presents the visitor with an admirable film on the Orient . . . Muslims and Jews continue to frequent Korbous: they appreciate the transformations we have undertaken to the spa, but they remain firmly attached to their millennial, ancestral habits, transmitted from father to son. It is the superposition of Oriental Korbous and European Korbous that gives such a unique flavor to the town." [70] If Korbous were a film, it was intended to convey a singular juxtaposition of Muslim and Jewish practice and French know-how; Muslim and Jewish rites, specificities, and cultures; and French urbanism and hydrotherapy.

Gaming

At virtually all the spas examined thus far (with the exception of Guadeloupe's smallest ones) casinos played a central role.[71] Only the archives concerning Korbous permit a reconstruction of the nexus of colonialism, gaming, and hydrotherapy present from Vichy to Salazie. Gambling has come under scrutiny as a site of tension and conflict in colonial contexts. A fine recent work on the British Raj has exposed multiple British anxieties: over the bazaar as a site of wagering, over the prospect that Indian kinship ties might render wager-based commerce an uneven playing field, and over the inability clearly to define legitimate trade in colonial terms.[72] A study of gambling in French colonial Indochina has revealed French fears of racial mixing and moral degeneration in and around gaming houses, and the effort of the French to distinguish their own *cercles*, or gaming establishments, from those of the ethnic Chinese.[73]

In Tunisia, the colonizers were not chiefly concerned with a supposed native obsession with gambling (as in Indochina) or with monitoring or restricting wagering in public commerce (as in India); rather, they were torn over the place of gaming in Islam. These concerns account in large part for the decision to ban gambling across the protectorate in 1939. Since 1904, gambling had been permitted by joint order of the French government and the Tunisian regency. Indeed, the Bey signed a decree in 1904 allowing Lecore-Carpentier's *Compagnie des eaux thermales et du domaine de Korbous* to manage gaming in practically all its forms, be it baccarat, poker, *"chemin de fer, petits chevaux* and its variants, or any other games that it could see fit in the future." [74] Gambling, of course, sat uneasily not only with many Muslims themselves, but also with the French image of Islam and with French cultural preservationists, authenticity buffs of all stripes, and cultural associationists opposed to assimilation schemes they equated with corruption or even cultural contamination.

More mundanely, gambling had, according to the management of Korbous's *compagnie des eaux thermales*, helped keep their enterprise afloat. In his response to the ban on gaming, Maillet explained, "By overturning the gaming economy, the government is irremediably compromising our financial balance. Our work achieved at Korbous—35 years of French toiling here—is therefore directly threatened . . . [for] it is the profit from gaming alone that has allowed us to continue our steady development of Korbous. Our accounting books . . . show this clearly."[75] Maillet presented Korbous's public service—medical, hygienic, and social—as directly dependent on the fruits of gambling, in a rather familiar argument for anyone cognizant of the lottery/social spending relationship. The public service in question was, however, explicitly tied to French prestige, modernity, hygiene, and business. Its connection to casinos revealed the spa's relative fragility.

A decade later, Tunisia's commissioner of tourism, J. L. Ferraton, broached the matter again, urging French and Tunisian authorities to "reestablish official gaming in Tunisia." New arguments were presented this time, extending well beyond the single case of Korbous. Ferraton noted the double standards created by gambling's simultaneous legality in Algeria and Morocco and illegality in Tunisia and by ongoing clandestine gaming in Tunisia.[76] Here, Ferraton identified multiple threats to Korbous: that its customers had deserted the spa for Hammam R'Hira and other establishments in the Maghreb and that underground gaming continued unabated in Tunisia, without profiting the *compagnie des eaux thermales* in the slightest. In the sensitive and emblematic arena of gaming, both colonial profitability and hydrotherapeutic/hygienic proselytizing had ironically been undermined by colonial control and preservationism.

Unrest and the Decline of the Colonial Spa

Like Antsirabe, Korbous found itself at the heart of decolonization struggles because of the privileged colonial position it had once occupied. The Cap Bon peninsula on which Korbous is situated was the scene of a French dragnet in January 1952 that aimed at quelling rising unrest, including a major strike and a series of assassinations of French officials. Insurgents in the Cap Bon region were well armed, having tapped into caches of military supplies left by Nazi Germany, which had made its final North African stand in the area in 1943.[77] Tunisia's path to independence should, of course, also be tied to global trends: not only Lybia's independence in 1949 and Morocco's in 1956, but also decolonization struggles across the French empire, from Indochina to Algeria, decisively influenced Tunisia's fate.

The year before Tunisian independence in 1956, Mrs. Maillet, the new proprietor of Korbous's *compagnie des eaux*, complained bitterly of a boycott against her establishment. The local administrator of Cap Bon relayed her grievance to Tunis: "The very significant drop in spa-visitors this year seems to have less to do with our economic difficulties than with a political movement aiming to boycott us. Articles published in the local Arab press a few months ago . . . are evocative of the final objectives of our detractors." [78] Tunisian nationalists had deliberately targeted Lecore-Carpentier's spa empire as a prominent symbol of French power.

In February 1956, a month prior to national independence, Korbous's management again addressed the French administration in Tunis. A letter of February 9, signed by the director of Korbous's *Hôtel des thermes*, reads,

> On the evening of February 8, around 10 pm., several individuals armed with revolvers and a machine gun erupted into my Korbous establishment. Wielding their firearms, these persons uttered threats, first against the pensioners, then the employees of my hotel. After investigation, it turns out that these gentlemen belong to your services. They had been asked to arrest a certain Taieb Chrea. While I can certainly understand the need to arrest people, I would be grateful if you could henceforth ensure that these gentlemen act with greater tact and discretion when undertaking their missions. My clientele is made up of honest Tunisian merchants and farmers, Muslims and Jews, most of them ill, and seeking treatment here at the spa. Many of them, scarred by these events, have left my establishment this morning.[79]

The spa thus found itself front and center in the cycle of independence actions and colonial reprisals. The hotel manager's mordant letter—sent only hours after these unsettling events—focuses largely on the spa's violated sanctity and serenity. But it is also replete with ironies: the very hotel once reserved for

European clients now catered primarily to Tunisian "merchants and farmers"; colonial police actions were undermining French economic interests at Korbous; "honest Arab patients" partaking in French hydrotherapy were presumed to be terrorists by the colonial *sûreté*; those Tunisians who had dared violate a boycott against the spa now found themselves menaced by colonial forces.

Epilogue

In 1966, a full decade after Tunisian independence, Dr. Z. Kallal and A. Djellouli edited an *ABC of Tunisian Hydrotherapy* on behalf of their institution, the national *Commissariat général au tourisme et au thermalisme* (CGTT). That Tunisia's ministry of tourism was twinned with a ministry of hydrotherapy is significant in its own right. The pamphlet contains other revelations. In spite of a scripture from the Koran on the frontispiece, the tome claims a strictly scientific Western approach—indeed stricter than that of the colonizers. The authors, for instance, reject out of hand the accommodations the French had made for Muslim bathers. One paragraph reads, "A new modern hydrotherapy establishment is nearly completed, and it will replace the decrepit so-called 'thermal apartments.' Indeed, we deem it necessary that bathers take their baths under full medical supervision, utilizing the techniques of modern hydrotherapy. That is why we decided to end the supplying of mineral waters to apartments." [80] Regarding Aïn Sbia, once so popular with Tunisian pilgrims and bathers, the guide explains: "Its proper tapping is rendered practically impossible because it opens into the mud and near the ocean; it is therefore polluted, and cannot offer a proper conduit. It shall thus not be developed." [81] Even the Dar-el-Bey's spring was revamped, tapped in a "rational manner since 1965." [82] Here, postindependence Tunisian hydrotherapists poured scorn on colonial segregation (under the guise of cultural exceptionalism), whether the designation of Aïn Sbia as a "spring for Tunisians" or the canalization of spring waters directly into "native apartments."

Korbous was subject to a host of shifting and concurrent cultural, social, political, religious, and medical uses and roles. That its internal contradictions failed to strike contemporaries constitutes perhaps its most remarkable feature. A popular precolonial site, it was appropriated by the colonizers as a cure for local diseases, while simultaneously stirring fear among the settlers for its reputation as a syphilis treatment center. A self-proclaimed site of science, its practitioners indulged in pilgrimage, gambling, votive offerings, and folk cures. A purported oasis of Frenchness and product of a French vision, to the point that it drew the ire of Tunisian nationalists, it was also vaunted as a "film of the Orient." Colonial doctors wrote with contempt of its famed twenty-one-day medbach and its local hammam, while never raising an eyebrow over the twenty-one-day Vichy cure or, for that matter, the introduction of a hammam at Vichy. Korbous, in short, served as a point of both contacts and tensions—tensions that persisted well after the decolonization process, as the *ABC of Tunisian Hydrotherapy* demonstrates. This Tunisian spa served as a colonial crucible, a site where science, identities, even modernities both jostled with and were conditioned by religions, rituals, and millennial legacies. The Dar-el-Bey's transformation from a precolonial princely retreat into a site of ultramodern hydrotherapy and back into a site of nostalgia or neglect speaks to both the elasticity of these appropriations and the inextricability of the postcolonial, colonial, and precolonial. Less readily visible today are Korbous's colonial functions and justifications: an enabler of settlement, a salubrious revitalizer, a beacon of French science, and a site where the exotic could be distanced, displayed, tamed, and modernized.

CHAPTER 7

Vichy: Taking the Waters Back Home

CLAUDE FOUET, NAMED VICHY'S FIRST INTENDANT of the waters by Louis XIV, was almost certainly the earliest to posit the effectiveness of Vichy waters in treating malarial fevers. His treatise of 1686, *Nouveau sistème des bains et eaux minérales de Vichy*, established this principle, which would serve as a crucial precedent for centuries to come: "Vichy water cures fevers that recur every four and every three days [that is, usually malaria][1] by correcting and blunting the bitter leavens that cause these periodic fermentations, much like Quinquina, which blunts and absorbs this same leaven that causes fevers."[2] Here Vichy's powers over malarial fevers were explicitly compared to those of quinquina, the new miracle bark of the era, recently "discovered" in South America and employed to combat malaria (the treatment had likely been borrowed from native healers some five decades earlier).[3] Already in the seventeenth century, we witness the juxtaposition of Vichy waters with the quinine's precursor, quinquina being the same bark that would ultimately yield this precious drug in 1820. Indeed, a careful reading of the passage reveals that Fouet believed Vichy waters to be superior to quinquina, insofar as they "correct[ed]" the root causes of malaria, while quinquina merely assuaged its symptoms.

To suggest that Vichy's colonial function began in 1686 would be teleo-logical. If anything, more metropolitan malarial patients than colonial ones would have come to take the waters in the late seventeenth century (one thinks of malarial ravages in France at the time, from the swamps of Sologne and Languedoc).[4] Nonetheless, a key concept had been coined: the effectiveness of Vichy waters over malaria. If one also factors in Vichy's growing reputation — well established by the nineteenth century — for treating liver ailments, then Vichy's emerging colonial role, assumed in earnest in the 1830s, is certainly more readily explained.

From Hamlet to *Reine des Villes d'eaux*

Vichy's colonial function in the nineteenth century and the twentieth cannot be understood independently from broader phenomena: the town's transforma-tion into one of Europe's premier spas and its related post-1860 reputation as a chic resort. Although the spa had been used since Roman times, Vichy had long remained a hamlet, dwarfed in the Middle Ages by nearby villages like Billy. By the seventeenth century, however, Vichy was beginning to attract powerful outsiders — elites looking to cure a variety of afflictions. The arrival on a single day in May 1676 of some ten French nobles to take the waters at Vichy shows that long before the rail era, transportation hurdles could be overcome, at least by the wealthy.[5]

Although Vichy's population remained small, its reputation in the early nineteenth century was fast becoming global. The town counted around nine hundred inhabitants in the 1820s. Some one thousand outsiders visited annu-ally to take the waters. According to Mackaman, Vichy in the 1820s "boasted a well-founded reputation for lively society in the summer season, as well as waters that were highly regarded by continental doctors. The combination of Vichy's reputation and the advantages it enjoyed as a state property placed it among the premier watering places of Europe."[6] Vichy cures were indeed being prescribed at an increasing rate both at home and abroad. They were dis-pensed for a broad range of afflictions, although especially for liver-related ills. As we have seen, this organ was widely believed to constitute the Achilles heel of the colonizers. But its swelling was also linked to excess and good living. In France, so-called *crises de foie* remain associated with overindulging in rich food, for instance. Here, standing, class, and colonialism converged around the French medical liver fetish.

Mineral water drinkers—for Vichy was first and foremost a site for drinking cures—queued over and over again at the town's many springs over the course of their twenty-one-day cure, in hopes of overcoming nagging afflictions. Soon crowds of medical penitents would turn this highly standardized ritual into a collective pilgrimage to a prescribed Vichy spring, be it Grande Grille, Chomel, Célestins, the Source de l'hôpital, and so on. Vichy offered no shortage of therapeutic options and a seemingly endless capacity for accommodating growing numbers of *curistes*.

Spa centers and towns sprang up across France in record numbers in the nineteenth century, transforming hamlets into thriving urban areas.[7] Historians agree that Vichy's explosion onto the national and international stage occurred in the 1860s. Its reputation as an elite destination was confirmed after Emperor Napoleon III graced the resort with his favor, spending five personal holidays there in the 1860s. Just as Vichy's star was rising in elite circles, crowds of emulators flocked to the scene, after the town was placed in the orbit of the French rail system (nearby Saint-Germain-des-Fossés was connected by rail in 1854; Vichy's own train station was inaugurated in 1862).[8] Between Napoleon III's first stay at Vichy in 1861 and his fifth and final cure there in 1866, the town's visiting summer population jumped from sixteen thousand to twenty-one thousand.[9] By 1934, Vichy's ratio of summer visitors to permanent inhabitants reached the staggering level of ten to one (twenty thousand inhabitants, two hundred thousand visitors).[10]

Vichy's elite, even noble, reputation was seemingly unaffected by the relative democratization brought about by rail access and the resulting manifest increase in middle-class drinkers and bathers. In fact, after the emperor's first cure at Vichy in 1861, the town's advertisers seized the image of an "aristocratic drinking/bathing class" to attract would-be emulators. The *Splendid-Guide* to Vichy of 1880, for instance, plainly stated, "Nothing was spared in the construction of Vichy's new casino to render it worthy of the aristocratic clientele, which makes up the majority of bathers at Vichy."[11] This is certainly an exaggeration, and Mackaman is undoubtedly correct in identifying Vichy as a space of bourgeois leisure. Still, Vichy did draw many aristocratic *curistes* and socialites, playing out their collective tension between extravagance and simplicity in a site that promised at once urbanity, clubbism, discipline, regularization, and ritual.[12] Indeed, Vichy was coded as a healthful site where elaborate normalizing tools and the elements themselves could overcome the symptoms of excess—whether their root cause was excesses of temperature, of food or drink, or of extravagance more generally.

An article in *L'Auvergne thermale et pittoresque* for July 1883 lists some 110 notables in attendance at a gala held at Vichy's *cercle* international club. They included, to cite only a small sample, "General du Bessol and his family, the Marquis of Villerslafaye, Admiral Thomasset, the marquise of Juigné, Wall de Loewenstein, Baroness Blanc, Mrs and Miss Lee, Count and Countess Luigi, Count Sternberg, Count and Countess Paraviscini, Princess Obolensky, Mrs Hennessy, Count and Countess de Casa Segovia, Lady Matheson, Marquis and Marquise Visconti Venosta, J. de Kaischewsky, Giacomo Profumo and his wife, General Hansler, Spahis Captain Abd-el-Kader, and many representatives of the army and navy."[13] The article ends on a flippant note: "Let us stop, for we will never end this column if we want to name everybody who attended." Although hardly representative of every Vichy soirée, this veritable who's who nevertheless sheds light on the cosmopolitan, indeed, truly international networks of influence established during Vichy's legendary summer seasons. Here, the great resister of colonialism and unifier of Algerians Abd-el-Kader rubbed shoulders with an international cast of Italian, Spanish, Polish, English, and French nobles as well as entrepreneurs, military figures, and the rich and famous more generally.

Colonial ties, like noble ones, were forged out of Vichy's growing role as a site of privilege, power, and networking. At the root of Vichy's specifically colonial function, however, lay a much simpler consideration: the reputation of its waters for treating colonial ills. This reputation was certainly tied in part to Vichy's notoriety for treating other excesses. The association seemed straightforward, given that, as we saw in chapter 1, the colonies were imagined as a distorted, moral- and sense-numbing, libidinous space.

A Colonial Specialization

In 1937, a Guadeloupe newspaper explained Vichy's dual role as an elite spa and a colonial haven: "Vichy has been rightly called the port of call of colonials everywhere. And if this quaint and welcoming little town has become every year the meeting place of part of the planet, it is mostly an oasis that draws all those who live in warmer climes, all of those whose long stays in distant lands require that they undertake a detoxification and regularizing of their digestive system. Many actually come spontaneously, without the necessary medical referral, simply to stay in good shape, so as better to endure tropical infections in the future."[14] The passage reveals Vichy's multiple colonial functions: meeting place, oasis, liver repair center, detoxifying agent, metabolic regulator, and prophylaxis. In this excerpt, as at Vichy itself, the medical, the social, and the cultural are intertwined. The latter two cannot be considered without a brief review of Vichy's clinical promise for colonials.

Augustin Alquier, a doctor with the rank of lieutenant colonel in the colonial forces, as well as the inventor of a new Vichy drinking glass (1931) designed to dispense both water and gaseous vapors,[15] asserted, "If Mont-Dore is a providence for asthmatics, then Vichy is the providence for colonials."[16] Being a colonial had become tantamount to suffering from a chronic medical condition, comparable to asthma. Alquier was not alone in formulating such reductions. Raymond Durand-Fardel, another famous Vichy hydrotherapist, concluded, "It is often said that the colony is a chronic disease; we can say today that it is a hepatic disease."[17] Here, the colony, at its very essence, was pathologized.

As early as 1862, Auguste Durand de Lunel had confirmed that Vichy waters excelled in treating "the chronic side-effects and consequences of intermittent fevers [that is, malaria], consequences that so often resist traditional treatment."[18] A series of stages led to the formula Vichy = colonies. By the 1870s, the very time when Max Durand-Fardel was calling for greater specialization in spas, Vichy had gained an international reputation as the liver treatment center par excellence. As a direct result, argued the military hydrotherapist M. Tamalet, "Vichy came to exert considerable attraction on the spirits of colonials."[19] The syllogism "Vichy = liver, liver = colonies, colonies = Vichy" had been fully established.[20]

In medical terms, Vichy's effects were summarized as follows: A properly designed (that is, through referral) drinking cure could, according to the former head clinician of the faculty of Paris, "rapidly shrink engorged livers [caused by malaria] and considerably relieve anemia."[21] Edmond Vidal, a doctor practicing at Vichy who doubled as head of a colonial hygiene review, went into greater detail: "When properly administered, Vichy water returns a malarial liver to its normal functions. Under the influence of Vichy water, the liver is profoundly modified, its functions are regularized, and after a 'crisis' usually occurring on the 8th or 9th day of treatment, the liver considerably decreases in volume."[22] Soon, Vichy's curative properties were transformed into prophylactic virtues. Indeed, doctors prescribed drinking cures at Vichy before, during, and after a stay in the tropics. In 1911, J. Gandelin vaunted the merits of a "preventive cure" at Vichy as well as admonishing colonials to return to Vichy after two years in the colonies.[23]

The step from Vichy's reputation as a repairer of colonial livers to its role as a colonial haven was a short one. Doctors like G. F. Bonnet conceded that patients could self-diagnose the need for a Vichy cure: "when they feel their liver."[24] And Vichy's operating company, the *compagnie fermière*, encouraged this simple association. In 1950, it claimed, "Vichy has always been a rallying center for patients residing in warm countries, whose influence on the liver is well known. Whether these alterations of the liver are due solely to climate, or to outbreaks of malaria, or even amoebic dysentery, they are always considerably alleviated by a Vichy cure."[25] Little wonder, then, that the Guadeloupe article of 1937 remarked, "Many [colonials] actually come [to Vichy] spontaneously, without the necessary medical referral."[26] Still, the most direct path from the colonies to Vichy ran through a doctor's office. It was doctors, after all, who had imagined Vichy's colonial function in the first place — in concert with hydrotherapy promoters and government agencies. A woman who grew up in Indochina recalls that upon her return to France in 1945, a family physician explained in the simplest of terms: "Coming from the tropics . . . [a Vichy cure] would be good for the liver."[27] Many a medical practitioner placed advertisements in the specialized colonial press. The former head doctor of Vichy's military hospital, Paul Velten, paid for an advertisement in Indochina's civil engineer bulletin inviting families to his private practice on the rue Royale, overlooking the park.[28]

Colonial Connections: Vichy as the "Hydrotherapeutic Capital of Overseas France"[29]

Vichy's rise and fall are coterminous with those of the second French imperial wave (1830–1962). A historian of Vichy writes that in the "1950s–60s, decolonization robbed Vichy of its best customers."[30] If Paris, Marseille, and Bordeaux played important roles in colonial affairs thanks to the presence there of the Ministry of the Colonies and sizable populations of colonial subjects, colonial exhibitions, and ports, Vichy fulfilled a positively critical and largely forgotten role at the heart of the French imperial matrix thanks to its curative specialization and the soon famous derivation "Vichy = colonies." [31] Unlike Marseille or Paris, which could lay claim to being "capitals of the colonies," [32] Vichy could thus boast of being the capital of the colonizers.

Although it is difficult to establish the precise number of colonial visitors to Vichy at any given time, it has been estimated that between the two world wars, 17 percent of all outside visitors to Vichy hailed just from North Africa — not counting the rest of the French empire — compared to 16.5 percent from the entire English-speaking world (often seen as one of the main customer pools for continental spas in this era). [33] By 1934, sufficient numbers of settlers from North Africa were undertaking the pilgrimage to Vichy to warrant the creation of a direct sea-rail link (involving an agreement between the Paris-Lyon-Marseille (PLM) train line and the Compagnie de Navigation mixte), taking customers from Oran to Vichy via Port-Vendres in southern France. [34] As we shall see, then, Vichy benefited immensely from the business of colonial entrepreneurs, soldiers, missionaries, settlers, and administrators.

This business, of course, had been carefully secured through the medical promises we have just examined. To quote Paul Jardet, who was practicing at Vichy: "The effects of the Vichy cure are well known, as are its specialization in the treatment of diseases like fevers, malaria, dysentery, Cochinchinese diarrhea, tropical anemia, and other colonial diseases. This reputation has attracted to Vichy both soldiers and administrators from our colonies. The activity of our military thermal hospital attests to this. In addition, many civilians consider a cure at Vichy to constitute a natural and necessary complement to a long stay in warm countries." [35] Colonials from all walks of life, horizons, and geographical origin congregated at Vichy. They did so, moreover, at different stages of their colonial careers. And, after years of frequenting Vichy on a seasonal basis, many ended up setting down roots there. In the words of one observer, writing in 1937, "On the banks of the Allier [Vichy's river] settlers, administrators, and missionaries all meet up. They have come here to replenish their strength before embarking on the trip to the colonies. Vichy has also become a preferred residence for many retired colonials, who continue to spread the word of French colonialism's achievements. Their associations have recently been merged into Vichy's Intercolonial association, whose headquarters is located at the Maison coloniale on the rue de l'Hôtel-des-postes."[36] Clearly, Vichy's reputation for curing colonial ills had transformed it into a kind of informal imperial hub—a site where colonials would not only mingle, but also retire.

Vichy positioned itself simultaneously as a preventative necessity, a stop-over, and a postcolony imperative. Roger Glénard observed in 1926, "Metro-politans considering a trip to the colonies come to Vichy to undertake a pre-ventative cure, in the event that their liver might have shown the slightest weakness. . . . Colonials come periodically to re-whiten[37] themselves at Vichy while on leave in France. And those who return for good to the motherland come to Vichy to rid themselves of the last hepatic traces of their colonial exis-tence."[38] Vichy thus played a critical role in the life cycle of every colonial—before, during, and after their colonial experience. It served explicitly as a re-whitening agent for those having lived so long among native others. Vichy was also believed to effect a powerful cleansing of the liver that could literally erase the internal scars of colonial life on French bodies.

In sociological and anthropological terms, Vichy ultimately became the metropolitan point of contact—a crucial interface to the motherland—for settlers, missionaries, soldiers, and administrators, whose years of expatria-tion in the colonies had "uprooted" them from their original metropolitan net-works—be they kinship or professional. To quote Glénard: "Having generally no fixed residence in France, coming to France in periods of holidays when citi-zens flee their large cities, colonials find more at Vichy than mineral waters and the finest therapies; they find the many distractions proper to the metropole."[39] Before settling down to retire on the banks of the Allier, these colonials had come for decades to take the waters to reaffirm their Frenchness—seasonally and ritualistically reimmersing themselves in a microcosm of France.

Who were these colonial *curistes*? Vichy's *Guide de l'étranger* for 1883 broke them down into sartorial categories: "From the original costumes [one sees Asians, Greeks, Levantines, and so on, at Vichy] let us move on to the serious. Here is the severe costume of Scottish clergymen . . . , of Lazarists, or Armenian priests, of ecclesiasts of the holy Roman church, of chaplains in our African army, in the colonies or the navy, with their long beards reminiscent of Russian Orthodox priests; all of this fits in rather well with the almost severe costume of magistrates, functionaries, army officers . . . some wearing brilliant Algerian uniforms, from the light blue tunic of the officer of indigenous *tirailleurs*, to the ample and picturesque costume of the spahis, illustrated by Jules Gérard, the lion slayer." [40] I shall return shortly to the overall divisions between exotic, paracolonial, colonial, and French visitors with which this passage opens. I wish to emphasize here the distinctions between the colonial actors considered: uniformed functionaries, military officers, missionaries, and chaplains composed some of the myriad colonial columns congregating at Vichy.

Some interesting recent scholarship has scrutinized imperial networks — involved in everything from Freemasonry to banking. Other studies have focused upon colonial fractures — rifts in colonial society, emblematized by the chasm between settlers and administrators in Madagascar, for instance. Others still have examined the construction of a colonial identity, cast against that of the colonized. Vichy does not fit in neatly with any of these approaches. On one level, Vichy did allow fragmented colonial entities to come together in a single site. But it also reveals odd traffic patterns. For at Vichy, although settlers and officers might rub shoulders under the arcades of the Source de l'Hôpital, they generally did not share either the same conditions (for example, reimbursements for their travel) or the same space. Vichy did, however, enable lateral encounters and networking that were impossible in the colonies themselves: officers stationed in Madagascar bunked with those from Tunisia; missionaries from every corner of the empire, though not colonial agents per se, could meet after years of perceived isolation; and, for that matter, an entrepreneur from Réunion could converse with a customs official from Indochina. Thus elites whether colonial or colonized, could mingle at Vichy. In short, although highly compartmentalized in some ways, in others colonial society at Vichy proved more fluid than in the colonies themselves. Five discrete groups of colonial constituents sojourned and took the waters at Vichy on a regular basis: settlers, colonial troops, colonial administrators, missionaries, and members of the colonized elites.

Profiles of the Colonial *Curiste*

SETTLERS

In his novel *45 degrés à l'ombre* (1936), set on a passenger ship returning home from the colonies, the novelist Georges Simenon sketches the motivations and personality of one Lachaux. This profoundly pessimistic and surly colonial plutocrat owns vast plantations in the Congo. But mostly, Lachaux seems to have developed a fetish for Vichy. He keeps a bottle of Vichy water by his side at night. And his reason for being on board the vessel in the first place is to return to France to take the waters at Vichy.[41]

Simenon's portrait is mostly lifelike: from the nineteenth through the twentieth century, a great many settlers made the journey home to France specifically to undertake a detoxification or liver cure at Vichy. Still, one should be careful not to generalize from Simenon's example. In particular, one has to consider variations in the wealth and social status of the colonial settlers (*colons*) who took the waters at Vichy. A touching exchange of letters from 1859 shows that laborers sent to Algeria likewise sought to improve their health by making the trip to Vichy. A certain Madame Barthelot had left Algeria with her seriously sick son, hoping he could be cured at Vichy. Instead, he perished there, and both she and her sister-in-law found themselves unable to afford the trip back to Algeria, where her husband awaited them. The prefect of the Allier seemed favorably disposed to helping pay for the trip back to Algeria, with the caveat that the Ministry of the Colonies was tightening restrictions on the entry of laborers into the colony. Indeed, the prefect noted that in a very similar and recent case, the minister of the colonies had advised, "Permits to go to Algeria are no longer being granted to workers, unless they can produce letters emanating from settlers, and certified by local authorities, showing that they have a stable job awaiting them in the colony."[42]

The vast majority of colonials sojourning in Vichy can be classified somewhere in between Lachaux and Barthelot, in that they were neither opulent nor destitute. A rich source sheds light on Vichy's role as a meeting place for colonials from every corner of the French empire and from many walks of life and horizons. The *Liste officielle des étrangers* registered, for police purposes, the name and origin of every single guest at a Vichy hotel. *Etranger* was taken here to mean any outsider, not merely "a foreigner," so that guests from nearby Roanne, Marseille, and Lyon but also those from more distant Algiers, Hanoi, St. Petersburg, or New York all featured on the list. Unfortunately, this source has its limits as a tool for measuring the colonial presence at Vichy. For one thing, because "place of domicile" was requested rather than "place of current residence," many colonials—be they settlers, religious, or military personnel—identified themselves as being from Paris or Toulouse rather than from the colonial outpost to which they were stationed. For instance, in 1896, a certain Father Rouet checked himself into Vichy's Hotel Rivoli under the category: "Missionary, Rennes."[43] Moreover, with the exception of soldiers (often posted at the Hôpital militaire), the profession of each guest was described only in the vaguest of terms, making it often unclear whether their trip to Vichy was funded by the administration or not. Indeed, settlers had to pay their own way to take the waters, unlike the military and administrative classes and even missionaries, whose way to Vichy was covered by the government until 1911.

In any event, the *Liste officielle des étrangers* does provide some valuable glimpses into colonial networks, patterns, and representation at Vichy. To take only a small sample, between June 29 and August 3, 1865 (the 1865 season, in other words) one can identify a legion of self-identified colonial guests checking into Vichy's hotels:

> From Algeria: Mr and Mrs Beaudoin, proprietors in Oran; Mr Chapouroti also from Oran; Mr Renier from Oran; Mr Durand, an interpreter from Constantine; the Rolands and the Mirands from Constantine; Mr Cabannon from Algiers; Mr Aumale from Algeria; Mr La Monta, a military doctor in Algeria; Mr Sarlande, the Mayor of Algiers; Mr and Mrs Pierrey, president at the imperial court, Algiers; Mr Begnier-Osseval, a proprietor in Algeria; Mr Aveline, a military pharmacist in Algeria; Mr Obitz from Algiers; Mr Belpaume, a landlord from Blidah; Mr Ballard, a landlord from Algiers; Dr Romana from Algiers; Mr Berelta, an entrepreneur from Blidah; Mr and Mrs Daboussy, military interpreter in Bône; Sid Seliman Ben Syame, from Muriam, Algeria; Mrs Sée from Algiers; Mrs Matheu and her daughter from Algiers; Mrs Abdelal, a colonel in Algeria; Mr Latil, a proprietor in Algiers; Si Sliman Ben Siam from Miliana, Algeria; Mr Meymac, a landholder in Algiers; Mrs and Miss Maschat from Oran; Mr and Mrs Millon from Algiers; Mr Pineau, a trader in Algiers; Mr Babert, a proprietor in Philippeville; Mr Savigny and son from Algiers; Mr Mercier from Constantine; Mr Chavagnac, a trader in Blidah; Mr and Mrs Hugo, a general in Algeria; Mr Matheu from Algiers; Mr and Mrs Bouscarin from Oran; Mr Bruyas from Constantine; Mr and Mrs Bastide from Algiers; Mr Chazotte a batallion leader from Constantine; Mr Mosnier, a landlord in Oran; Mr Abda-La-Ben-Msahoud from Gelma; Mr and Mrs Corre from Algiers.

In addition, twenty officers from Algeria checked into the hôpital militaire, which is listed even though it is not strictly speaking a hotel.

From other colonies:

Mr and Mrs Spielmann and their son, traders in Pondichéry; Mr Lemerle from
Martinique; Mr and Mrs Moreau from Réunion; Mr Navaizard, a policeman in
Sénégal; Mr Tessière, a trader in Sénégal; Mr de Vilier, a landlord in Bourbon
(Réunion Island); Mr Laugié, a proprietor in Martinique; Mr Manès, a landlord
in Réunion.[44]

The makeup of this representative sample calls to mind several points. First
of all, colonial elites clearly hobnobbed at Vichy. The mayor of Algiers, a general, a host of notables (including three Algerians), and a plethora of landed
magnates all met and socialized in the halls of Vichy's baths, arcades, and
drinking queues. Second, and perhaps paradoxically, these encounters sometimes transcended the administrative divides of colonial society: translators
rubbed shoulders with traders, landlords, police officers, and rural settlers.
Third, they definitely breached geographical boundaries, with colonials from
Pondichery entering into contact with others from Senegal, Martinique, and
Algeria. Finally, Algeria was, of course, significantly overrepresented here,
compared to other colonies, in an era before the second great French wave of
colonial expansion, launched after 1871.[45]

Subsequent *Listes des étrangers* provide additional insights. That of 1899 reveals patterns of hotel loyalties. In trying to respond to Vichy's ever-growing
cosmopolitanism, some establishments had begun catering to specific ethnic or
religious groups. Thus the aptly named Cosmopolitan Hotel featured a Hebrew
inscription within the *Liste des étrangers* and appears to have attracted a predominantly Jewish clientele. A similar phenomenon appears to have emerged
for colonials: the Hôtel britannique (which would, under the Vichy regime between 1940 and 1944 come to house the Ministry of the Colonies), and the
Hôtel de la Cloche, seem to have secured at the very least a returning colonial clientele. In late July 1899, the Hôtel de la Cloche welcomed eight guests
from Algeria. In early August of that same year, another three colonial guests
checked in — one from Oran, another from Guadeloupe, and a third identified
only as "from the colonies." A week later, two guests arrived from Dakar. In
early September, another arrived from Oran, and another yet from Dakar.[46]
Imperial networks were being knotted in the halls and at the breakfast tables
of Vichy's hotels.

Beyond socialization and the obvious quest for better health, what did these settlers seek at Vichy? The history of intentions is not an easy one to map. Yet certain sources confirm that coming to Vichy had become part of a complex ritual of periodic cultural reimmersion for colonials. Take, for example, the text on a Vichy postcard, sent from an Algerian settler to his friend in the gendarmerie in Biskra, Constantine, in 1912: "Be certain that I will do my utmost to bring you some French air, for here it is cool. I'm getting my money's worth of it, and will only be returning to Algeria in early October . . . All is well, and I have rebuilt my health a little, as has my wife, who sends you a gracious hello."[47] If one scratches beneath their formulaic civilities, such messages reveal the belief that ethnic French—no matter the number of generations they might have inhabited Algeria—must from time to time return to their climes, where they must undertake elaborate, lengthy, and prescribed cures to reconstitute their fragile health. If fragility stemmed from alienness, then it followed that good health could be derived from the familiar. And Vichy thrived on producing the familiar—on actually generating it—through rituals, returns, rules, and regulations surrounding the famous twenty-one-day cure.

COLONIAL TROOPS AND THE HÔPITAL MILITAIRE

Vichy's military-colonial connection began in earnest with the French conquest of Algeria in 1830. Thirteen years later, some thirty officers received authorization to come to Vichy, where they were granted free baths and drinks for their patriotic efforts. Oral history has it that in 1844, upon seeing a simple soldier taking the waters "dressed as a pauper," Baron Dubouchet, the military intendant at Vichy, requested "an official position worthy of men who have sacrificed their health to defend the honor of their country and the interests of the nation." The minister of war agreed and ordered the founding of Vichy's military hospital on July 1, 1847. Its purpose was to "receive all troops, but especially those who have returned from Africa and the colonies."[48]

A vital principle had been established: the right of military personnel to be transported to, lodged at, and administered the waters at Vichy for free. Very quickly, military personnel afflicted with malaria rushed to Vichy for treatment. The proportion of colonials at Vichy was already substantial. Indeed, the military hospital opened that year could accommodate 50 officers and 44 soldiers, although one source speaks of 30 officers and 70 soldiers.[49] In 1855 a new structure was built behind the neoclassical facade of the old Hôtel Cornil, bringing the total number of beds to 94 for officers and 157 for soldiers and noncommissioned officers. By the twentieth century, the premises had once again expanded, this time to accommodate 175 officers. An elaborate rotation system was implemented in 1919 to ensure that any malarial soldier or other serviceman victim of tropical disease could have access to the facility: 23 seasons of 100 patients each were established, each season lasting, not surprisingly, the twenty-one days of the standard Vichy cure.[50] In 1930, 2,325 patients were treated at Vichy's hydromineral military hospital.

The hospital was known as the *hôpital militaire thermal de Vichy*. Hydrotherapy rested at its very core. By 1931, the establishment boasted 22 individual bathing compartments for immersion in naturally warm waters, three "horizontal intestinal shower installations" for more intrusive treatments, one underwater shower system, one shower device connected to a bed, two underwater massage tables, and so on. In 1930, the hospital dispensed 21,625 "hepatic showers," 14,483 "thermal baths," 1,321 underwater massages, and 77 intestinal showers.[51] The empire was certainly keeping the staff of Vichy's military hospital busy.

This considerable military colonial presence did not go unnoticed at Vichy. A local newspaper, *Vichy thermal*, wrote with wonder in 1899, "Under the foliage of the old park, there they come strolling down the asphalted path. They are no longer in some jungle full of tropical creepers, of mysteries and ambushes, sweating fever and death. No, they are in the thermal city whose miraculous springs cure afflictions contracted in Tonkin or Madagascar. And from morning to evening, indistinguishable from the crowd of drinkers, our officers bring a patriotic note to the high society and the gentlemen who queue to take the waters."[52] In the last decade of the nineteenth century, at the height of French imperial expansion, troops on sick leave from colonial campaigns had become so commonplace at Vichy that a local journalist pondered in 1895, "We have been asked whether the colonial medal should be worn on civil costume [at Vichy]. The colonial medal is certainly a great honor for those on whom it is bestowed, but we may be pushing our love of ribbons too far by wearing it on jackets in civil life. It is after all not a distinctive sign of honor or courage, like the *médaille militaire*; it simply proves that one has gone on campaign in the colonies, and mostly that one has returned alive, which is admittedly a fortunate thing." [53] Clearly, at Vichy it had come to be seen as outré and indecorous to display something that such a large percentage of visitors could wear if they so chose. What might have constituted a rarity in some rural backwater or a conversation piece in the capital was simply commonplace at a site that colonial troops considered their home away from home. For like administrators and settlers, many veterans ultimately set down roots at Vichy. Vichy in essence became the colonial serviceman's equivalent of the Parisian Val de Grâce Hospital and the Invalides, wrapped into one.

ADMINISTRATORS

While French colonial soldiers and officers were able to stay gratis at a dedicated institution, colonial administrators, conversely, had to seek out their own transportation to and accommodation at Vichy. Their lot was nevertheless considerably more enviable than that of settlers. Indeed, their voyage and stay were substantially subsidized thanks to a number of measures and laws that allowed members of the colonial service posted in the colonies regular furloughs to France and substantial monies for staying at Vichy proper. A decree of January 28, 1890, mandated that the government pay a significant proportion of the costs incurred for colonial administrators to return to France specifically "to take the waters." [54]

In 1893, under the direction of the undersecretary of the colonies Théophile Delcassé, a bold new project was initiated to bring colonial administrators completely in line with military personnel at Vichy. The plan involved purchasing a building in central Vichy to house a colonial administrator's hospital. The rationale was simple: "The number of officials, functionaries and agents belonging to different bureaus in the colonies coming to Vichy has been increasing notably in recent years, draining both local budgets (of individual colonies) and the colonial budget (in Paris) itself. These functionaries and agents are taking the waters at Vichy, of course, because of their renowned curative virtues against most diseases contracted overseas." [55] In addition to creating a budget crunch, the administrative rush on Vichy waters had strained the limits of Vichy's accommodations. The Ministry of the Colonies noted bluntly that the army had not opened sufficient rooms at Vichy's military hospital for administrators, simply because their own hospital rooms and hydrotherapy center were already overcrowded. And the Ministry of the Colonies worried that unlike soldiers, who were routinely examined by experts in tropical medicine, administrators seeking individual consultations at Vichy were being treated by nonspecialists. Finally, noted the report, colonial administrators still ended up paying part of their Vichy stay out of their own pockets, in part because they often traveled with their families and in part because while in France they were not able to collect their colonial bonus—the bonus granted for the time one spent in the colonies.[56]

At Delcassé's request, in 1893 the head of the Colonial Bureau's second office, Billecocq, traveled to Vichy to find an appropriate site for the future hospital. He was accompanied by none other than Georges Treille, the leading authority on tropical hygiene. They noted the exorbitant cost of the villas and hotels where administrators had heretofore tried to find a room. Billecocq and Treille settled on the Hôtel Maussant et de Madrid to house the future administrators' hospital. It stood conveniently across from the Hôpital militaire, and, Treille noted, it could easily be provided with mineral water from Vichy's *compagnie fermière*. Both men were persuaded after negotiations that they could obtain free water from the *compagnie fermière*. Transformed into "a model colonial hospital," the building would house state-of-the-art hydrotherapy equipment and could provide eighty administrators with comfortable individual convalescence rooms.[57]

The overall goal of this project was plain: to assist the "administrator sapped by colonial climates . . . to follow the treatment necessary to him."[58] The blueprints seem to have responded to a very real demand that was reaching a fever pitch in the 1890s, at the zenith of empire. Interestingly, unlike the Hôpital militaire and the Maison du missionnaire, this project never materialized, in part because colonial governors seem to have balked at the costs imposed on each colony.[59]

MISSIONARIES

Like soldiers and administrators, missionaries prior to 1911 had been able to undertake periodic trips to Vichy—and indeed treatment itself at Vichy—at the French taxpayer's expense. The formal separation of Church and State in France in 1905 would soon change this. In 1911, under a new minister of the colonies intent on applying secularism both in spirit and to the letter, missionaries suddenly found themselves unable to take the waters back home without incurring substantial costs — well beyond most of their personal budgets. To be precise, the turnaround came on March 15 1911, when Minister Adolphe Messimy released a circular ending free trips for missionaries on board the vessels of the Messageries Maritimes, the lifeline of colonials.[60]

A Lazarist missionary who had spent years in China, Father Henry Watthé would dedicate the second part of his life to rectifying the "injustice" of 1911. Watthé had returned to France during the Great War — clergymen being subject to the draft since the late nineteenth century. In France, he had first served as a translator for Chinese workers and troops fighting for France, before finally leading a unit of some five hundred Chinese men between 1917 and 1919. He arrived at Vichy later that year, on the advice of one Dr. Rendu from the Hôpital Saint-Joseph in Paris, who predicted dire consequences if he chose to return to China.[61] Given the rather draconian alternative of either good health at Vichy or certain death in China, Watthé quite sensibly opted for the former. At Vichy, he began giving lectures on China and meeting fellow missionaries. Most lived in precarious conditions, "staying in discount hotels, or lodged in attics . . . unable to afford the luxury of a room." He soon encountered a host of fellow missionaries, from different orders, posted on different continents. In his words, "At Vichy I met many missionaries from Africa — something entirely new for me. My thesis was only reinforced: missionaries are . . . shown no gratitude . . . they die like flies, because of an absence of even basic health care."[62] After consulting with local specialists in colonial medicine, Watthé hatched the idea of founding a missionary house, which would lodge missionaries gratis during their twenty-one-day hydrotherapy cure. Thanks to his contacts with local doctors, he was even able to offer free cures for all missionaries staying at his establishment. In so doing, Watthé believed, "he could prolong the life of a missionary by some 20 to 30 years."[63]

Opened in 1923, Watthé's Maison du missionnaire soon proved immensely popular and successful. Between 1923 and 1931 alone, sixteen hundred missionaries were lodged and fed at Watthé's center.[64] Watthé demonstrated considerable skills as a fundraiser for and promoter of his brainchild. He benefited from both political and press connections.[65] The Maison soon featured regular lectures on colonial topics — to which all of Vichy was invited. It also housed a small museum of "exotic artifacts," built from Watthé's original collection of Chinese pieces and subsequent donations from visiting missionaries (like the missionary from the Congo who wrote in 1933 that on his travels he "would think of finding some pieces for your museum").[66] The collection remains in place today—although a recent effort has been made to modernize the displays and museography behind them, hence its reinvention as the Musée des arts d'Afrique et d'Asie. All of these imperial by-products added to Vichy's growing colonial scene. But at its core, the Maison du missionnaire was intended to make cures at Vichy possible. Its mission statement was unambiguous: "Prolong the strength, health, and life of missionaries, through hydromineral cures and appropriate treatments."[67]

Like all colonial hydrotherapy ventures, this one was framed as a vital necessity. Monseigneur Guichard, in the French Congo, noted, "Our climate in Equatorial Africa is murderous, and there is not a single missionary having lived here several years, who does not require a cure at Vichy."[68] Rationales for cures were sometimes presented more piously. Marc Faure wrote of Watthé, "This apostle has understood the value of Vichy waters for the treatment of so-called colonial diseases."[69] Alquier, for his part, spoke of Vichy waters effecting resurrections among missionaries.[70] A journalist added somewhat turgidly, "The missionary, enflamed by his faith, consents to martyrdom, pushing and dragging himself through burning climates, where swamps teeming with miasmas attack his indefatigable apostle's body."[71] Vichy emerged as a kind of more reliable Lourdes—a dual medico-religious cure against ills still framed at least residually in miasmatic and moral terms.

The letters of gratitude expedited to Watthé and his Lazarist successor Cyprien Aroud display some interesting patterns. Many insist on the dual action of their stay at the Maison du missionnaire—a duality involving the curative action of Vichy's waters and the moral influence of the Maison itself.[72] Thus, a missionary about to return to Cambodia wrote in 1931, "You have understood that the missionaries require . . . moral comfort as much as a water cure."[73] Crucial to this moral comfort was the spirit of camaraderie fostered at Bethany, as the Maison du missionnaire was often called.

The Maison du missionnaire contributed in its own way to the powerful common identity emerging among French Catholic missionaries certain of performing both patriotic and religious deeds in the colonies. French missionaries considered themselves underappreciated agents of empire and nation as much as agents of the Church.[74] Watthé's initial efforts to aid ailing missionaries earned the support of the notorious ultranationalist Maurice Barrès, who lent his time and energy to the creation of the Maison du missionnaire.[75] Barrès wholeheartedly endorsed the strong nationalist streak in Watthé's discourse, evident most notably in Watthé's initial plea for a missionary house:

> An army of missionaries, of French race, is engaged in the work of missions. Two-thirds of missionaries in the world are French.[76] They represent our honor and the moral force of our empire. . . . We have established the principle of a right to health care for the most obscure roadman in the French colonial service, of the last stable-man in our consulates, without ever caring about our missionaries. . . . The war (1914–1918) has deprived us of our best missionaries, some having lost their lives for the nation, others working themselves to death to replace those mobilized. The war also took from us aspiring missionaries, future recruits; they fell in large numbers in the fields of honor, and leave a void today that will only be replaced *by foreigners*.[77]

Here Watthé and Barrès found common ground on the greatness of the French "race," the errors of secularism, and the importance of keeping France's imperial auxiliaries — that is, missionaries — French. To Watthé and Barrès, missionaries were not merely the quintessential foot soldiers of empire and nation, but also terribly underappreciated martyrs, whom an ungrateful secular nation chose to leave crucified by disease in their hour of need. The Maison du missionnaire was intended to remedy this situation, while also fostering the missionary spirit and saving those who served the empire.

For all of their imperialist rhetoric, missionaries also staked out points of uniqueness: unique skills and a special esprit de corps that only the marriage of apostleship and empire could produce. In a letter written to Watthé in 1924, Father Joulord, a former missionary in Dahomey who had subsequently become bursar of the Missions Africaines in Lyon, said, "By prolonging the life of missionaries, who know the usages and languages of the peoples they must evangelize, you have admirably served the cause of religion and the nation."[78] Not only did missionaries serve as foot soldiers of nation, empire, and God, they were, as Joulord reminds us, a precious commodity thanks to their unique linguistic and cultural skills, acquired through years of work in the field. Anything that could prolong their lives would thus reap exponentially positive benefits for both France and Catholicism. And missionary letters seemed to prove Watthé right: One J. Pagès wrote from Tunisia that his cure at Vichy "had turned the clock back. Without Vichy, you would long ago have read my name in the obituaries." [79]

Fellowship might at first seem a self-evident characteristic of missionaries, if one were to overlook how divided they were by orders, nationalities, and place of posting. The Maison du missionnaire, like Vichy's military hospital and its hotels, served to facilitate encounters. One grateful missionary conveyed this message in a poem dedicated to the Maison:

> They come at present from India and Japan
> From Patagonia and Gabon
> Our Apostles from all points on the horizon.
> They rush to this modern Bethany
> Under the healthful skies of the motherland
> To find new life at Vichy.[80]

Networking extended beyond traditional imperial fault lines.[81] Most obviously, neither Patagonia, nor India, nor Japan were French colonies. Although the vast majority of missionaries staying at the Maison du missionnaire hailed from tropical regions (40.65 percent from Africa, 15.3 percent from Asia — and within these categories Cameroon, Madagascar, and Indochina, all French territories by 1919, were most represented), a handful came from colder climes.[82] Father Portier is a case in point. He wrote in 1929 from North Battleford, Saskatchewan (Canada), "My stay at Vichy undeniably helped me immensely thanks to your hospitality and the [water] treatment. . . . But I don't know how much longer my system can take the cold, the miseries and the travels. I fear I will soon have to leave the savages and immensities of this land." [83]

The national divide was important as well. In a letter to Watthé, a Dutch missionary named Paulissen reveals the globalization of Vichy's reputation as a colonial cure: "When I was in the tropics, and I had liver attacks, I took Vichy candy or some of the Vichy salts that were sent to us from Europe, and this helped. . . . Only the cost kept us from taking a cure at Vichy itself." [84] And in 1929 the British missionary Henri Gabriel wrote of needing to take the waters, in view of a forthcoming trip to India.[85]

Missionaries seem to have taken cures before, during, and after their stays in the colonies. One wrote in 1933 of needing to undertake a cure at Vichy on doc-

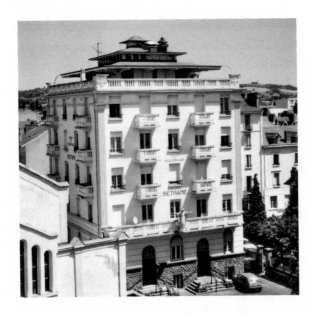

FIGURE 17.
The Maison du
missionnaire, Vichy.
Note the Chinese
influence on the roof.
The Maison's museum
is located on the
lower left. Author's
photograph, 2003.

tor's orders before returning to Cameroon, even though he "had spent eight years there in relatively good health."[86] Here one finds Vichy used as a precautionary prophylaxis. Another father mentioned "requiring a cure" simply because of "my eight years in the Congo."[87] Others wrote of needing a cure to combat chronic ailments, like the "benign but inveterate congestion of the liver" suffered by Alfred Jarreau after twenty-eight years spent in China.[88] Another missionary, recently posted in Haiti, wrote of needing to decongest his liver after "nearly 30 years spent in warm countries."[89] Each wore his years in the colonies as both a badge of honor and a yardstick of hepatic weakness. A missionary posted in Togo wrote of having "gotten rid [at Vichy] of the toxins that sapped [my] health."[90] Father Jérôme, for his part, believed that only through his cure at Vichy had he been able to convince his superiors to send him back to the Congo, so worried had they been previously about his fragile health.[91] Here, Vichy provided leverage for undertaking further abnegation, suffering, and duty. Cures seem to have had lasting effects. In September 1925, a missionary wrote back from Hué (Indochina) that his cures at Vichy in 1922 and 1923 "are still leaving visible benefits. I can now withstand physical and intellectual fatigue stemming from the tough climate."[92] A single reimmersion at Vichy could thus recharge a missionary's batteries, allowing him to function for several years in the tropics.

In colonial terms, Vichy served first and foremost as capital of the colonizers. But it also attracted, as we have seen, some indigenous elites, like Abd-el-Kader. This trend, begun in the mid-nineteenth century, in many ways defied the logics of climatic determinism and *mésologie*. After all, a strict reading of climatic determinism would have dictated that Frenchmen would find health at Vichy, while Indochinese would have been healthier in Indochina, Algerians in Algeria, and so on. And yet, Vichy promoters like Raymond Durand-Fardel, the head of Vichy's society of medical science, argued in 1932 that Vichy would benefit "all colonials, in the largest sense of the term, regardless of whether they be metropolitan or native, whose organisms has by definition suffered from the detrimental effects of tropical weather."[93] In this interpretation, Vichy waters could prove salutary for all inhabitants of the tropics, recent or not, regardless of race.

Class undeniably plays an important role in explaining this exception to the so-called laws of climatic determinism. Local newspapers trumpeted the arrival of emperors of Annam and sovereigns and princes from French North Africa. Columnists did this with no great regard for empire per se, since the Shah of Iran and emperor of Brazil received coverage more or less identical to that of crowned heads from the French imperial sphere. Vichy, it seemed, had quite simply emerged in the mid-nineteenth century as one of Europe's most cosmopolitan and worldly spas. Napoleon III's legendary predilection for Vichy cannot in itself explain the remarkable vogue of the spa among international elite circles in the late nineteenth century and early twentieth.

The colonial sovereigns who arrived to take the waters were not all at the summit of their power. One interesting category involved former monarchs replaced or squeezed out by the French. Sultan Moulay Hafid came to take the waters at Vichy in 1912 after having been passed up in favor of his brother for the throne of Morocco by Marshal Lyautey.[94] Similarly, Emperor Ung Lich of Annam stayed at Vichy's Hôpital militaire in 1889 after having been deposed by the French in 1885 and exiled to Algeria in 1888. At Vichy, he was lodged next to one J. Loubens, an official working in the customs service in Indochina.[95] Informal elite imperial networks thus quite logically incorporated indigenous sovereigns, whether left in place or removed from power by the colonizer.

This increasing worldliness was occurring in what was still, in terms of population, a small village in the French heartland.[96] Vichy numbered under one thousand permanent inhabitants in 1831,[97] roughly two thousand in 1847, three thousand by 1861, and eight thousand by 1880.[98] Robert Aldrich has recently underscored the pervasiveness of colonial sites and "vestiges" across the *la France profonde*, and not merely in imperial hubs like Marseille or Bordeaux.[99] The encounter between colonized peoples on cure and local inhabitants of Vichy struck a cartoonist in 1882 (see figure 18). The drawing shows two local women, a milkmaid and a laundress in their clogs. Each is presumably employed by Vichy's hotel industry, itself obviously a spin-off from the hydrotherapy business (more than 10 percent of Vichy's inhabitants were employed in the spa sector).[100] The two women are discussing the vaguely North African men — spahis or colonial soldiers perhaps — standing in the background. The women's worries reflect in part the site of this colonial encounter. It took place in the French heartland, at a site theoretically more isolated from things imperial than most French port towns. One asks, "My god, my dear, what country are they from?" The other responds, "From a country where each man has five women apiece." And finally, "Ah, my lord! Let's hope they do not bring this fashion to Vichy."

The Daumier-inspired cartoon conveys multiple and ambiguous messages. It hints at once at the parochialism of local working-class women and at their common sense for wanting to maintain French gender relations in the face of a freshly discovered, menacing other model. This particular culture shock is at once gendered, classed, and racialized. Here, turning imperial logic on its head, the local working women, not the North African men, embody the clichéd "bewildered native" in the colonial–colonized encounter (in large part because of their sex and class).

This reverse encounter occurred at the very time when, Eugen Weber argues, Paris was busily colonizing provincial France. Departments like the Allier and regions like the Bourbonnais, where Vichy was located, were indeed undergoing profound transformations in this period, transformations tied in part to the proliferation of new rail lines.[101] Guidebooks to Vichy and the Auvergne drove home the association between Auvergnats and colonial natives. A guide from 1901 began by discussing Paul Brocca's anthropometric measurements of local people in the Allier, before waxing about regional folklore and clothes:

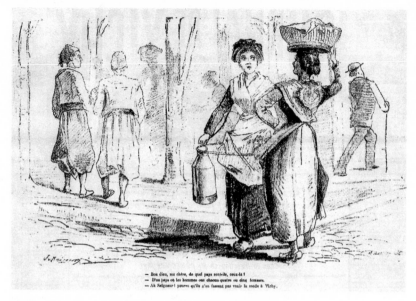

FIGURE 18. Cartoon in the *Journal de Vichy*, June 3, 1882.

"Of these old costumes, only the clog will soon remain . . . and even then in a modernized form. Bathers and tourists at Mont-Dore and La Bourboule may still see, for a few more years, the singular hairstyles of local mountain women."[102] The disappearing authentic native was a trope shared by early-twentieth-century travel guides to colonial Africa and the Massif Central. But in the cartoon seen here, the "civilizing" of the French countryside, described by Weber, is complicated by the growing presence of indigenous elites at Vichy, presenting locals with other, decidedly non-Parisian cultural ways at the zenith of Parisian influence over the French provinces.

PARACOLONIAL ELITES AND VICHY COSMOPOLITANISM

The presence of colonized elites seems to have contributed to a second Vichy identity—coexisting with that of "capital of the colonizers." This second identity was, as we have seen, quintessentially cosmopolitan. "All the peoples of the universe are represented [in the *grande allée du parc*]," proclaimed *Vichy's Guide de l'étranger* for 1883.[103] This Babylon was in many ways supraimperial, as the cover of *Vichy's Guide de l'étranger* in 1901 suggests. The drawing shows a French officer drinking the waters in the company of two young women, one presumably French, the other Japanese, who are surrounded in turn by *curistes* from North Africa as well as the Near and Far East. The cover was almost certainly designed to vaunt the affluence of women at Vichy — exotic women no less — while simultaneously extolling French *galanterie*, expressed allegorically by France's offering a drink of mineral water to Asia.

In a brochure from 1950, the *compagnie fermière*, boasted,

> Vichy, international hydrotherapy capital, has come into contact with so many civilizations, it has seen so many different peoples walk down its *Hall des sources*, it has received so many monarchs, fed so many glories, that, like bygone Byzantium, it no longer seems to recognize what is its own, and what it has borrowed from others. . . . After the war of 1914–1918, sovereigns of Portugal, Egypt, Tunisia, Romania, Morocco, and Annam mingled here with American millionaires rediscovering Europe. No one feels homesick here. . . . In the geographical center of France, Vichy, the international hydrotherapy and tourist mecca, is always remembered fondly by all.[104]

Here Vichy took on an almost ancient Roman capacity for simultaneous absorption and purported pluralism. While settlers, colonial administrators, and missionaries flocked there to "rewhiten," to escape homesickness, to cure themselves and recharge their batteries in the center of France, indigenous elites from both France's formal empire (Annam, Tunisia, Morocco) and from its less formal web of international influence (Romania, Portugal, Egypt, Brazil) congregated there as well, as much to network and socialize as to take the waters. The *Splendid-Guide* to Vichy explained in 1880, with its special brand of humor, that Brazilians were so numerous at Vichy that one should think twice before labeling "that jaundiced gentleman you just passed" a liver patient due to his peculiar copperish or yellowish hue. He might well be Brazilian, rather than hepatic.[105]

Colonials and missionaries were not the only ones defining the contours of their collective identities at Vichy: so too were an international array of crowned princes, nobles, and the bourgeoisie that sought to mimic them. Although they were certainly seen as "sticking out," curiously elite non-European visitors were somehow considered immune from the laws of *mésologie*. French sources suggest that at Vichy they managed to avoid homesickness and even to thrive in a cosmopolitan atmosphere. While Vichy could incarnate the goodness of the motherland for some, it could just as unproblematically embody a hybrid cosmopolitanism for others.

A Colonial Aura

As the visits of sovereigns—some Brazilian, others Vietnamese—suggest, it is sometimes difficult to parse the doses of exoticism, orientalism, and outright imperialism present at Vichy. To be sure, direct formal colonial connections abound, especially when one focuses on social or economic ties. In 1954, for instance, a company known as the Brasseries et Glacières de l'Indochine (BGI) purchased Vichy's famous *compagnie fermière*.[106] The BGI, anticipating the worst in the wake of the battle of Dien Ben Phu that very year, decided to withdraw from Indochina and to invest in the metropole. And what more logical an investment than Vichy for a colonial enterprise?

Culinary and material cultures also attest to Vichy's complex colonial connections. An Internet search for the terms *Moroccan* and *Vichy* yields a surprising mix of results: Some discuss the overlooked role of Moroccan troops in the liberation of France in 1944 from the clutches of Marshal Pétain's Vichy regime; others focus on a caramel specialty found only at the town of Vichy. The caramel was given its name, Marocains, in the wake of World War One, in honor not of Moroccan troops, but rather of "the assiduous frequentation of Vichy by *curistes* coming from North Africa."[107] The flavorful candy remains popular to this day. The two examples of Marocain boxes I was able to uncover, one likely from the interwar years, the other from the present day, are shorn of any colonial referent per se (figs. 19 and 20). The older one displays local inhabitants of the Allier in their clogs and traditional costume and speaks more to a colonial relationship with local peoples than to the outside world. The present-day model seems to hint at the good life enjoyed by settlers melting into Vichy's high society. This caramel connection, like its missionary house, its former military hospital, its colonial investment patterns, and its evocative hotel names, like the Algeria Hôtel and the Villa tunisienne, certainly reflects Vichy's deep colonial ties. But while the candies themselves bear affinities with North African sweets, their box designs eschew explicitly colonial motifs. No doubt some settlers on a furlough/cure in France wanted least of all to be reminded of the colony.

More delicate still is the task of deciphering colonial influences inscribed on the very face of Vichy—most notably in its architecture. The brasserie formerly known as the Alhambra (nowadays transformed into a bookstore) smacks of Moorish exoticism. But as its name suggested, it was meant to evoke Anda-

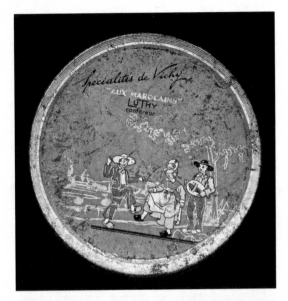

FIGURE 19. A box of
Marocains, circa 1930.
Author's collection.

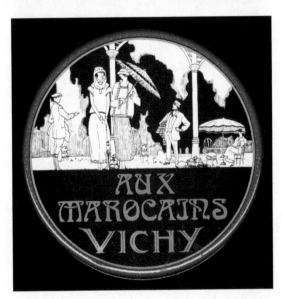

FIGURE 20. A modern-
day box of Marocains.
Author's collection.

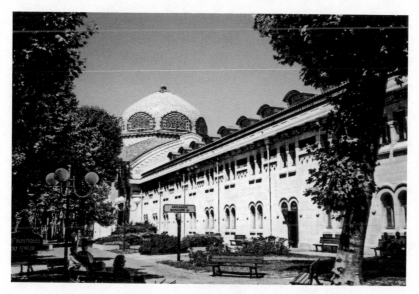

FIGURE 21. Vichy's main *établissement thermal* (*des dômes*). Author's photograph.
All rights reserved.

lusia more than French colonies. Likewise, the grandiose domes of Vichy's
main thermal establishment, constructed in 1903 (figure 21), suggest an impre-
cise orientalist influence[108] — the kind of hybrid modern-colonial pastiche that
would soon be in vogue in Lyautey's Morocco[109] — without explicit reference
to a single colony, protectorate, or overseas territory. Pascal Chambriard's detailed study of Vichy shows that architects had first toyed with classical and
Byzantine-style domes before settling on the oriental blueprint. Chambriard
also draws attention to the much more explicitly Algerian or Moroccan design
of two nearby springs. The revealingly named *sources du Hammam* in neighboring Hauterive featured explicitly North African mosaics, doorways, and so
on. And in nearby Saint-Yorre, one finds a *source du minaret*, a spring enclosed
within a minaret replica, erected circa 1930.[110] Vichy and its suburbs abound
with exotic architectural motifs, from the Byzantine to the Moorish. Although
it is tempting to consider such sites examples of "Orientalism in the French
provinces,"[111] the fact remains that such exoticism, although certainly contributing to Vichy's colonial aura, cannot be completely or easily conflated with
any single colonial project.

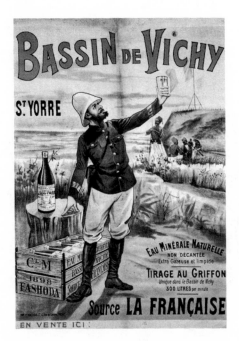

Spin-off

While colonial motifs in Vichy's architecture display varying degrees of imprecision, the colonial themes used to market Vichy products could not have been clearer.[112] No elaborate semiotic analysis is required to see how Vichy hydrocrats brazenly exploited the image of Marchand confronting Kitchener at Fachoda to sell bottled waters (figure 22). Marchand's French column had met Kitchener's British force at Fachoda in the Sudan in 1898, leading to an epic, though brief and, for the French, disappointing confrontation of the two colonial superpowers of the nineteenth century. The idea behind the advertisement, no doubt, was to simultaneously profit from patriotic fervor generated by Fachoda in France and to strengthen sales of bottled Vichy water to colonials.

Astute developers seeking to tap into mineral water exports to the colonies dubbed one of the Vichy area's springs dedicated to bottled water Colonial. The brand registration notice of "St. Yorre Coloniale" (figure 23) extolled the water's virtues against stomach, intestinal, bladder, and liver ailments. This proved a clever strategy because bottling an explicitly "colonial" Vichy water answered the obvious demand not only of those who wished to continue their

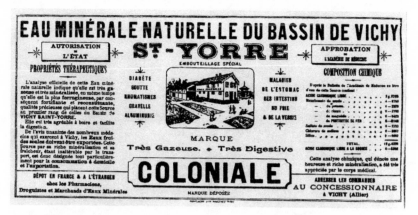

FIGURE 23. "Eau minérale naturelle . . . coloniale." Registered brand name for a "colonial" Vichy bottled water.

cure upon returning to the colonies, but also of those who could not afford to come to Vichy. In the words of Dr. Glénard, "a proper diet, hydrotherapy and a change of climate complete the favorable effects of a Vichy drinking cure. The subsequent continued consumption of bottled Vichy water will ensure the cure's lasting effects."[113] Already in 1859, a Vichy hydrotherapist had asserted,

> [Bottled] Vichy waters are the most exported of all mineral waters, both in France and overseas. . . . [Despite being less potent than at the source] bottled mineral water is nonetheless a precious medication for patients, who for diverse reasons and circumstances find themselves unable to travel to Vichy. This concerns especially inhabitants of French and English colonies or inter-tropical regions, who, because of negative climatic conditions find themselves victims of . . . liver and spleen engorgements. . . . All of these patients who are too far away to take a Vichy cure on location will find in the continued use of transported waters a precious medication, not only to destroy the different morbid causes of their disease, but also to combat the pernicious influence of climate which poses a constant threat to them.[114]

It was but a small step, in other words, from a Vichy cure on location to a bottled and hence portable version of the same product.[115] Again, the product was pitched specifically to colonials, as a tonic agent against both the heat of the tropics and tropical diseases.

Vichy water imbibers in the colonies were not all imperial heroes or poster

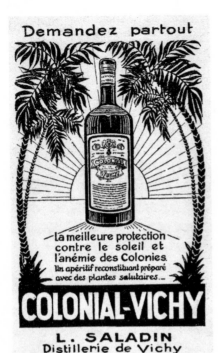

FIGURE 24. Colonial-Vichy liqueur.
Advertisement in *Saison Vichy*, 1929.

children like Marchand. In 1895–96, the pro- and anti-Dreyfusard camps waged a press battle over the bubbly drink sipped by Captain Alfred Dreyfus on Devil's Island. The fizzy beverage, granted to him for a short time on medical grounds, proved to be none other than Vichy water (and not champagne, as the anti-Dreyfusard *Libre parole* suggested).[116]

Throughout the Second Empire and Third Republic, the Vichy name was notoriously and gratuitously appropriated for unrelated ends. Consider, for instance, the commercialization of Vichy candles and Vichy cigarette papers.[117] The liqueur illustrated above (figure 24), however, retains, or rather profits from, at least one fundamental link to Vichy: the idea that a Vichy product could by definition protect a French person from the tropics. The producers of "Colonial-Vichy" claimed that its ingredients ("salutary plants") rendered it "the best protection against the sun and anemia in the colonies." But mostly, this distillery located at Vichy was evidently trying to benefit from the popular association Vichy = colonies. Although capitalizing on the Vichy name and the Vichy–colonial connection makes perfect business sense, the idea of selling a curative alcohol for colonials does not pass medical muster. Indeed, colonial doctors frequently railed against the abuse of alcohol in the colonies, insisting that its deleterious effects were amplified by the tropics. Some skeptics had long wondered whether the liver afflictions for which colonials sought treatment at Vichy were caused by the ravages of malaria or those of alcohol. At the zenith of the Vichy regime's moral order in 1942, an air force pilot, a certain Commandant Gaudilière, noted wryly, "I have met so many colonials who blame the climate for their liver disease. They neglect to mention that they drank twenty whiskies a day in the colonies."[118]

Epilogue

Most inhabitants of Vichy deplore that their town's name still evokes Marshal Philippe Pétain's collaborationist, xenophobic, and far right Vichy regime, which suddenly propelled the spa town into the French administrative capital between 1940 and 1944.[119] There, in 1940, French officials transplanted from Paris discovered firsthand Vichy's deep ties to the colonies. The Ministry of the Colonies set up shop in a hotel—the Hôtel britannique—adjacent to the Hôpital militaire, where troops had recovered from tropical afflictions since 1847. The notorious Commissariat général aux questions juives settled into the Algeria Hôtel, directly across from the Villa tunisienne.[120] Pétain's entourage attended lectures dealing with the peoples of Madagascar and Indochina and visited folkloric displays and colonial exhibits at the missionary house and elsewhere. Pressure groups of retired colonials weighed on the government, concerned about overseas issues.[121] Today, long after the seat of government power shifted back to Paris in 1944, the shadow of the Vichy regime still largely obscures the legacy and memory of this far more deeply rooted and longer-standing Vichy function—the town's role as de facto capital of the colonizers.

Between roughly 1830 and 1962, colonials of all walks of life and from all corners of the empire—even from rival empires—thronged to Vichy, seeking to improve their health and to reimmerse themselves ritualistically into the motherland. So too did colonized elites make the voyage to Vichy, where they rubbed shoulders with a variety of colonizers, from plantation magnates to administrators, military personnel, and missionaries. All answered the call of French hydrotherapy. It promised colonials to restore their livers, assuage their recurring malarial symptoms, and lift their spirits. The vaunted, almost alchemical workings of hydrotherapy against tropical disease ultimately succeeded in transforming a metropolitan village into an imperial hub.

Conclusion

FRENCH IMPERIAL HYDROTHERAPY AND CLIMATOL-
ogy cannot be understood independently from the dual
quest for authenticity and *ressourcement* on the one hand
and for overcoming chronic tropical afflictions on the other
hand. More was at work here than simple settler nostalgia
(although that played a considerable role, as at Antsirabe,
which seemed to evoke home for all settlers, regardless
of origin). Colonial spas were, of course, firmly believed
to treat colonial ills—ills whose etiology remained unexplained and whose treatment was otherwise tenuous
well into the twentieth century in many cases. Indeed, the
threat, which we would now designate as disease, was long
defined (even after the Kochian turn) as "the colony itself."
The legendary "colonial liver" constituted one of its supposed symptoms. In short, the colonial body, or the French
organism, as so many of my sources call it, was perceived
to be under constant assault in the colonies.

It should come as no surprise that the nineteenth century marked the golden age of both French spas and French
imperialism. In a nineteenth century obsessed with degeneration, spas seemed to promise a measure of highly ritualized salvation. Spa medicine was transformative in its
logic, predicated on immersion or repeated consumption

of site-specific suspended minerals. As theories of environmental determinism hardened in the nineteenth century—emblematized at their apex by the science of *mésologie*—colonial scientists hoped that spas could help keep colonials not just free of disease, but also French. Those who asserted the simultaneous fixity and precariousness of racial purity sought, through a science at once ancient and thoroughly modern, to manipulate the environment so as to level the uneven climatic playing field. This is precisely where geography, topography, hydrology, hydrotherapy, and *climatisme* could intervene to save the colonial body. Given the powers imputed to hydrotherapy and climatology—their therapeutic range, their transformative virtues, and the principle of immersion or even *mésologie*—it followed that they could be thought to condition identities.

Colonial spas thus proved instrumental in the construction of the "artificial environment" that the imperial hydrotherapist Serge Abbatucci saw as critical for colonial survival. But in order to establish this whitening, Frenchifying function, colonial scientists were forced time and again to distance their practice and knowledge from those of precolonial societies. In Guadeloupe this meant negating and condemning the "Mulatress' treatment" for yellow fever. In Réunion it involved eliding pre-1848 maroon and slave uses of the waters. In Madagascar and in Tunisia, colonial doctors adopted a two-pronged approach, placing spas at the heart of their "civilizing mission" toward natives, while systematically disassociating hydrotherapy from indigenous forms of balneology or spirituality related to springs—*vazimba* meanings and the *hammam* and *medbach*, respectively. In the colonial era, the malleability of imperial spas was put to the test: ancestral sites of worship or pilgrimage were coded as medical, French, and modern. And in a supreme postcolonial irony, after decolonization some scientists in formerly colonized lands subsequently poured scorn on the colonizers for not having followed a sufficiently medical and universal hydrotherapeutic policy. Such was the case at Korbous, most notably.

Colonial spas had once served as oases of Frenchness. These fruits of colonial segregation, however, proved fallible in their social and cultural functions as symbols of power. Colonials were forced to relinquish their goal of making Antsirabe Madagascar's capital. Sites that were intended to project modernity, cleanliness, rationality, and supremacy were often rife with intrigue, discord, and transgressions. Mixity at Antsirabe's brothel challenged the municipal council's apartheid objectives; Cilaos's dirtiness and Spartan amenities undermined its claims to modern hygienic standards; competition between Guadeloupe's spas threatened the sector; Korbous's association with syphilis drove away prospective colonial bathers; and Vichy's cosmopolitanism cast doubts on its ethnically specific restorative powers.

The constant reinvention of the spa—redefined in some cultures today as a salon, in which only the notion of detoxifying has been retained—should not be allowed to erase hydrotherapy's long complicity with French empire: from Fouet's first association of quinine and Vichy waters in 1686, through the zenith of the colonial spa between 1870 and 1940, to the loss of Algeria and the twilight of French imperialism in 1962. Much as ancient Roman, Ottoman, and even Russian conquerors had established spas and baths as staples and symbols of their empire, so did French colonial doctors attempt to make colonial spas a feature of a global Pax Gallica. Like these other imperial baths, French colonial spas served not only as potent reminders of home, as interfaces between metropole and colony, but also as rallying points and sites of networking, as at Vichy. They likewise crystallized power and civilization, modernity and knowledge. And finally, they all featured a very similar combination of ritual, medicine, pilgrimage, and socialization. Where French colonial spas differed from Roman, Ottoman, or Russian ones, of course, was in their raison d'être: derived as they were from profound fears over European fragility in the tropical world, reinforced by the debate over the possibility of empire, they came to be conceived as necessities and even enablers of modern colonial life.

In their postcolonial afterlife, these spas reveal something quite different. The very places once considered replicas of France, sites of ritual at the heart of the colonial catechism, have subsequently been reinvented. In Guadeloupe and Réunion, the highland spas that once dwarfed seaside resorts have lagged behind and now cling to a local clientele. They are simultaneously positing a freshly invented indigenousness, in hopes of attracting metropolitan French curistes. Ellen Furlough has captured the irony of European postwar tourists, avid for "heightened exoticism," luxury, and évasion, embarking in 1948 upon an "adventure" to the Antilles—which had become constitutionally part of France two years earlier.[1] In Korbous, Tunisia, meanwhile, postindependence doctors have rejected colonial attempts to cultivate difference through hydrotherapeutic differentiation and preservationism; they seem to have wholeheart-edly embraced the science of the onetime colonizers. In its own way, this appropriation mirrors the inversions that have taken place in Guadeloupe and Réunion. As colonial tourism entered its twilight, the polarity of authenticity was simply altered.

Archival Abbreviations

ADG   Archives départementales de la Guadeloupe

ADN   Archives diplomatiques de Nantes (Tunisian Protectorate)

ADR   Archives départementales de la Réunion

AIP   Archives de l'Institut Pasteur (Paris, France)

AMM   Archives de la Maison du missionnaire, Vichy

AMV   Archives municipales de Vichy

AN   Archives nationales (Paris, France)

ANM   Archives nationales de Madagascar (Antananarivo)

CAOM   Centre des Archives d'outre-mer (Aix-en-Provence)

NMSI   Norwegian Missionary Society Archive, Isoraka, Antananarivo

NMSS   Norwegian Missionary Society Archive, Stavanger, Norway

Notes

Introduction

1. Abbatucci, *Le parfum de la longue route*, 240.
2. On French colonial fragility and health anxieties, see Michael Vann, "Of le Cafard and Other Tropical Threats," 95–106.
3. "La saison de Vichy, 1937," *Le Nouvelliste de la Guadeloupe*, May 26, 1937, 3 (full quote in chapter 3).
4. Said, *Culture and Imperialism*, 7.
5. A fascinating panel at the 2002 meeting of the Society for French Historical studies was devoted to such imperial networks.
6. Literature on colonial hill stations includes Kennedy, *The Magic Mountains*; Kenny, "Constructing an Imperial Hill Station"; Kenny, "Climate, Race and Imperial Authority"; Kanwar, "The Changing Profile of the Summer Capital of British India"; Aiken, "Early Penang Hill Station"; Aiken, *Imperial Belvederes*; Reed, "The Colonial Genesis of Hill Stations"; Crossette, *The Great Hill Stations of Asia*; Bhasin, *Simla, the Summer Capital of British India*; Mitchell, *The Indian Hill-Station: Kodaikanal*; Goerg, "From Hill Station (Freetown) to Downtown Conakry (First Ward)."
7. On French spas, see Mackaman, *Leisure Settings*; Weisz, "Spas, Mineral Waters and Hydrological Science in Twentieth-Century France"; Weisz, "Water Cures and Science"; Jamot, *Thermalisme et villes thermales en France*; Chambriard, *Aux Sources de Vichy*; and Penez, *Histoire du thermalisme en France*.
8. Except by the novelist Erik Orsenna, who broached the question in 1988, as we will see in chapter 2.
9. See, for example, Vaughan, *Curing Their Ills*; Arnold, *Colonizing the Body*; White, *Speaking with Vampires*.
10. Vaughan, *Curing Their Ills*, 8.
11. Kennedy, *The Magic Mountains*.
12. On the intimate, see Stoler, *Race and the Education of Desire*; and Stoler, *Carnal Knowledge and Imperial Power*. On the sartorial, see Cohn, *Colonialism and Its Forms of Knowledge*, chapter 5, and Edwards, "Restyling Colonial Cambodia." On the experimental, see

Mitchell, *Rule of Experts*; Rabinow, *French Modern*; and Wright, *The Politics of Design in French Colonial Urbanism*.

13. De Certeau, *The Practice of Everyday Life*; Corbin, *The Lure of the Sea*; Vigarello, *Le propre et le sale*.

14. Ross, *Fast Cars, Clean Bodies*, 77.

15. Stoler, "Rethinking Colonial Categories."

16. "Antsirabe, le Vichy malgache," *La quinzaine coloniale*, July 10, 1934 (full quote in chapter 5).

17. Fisher, *The First Indian Author in English*, 321–22.

1. Acclimatization, Climatology, and the Possibility of Empire

1. Much recent work has been devoted to acclimatization, climatology, and fears of hot climes. See Livingstone, "Race, Space and Moral Climatology"; Livingstone, "Tropical Climate and Moral Hygiene"; Livingstone, "Human Acclimatization"; Kupperman, "Fear of Hot Climates in the Anglo-American Colonial Experience"; Kennedy, "The Perils of the Midday Sun"; Arnold, *Warm Climates and Western Medicine*, introduction; Anderson, "Climates of Opinion"; Harrison, "The Tender Frame of Man"; Grosse, "Turning Native?"

2. Porter, "Introduction" to *The Medical History of Waters and Spas*, viii.

3. Ehrard, *L'Idée de nature en France*, 691.

4. Anthony Pagden has underscored how climate, though important for Diderot and Montesquieu, was merely a "limiting condition." For Hume, it barely mattered at all. Pagden, *European Encounters with the New World*, 146. Robert Young argues that Herder combined climatic determinism with an even more ominous doctrine: "Herder claims that individuals, and the character of nations, develop not only in relation to local climate (a common Enlightenment assertion) but also in intimate connection to the land and the specific popular traditions that develop out of it." Young, *Colonial Desire*, 38.

5. Diderot and d'Alembert, *Encyclopédie* definition of "women." Anne McLintock has written, "Within this porno-tropic tradition, women figured as the epitome of sexual aberration and excess. Folklore saw them, even more than the men, as given to a lascivious venery so promiscuous as to border on the bestial." McLintock, *Imperial Leather*, 22.

6. Montesquieu, *De l'Esprit des lois*, 507.

7. Cohen, *The French Encounter with Africans*, 19, 67.

8. Montesquieu, *De l'Esprit des lois*, 449, 764.

9. Ibid., 567.

10. Cheney, "The History and Science of Commerce," 114.

11. Ehrard, *L'Idée de nature en France*, 691, 713, 715–17.

12. Chamley, "The Conflict Between Montesquieu and Hume," 281.

13. See, for example, Dariste, *Conseils aux Européens qui passent dans les pays chauds*, 6–7.

14. Montesquieu, *De l'Esprit des lois*, 693.

15. Pagden, *European Encounters with the New World*, 146.

16. Williams, "The Science of Man," 30.

17. Ibid., 33.

18. Staum, *Labeling People*, 26. Grosse, "Turning Native?" 187. For a deconstruction of "going native," also see White, "The Decivilizing Mission."

19. Cohen, *The French Encounter with Africans*, 98.

20. Dr. Rochard spoke of a "pathology of races." In the 1880s, Alphonse Bertillon remarked upon the pathological variations between "Aryans" and "Semites," noting, "Imagine then what would be revealed if we could compare the pathological variations—so uniformly cited by medical practitioners in the colonies—between Negroes and Europeans." Quoted in Orgeas, *La pathologie des races humaines et le problème de la colonisation*, vi.

21. Orgeas, *La pathologie des races humaines*, 285.

22. Harrison, *Climates and Constitutions*, 3, 11–12.

23. Moulin, "L'Apprentissage pastorien de la mosaïque Tunisie," 377.

24. Daniel Pick has argued much the same point regarding heredity theories, which "hardened into a key term . . . [over] several decades" in the mid-nineteenth century. Pick, *Faces of Degeneration*, 48.

25. See Claude Blanckaert, "Of Monstrous métis? Hybridity, Fear of Miscegenation and Patriotism from Buffon to Paul Broca," in Peabody and Stovall, *The Color of Liberty*, 50–53.

26. *Bulletin de la Société d'Anthropologie de Paris*, séance du 4 juillet 1861, 489–90.

27. The tension between morphological and teleological models extended well beyond the realm of climate and racism. It arguably reached its apex in the field of zoology during the famous Cuvier-Geoffroy debate of 1830. See Appel, *The Cuvier-Geoffroy Debate*.

28. Bewell, *Romanticism and Colonial Disease*, 283.

29. Livingstone, "Tropical Climate and Moral Hygiene," 94.

30. On tropical Edens, see Grove, *Green Imperialism*.

31. Gregory, "(Post)Colonialism and the Production of Nature," 101.

32. Duvivier, *Solution de la question de l'Algérie*, 49.

33. These two examples are drawn from Jean Boudin, "Sur le non-cosmopolitanisme de l'homme," in *Bulletin de la Société d'Anthropologie de Paris*, séance du 16 juillet 1863, 370.

34. Curtin, *Disease and Empire*, 151.

35. Osborne, *Nature, the Exotic and the Science of French Colonialism*, xiv.

36. Bonneuil, *Des savants pour l'empire*, 29.

37. Osborne, "Acclimatizing the World," 135–51.

38. Anderson, "Climates of Opinion," 147.

39. Dariste, *Conseils aux Européens*, 18.

40. Dariste would later be elected deputy of the Gironde in 1830 (*Archives biographiques françaises*).

41. Dariste, *Conseils aux Européens*, 14.

42. Huillet, *Hygiène des Blancs, des Mixtes et des Indiens à Pondichéry*, 6.

43. Nicolas, Santa, et al., *Manuel d'Hygiène coloniale*, 49–50.

44. Treille, *De l'acclimatation des Européens dans les pays chauds*, 3.

45. Ibid., 8.

46. CAOM, Généralités 29 (256), August 10, 1820, debate within the "Commission nommée en 1820 pour l'examen du régime commercial des colonies."

47. CAOM, Série géographique, Guyane 59 (16), Interim Governor Burgues de Missiessy, July 12, 1826.

48. CAOM, Généralités 29 (256), August 10, 1820, debate within the "Commission nommée en 1820 pour l'examen du régime commercial des colonies."

49. Ibid.

50. CAOM, Série géographique Guyane 60 (17), Governor Milius to Minister of the Colonies, January 12, 1825.

51. CAOM, Série géographique, Guyane 60 (18), Minister of the Colonies to the Governor of Guyane, August 30, 1831.

52. Anonymous, *Précis sur la colonisation des bords de la Mana*, 42–43, 70.

53. On the articulation of this doomsday scenario in the French case, see Jennings, *French Anti-Slavery*, 78.

54. Fallope, *Esclaves et citoyens*, 172–73; "Seasoning," in Joseph Miller and Paul Finkelman, eds., *MacMillan Encyclopedia of World Slavery* (London: Simon and Schuster, 1998), 793; Tardo-Dino, *Le collier de servitude*, 106–7.

55. Stewart, "Climate, Race and Cultural Distinctiveness," 248–49.

56. For a kind portrait, see René Bonnet, "Le Docteur Louis-Daniel Beauperthuy, pionnier de la Médecine tropicale, précurseur de Carlos Finlay, de Louis Pasteur et de Robert Koch, 1807–1871," *Bulletin de la société d'histoire de la Guadeloupe* 112–13 (1997): 3–7.

57. Beauperthuy, "De la climatologie," 1837, 5.

58. Ibid., 8.

59. Ibid., 12.

60. Ibid.

61. Ibid., 27.

62. Beauperthuy, *Travaux scientifiques*, 75.

63. Bewell, *Romanticism and Colonial Disease*, 279.

64. Ibid., 280.

65. Osborne, *Nature, the Exotic and the Science of French Colonialism*, 86.

66. Ibid., 91, 198.

67. Cohen, *The French Encounter with Africans*, 260

68. Arnold, *Colonizing the Body*, 35–36. This same point is made by Mark Harrison with regard to the Raj. Harrison, *Climates and Constitutions*, 204.

69. "Moralistic descriptions of climate — enervating, monotonous, lazy, indolent — were still being presented as settled scientific maxims [in 1957]." Livingstone, "Race, Space and Moral Climatology," 173.

70. Ibid., 168.

71. Pick, *Faces of Degeneration*, 50–51.

72. Ibid., 45.

73. *Bulletin de la Société d'Anthropologie de Paris*, séance du 4 juillet 1861, 484–90. French anthropology was then dominated by physical anthropology and its craniometric strand. As Alice Conklin points out, a more philosophical or cultural current was gradually emerging in the late nineteenth century and started overtaking the discredited craniometric branch around 1914. Conklin, "What is Colonial Science?"

74. Thibaut, *Acclimatement et colonisation*, 2.

75. Ibid., 5.

76. Ibid., 9.

77. Ibid., 10.

78. Ibid., 145.

79. Rochoux, *Recherches sur les différentes maladies qu'on appelle fièvre jaune*, 37.

80. Gros, "Modifications physiologiques de l'Européen en pays chaud salubre," *Archives de Médecine navale et coloniale* 57 (1892): 262–73.

81. Anderson, *The Cultivation of Whiteness*, 4.

82. George Treille, "Questions d'hygiène coloniale," *La quinzaine coloniale*, April 25, 1897, 225. Such logic was equally prevalent in Britain in the 1890s. Thus, Sir John Kirk argued as follows before the Sixth International Geographical Congress of 1895: "*Climate* is the most important of all considerations in the choice of a home for Europeans in Central Africa." Livingstone, "Tropical Climate and Moral Hygiene," 99.

83. Livingstone, "Race, Space, and Moral Climatology," 178.

84. Navarre, *Manuel d'hygiène coloniale*, 46.

85. Ibid., 44.

86. Ibid., 63.

87. Young, *Colonial Desire*, 118.

88. See Orgeas, *Guide médical aux stations hivernales*.

89. Orgeas, *La pathologie des races humaines*, 290.

90. Ibid., 291.

91. Ibid., 388.

92. Ibid.

93. Ibid., 410.

94. Osborne, *Nature, the Exotic and the Science of French Colonialism*, 95.

95. Jousset, "De l'acclimatement et de l'acclimatation," 447–48.

96. Richard Fogarty and Michael Osborne, "Constructions and Functions of Race in French Military Medicine, 1830–1920" in Peabody and Stovall, *The Color of Liberty*, 207–9.

97. Paul, *From Knowledge to Power*, 69–70.

98. Jousset, "De l'acclimatement et de l'acclimatation," 448.

99. Harvey, "Races Specified, Evolution Transformed," 131–32.

100. A membrane enveloping the bones.

101. A. Bertillon, "Mésologie," in *Dictionnaire encyclopédique des sciences médicales* (Paris: G. Masson, P. Asselin, 1873), 219–20, 228.

102. Deborah Neill has recently exposed this previously overlooked complicity: Neill, "Transnationalism in the Colonies."

103. Interestingly, Joy Harvey notes that some French contemporaries took Virchow to task for allowing anti-Semitism to infiltrate German anthropology. She writes, "Mortillet . . . accused Virchow of having led this 'anti-liberal, anti-scientific and anti-anthropological' movement in Germany, but published a retraction in the following number of the journal, expressing satisfaction that Virchow had begun objecting to the increasing anti-Semitism in the Universities." Harvey, "Races Specified, Evolution Transformed," 311.

104. Boyd, *Rudolf Virchow*, 204, 244. Boyd even mentions that Virchow would later be condemned by the Nazis (178). Also see Ackerknecht, *Rudolf Virchow*, 209, 215, who argues that "[Virchow] did not feel that there existed any proof for the superiority of any race or nation" (215). Benoist Massin writes that "in Berlin, Virchow was the main political opponent of the notorious anti-Semite Stöcker, twice defeating him for office. Virchow was so opposed to the new political anti-Semitism that a legend spread in anti-Semite

circles that he was himself a Jew." Massin, "From Virchow to Fischer," 89. Recently, Ian McNeely has hailed Virchow as being imbued with classic liberalism. See McNeely, *Medicine on a Grand Scale.*

105. Massin, "From Virchow to Fischer," 86–87.

106. A reappraisal of Virchow already seems under way. George Mosse, Stanley Payne, and Sander Gilman have all pointed to Virchow's use of racial categories as having legitimized racial taxonomies—sometimes, paradoxically, in the name of antiracism. Mosse, *Toward the Final Solution*, 90–91; Payne, *A History of Fascism*, 30; Gilman, *The Jew's Body*, 177.

107. Virchow, "L'acclimatement et les Européens aux colonies," 742.

108. Ibid., 742–46.

109. Ibid., 743.

110. On this topic, see Brechtken, *Madagaskar für die Juden.*

111. Virchow, "L'acclimatement et les Européens aux colonies," 746.

112. Navarre, "Manuel d'hygiène coloniale," 54.

113. Virchow, "L'acclimatement et les Européens aux colonies," 746.

114. Jousset, "De l'acclimatement et de l'acclimatation," 307.

115. Lémure, *Madagascar, l'expédition au point de vue médical et hygiénique*, 82–83.

116. Mac-Auliffe, *Cilaos pittoresque et thermal*, 202, 206, 212.

117. Sambon, "Acclimatization of Europeans in Tropical Lands," 590.

118. Ibid., 594.

119. Dane Kennedy has shown how practices influenced by climatic determinism continued unabated in twentieth-century British India, in spite of the dominance of bacterial medicine. Kennedy, *The Magic Mountains*, 19–38.

120. Similarly, the entire field of (tropical) medical geography, Warwick Anderson has suggested, proved quite resilient around this time, "even if increasingly constructed of straw." Anderson, "Disease, Race, and Empire," 65.

121. Latour, *The Pasteurization of France*, 141.

122. Ibid., 143–44. On the multifront war and the recipes and precautions with which to wage it, see ibid., 20.

123. Moulin, "Expatriés français sous les tropiques," 224. Religious metaphors were legion in the field of tropical medicine and hygiene. The quintessential guide to hydrotherapy for colonials, written by Serge Abbatucci and J. J. Matignon, was, after all, entitled *The Colonial's Hydrotherapeutic Breviary.*

124. Faure and Moll-Weiss, *La vie aux colonies*, 40.

125. Ibid., 168.

126. For a fine overview of this expansion, see Aldrich, *Greater France*, 24–88.

127. Cohen, "Malaria and French Imperialism," 25. On comparative European casualty rates in colonial campaigns, see Curtin, *Disease and Empire.*

128. Ibid., 229.

129. Philip Curtin and William Cohen provide different answers to the chicken or egg question: "Did tropical medicine make empire possible, or did empire make tropical medicine possible?" Curtin suggests that doctors had shifted from "possibility of empire" debates in the 1820s to discussing how best to protect settlers and soldiers by the 1840s. Ibid., 27.

130. Metcalf, *Ideologies of the Raj*, 172.

131. Lémure, *Madagascar, l'expédition au point de vue médical et hygiénique*, 81.

132. Kermorgant, "Sanatoria et camps de dissémination de nos colonies," *Annales d'hygiène et de médecine coloniales* 12:3 (July–September 1899): 345.

133. Curtin, *Death by Migration*, 28.

134. Faure et al., *La vie aux colonies*, 57.

135. Pretceille and Levaré, *Le confort aux colonies*, 64–66, 298.

136. Ingold, *Veillons au salut de l'Empire*, 91–92.

137. Dryepont, *La question des sanatoria dans les colonies*, 18.

138. Marcel Léger, "Le déterminisme de la guérison des paludéens: Relation possible avec le chimisme sanguin, climato et crénothérapie," *Bulletin de la société de pathologie exotique* 23 (1930): 834.

139. Carole Carribon, "Thermalisme et corps médical en France, 1919–1939," in Jacquart, ed., *Villes d'Eaux: histoire du thermalisme*, 138–39.

140. Ibid., 144.

141. Weisz, "Spas, Mineral Waters and Hydrological Science in Twentieth-Century France," 475. Weisz sees the complicity between climatology and hydrotherapy as coming much later, at the beginning of the twentieth century.

142. See Jérôme Penez, *Histoire du thermalisme en France*, 180.

2. Colonial Hydrotherapy

1. Advertisement entitled "Et puisque nous parlons de Vichy," in *L'Afrique du Nord illustrée*, special issue "La France thermale et pittoresque" 159 (May 17, 1924): 13.

2. See, for instance, Rockel, *Taking the Waters: Early Spas in New Zealand*; A. Katsambas and C. Antoniou, "Mineral Waters and Spas in Greece"; and Seung-Kyung Hann, "Mineral Water and Spas in Korea," in *Clinics in Dermatology* (Special issue on hydrotherapy) 14 (November–December 1996): 615–18, 633–36; on hydrotherapy in Britain, see Price, "Hydrotherapy in England," 269–80; N. Coley, "Physicians and the Chemical Analysis of Mineral Waters in Eighteenth-Century England," *Medical History* 26 (1982): 123–44.

3. Mackaman, *Leisure Settings*, 110–17, 143.

4. On the spa as pilgrimage, see Jean-Michel Belorgey, "Au plaisir de l'eau," in Grenier, ed., *Villes d'eaux en France*, 9, and in the same volume, Michel Craplet, "La médecine thermale: du plaisir à la cure," 207. On the spa's cure as "miraculous," see Penez, *Histoire du thermalisme*, 263.

5. Jamot, *Thermalisme et villes thermales en France*, 30.

6. This point has been made eloquently by Tamarozzi in "Retour aux sources," 415, 422.

7. Christian Jamot distinguishes between nineteenth-century terms for spa-practitioners, like "baigneur" and "étranger" and the post-1939 meaning of the word *curiste*, which had come to include a host of practices, including drinking the waters or even merely frequenting spa towns. Jamot, *Thermalisme et villes thermales en France*, 17–18.

8. AN F 12 8800. Conseil National Economique, le tourisme, le thermalisme et le climatisme, "Conclusions adoptées par le Conseil national économique dans sa session du 12 avril 1935."

9. Dominique Jarrassé and Lise Grenier, "Les thermes," in Grenier, ed., *Villes d'eaux en*

France, 53–81. Flaubert's quote, 53 (drawn from Gustave Flaubert, *Voyage aux Pyrénées et en Corse*, 1840).

10. Mackaman, *Leisure Settings*, 101.

11. To quote Mackaman, "To the partly cocky, partly timid, somewhat risen, and somewhat nascent social group that was the French bourgeoisie, spa medicine offered precise prescriptions according to which leisure was to be practiced. Thus medicine let the bourgeoisie have its rest, all the while making that rest impermeable to waste, indecency, excess, sloth, and the other social attributes the still forming bourgeoisie took to be antithetical on the dual guises of productivity and respectability." Mackaman, *Leisure Settings*, 6.

12. L. W. B. Brockliss, "The Spa in Seventeenth-Century France" in Porter, ed., *The Medical History of Water and Spas*, 46–47.

13. Weisz, "Water Cures and Science," 394.

14. Mackaman, *Leisure Settings*, 29–30.

15. On sauntering, mobility, and promenades in French hydrotherapy, see Cécile Morillon, "Lumière et déambulation dans le grand établissement thermal de Vichy," in Jacquart, ed., *Villes d'eaux: histoire du thermalisme*, 458.

16. Mackaman, *Leisure Settings*, 127.

17. Federica Tamarozzi, "Retour aux sources," 423.

18. Mackaman, *Leisure Settings*, 127.

19. Hérault, "Les eaux minérales de Madagascar." *Revue de Madagascar* (October 1899): 245.

20. Weisz, "Spas, Mineral Waters, and Hydrological Science," 457.

21. Glénard, "Hépatisme colonial et crénothérapie," *La presse thermale et climatique* (March 1, 1927): 148.

22. Rakotozafiarison, *Encausse-les-Thermes*, 35.

23. Verdalle, *La Bourboule*, 54.

24. Bestial metaphors play a prominent role in tropical medicine. In relation to malaria, Sir Ronald Ross spoke of discovering "the beast in the mosquito." Bynum and Overy, *The Beast in the Mosquito*.

25. Du Clos, *Observation sur les eaux minérales*, 171–72.

26. Durand de Lunel, *Traité dogmatique et pratique des fièvres intermittentes*, 438.

27. Ibid., 456.

28. Anonymous, *De l'usage des eaux minerale naturelles de Vichy dans l'Algérie. . . .* , 12.

29. Durand-Fardel, *Traité Thérapeutique des Eaux minérales*.

30. Quoted in Tamalet, "Les suites éloignées des affections des pays chauds," 99.

31. Gandelin, *Vichy pour les Coloniaux*, 13.

32. Edmond Vidal, *Le paludisme chronique et son traitement par la cure de Vichy*, 5.

33. Alquier, quoted in *Le Bulletin du Missionnaire (Vichy)* (1923–24): 29.

34. Vigarello, *Le propre et le sale*, 7.

35. Laure Adler, *Marguerite Duras*, 39.

36. AIP. IPO-RAP 28, Madagascar, Report from 1913, 24.

37. Gouzien, "A propos du *bréviaire thermal des coloniaux*," 29–30.

38. On specialization, see Weiss, "Spas, Mineral Waters," 465, and Penez, *Histoire du thermalisme*, 148–49.

39. Pascal Chambriard shows how the state's claim to Vichy waters goes back to 1523, when the region came under the control of King Francis I. Chambriard, *Aux sources de Vichy*, 48.

40. James, *Guide pratique aux eaux minérales*, 461.

41. Both quotations are from Abbatucci and Matignon, *Le bréviaire thermal des coloniaux*, 1.

42. Ibid., 59.

43. Arnold, *Colonizing the Body*, 36.

44. Chesterman, *Manuel du Dispensaire tropical*, 110.

45. Abbatucci and Matignon, *Le bréviaire thermal des coloniaux*, 64.

46. Ibid., 69.

47. Serge Abbatucci, the most prominent French advocate of colonial thermalism, was also a staunch proponent of the colonial helmet, Abbatucci, "L'Habitation coloniale," in Faure, ed., *La Vie aux colonies*, 65–66.

48. Abbatucci and Matignon, *Le bréviaire thermal des coloniaux*, 2.

49. Glénard, "Hépatisme colonial et crénothérapie," 146.

50. Fleury, "Cours clinique d'hydrothérapie donné à l'Hôpital militaire de Bruxelles."

51. Dobieszewski, "Sur le traitement par les eaux de Marienbad de la fièvre paludéenne," 1.

52. Ibid., 2–4.

53. National Archives of Vietnam, Archives number 2, Ho Chi Minh City. Cochinchine, 5589, 1A-8/1813, "Séjour des malades dans les villes d'eau du Japon."

54. Gouzien, "A propos du *bréviaire thermal des coloniaux*," 109.

55. Circular from the minister of the colonies on the Dax spa, Paris, September 21, 1909, *Journal officiel de Saint-Pierre et Miquelon*, 1909, 549.

56. ADR, 5M 20, circular dated February 18, 1929, from the Ministry of the Colonies.

57. Carribon, "Thermalisme et corps médical en France," in Jacquart, ed., *Villes d'eaux: histoire du thermalisme*, 145.

58. Orsenna, *L'Exposition coloniale*, 144–45, 262.

59. See Musée de la Corse, *Corse-colonies*.

60. *Le Topo, Bulletin mensuel de l'association amicale du personnel des travaux publics de l'Indochine*, October 1923, 250, December 1923, 302, and October 1924, 208–9.

61. H. Verdalle, *La Bourboule*, 54.

62. Mangin in "Les relations franco-allemandes et les bains mondains d'outre-Rhin," 649–75, has shown how in the wake of the Franco-Prussian War of 1870, the French government expended considerable effort to encourage the frequentation of French over German spas. Weisz ("Water Cures and Science," 397) and Mackaman (*Leisure Settings*, 65) likewise stress the competition between French and German spas after 1870. In his probing book on Michelin, Stephen Harp has rightly noted in respect to tourism more generally, "Douce France [was presented] as so truly unique that the French would be crazy to ever leave, and it was only natural that foreigners would want to come." Harp extends this concept to the empire as well. Harp, *Marketing Michelin*, 228.

63. CAOM, Fonds ministériels F80, 607. My thanks to Caroline Douki for this information.

64. CAOM, Fonds ministériels F80, 601.

65. "Instruction ministérielle relative à l'admission et au traitement des fonctionnaires coloniaux dans les établissements thermaux du Service de santé," *Journal officiel de l'Indochine française*, February 18, 1931, 626.

66. Ibid., 627–28.

67. *Action* (Guadeloupe), December 25, 1920, 1.

68. "Congés d'agrément," *La quinzaine coloniale*, March 10, 1900, 131.

69. *Bulletin de l'Académie de Médecine* 1 (1836–37): 308–9.

70. CAOM, Série géographique Réunion, carton 553, dossier 6592.

71. This commission was established by decree on June 16, 1932. Cited in *Annuaire du Ministère des Colonies*, 1942, 45.

72. ADR, 5M 17, Cable 251 dated April 17, 1941.

73. Ibid., Governor Aubert's response, April 26, 1941.

74. Much has been written recently on colonial nostalgia, homesickness, or *le cafard* among French colonizers. See, for example, Vann, "White City on the Red River"; Bullard, *Exile to Paradise*; Slavin, *Colonial Cinema and Imperial France*, 169–70.

75. On malaria and degeneration theories, see Arnold, " 'An Ancient Race Outworn,' " 123–43.

76. See Honigsbaum, *The Fever Trail*, 63–64.

77. Cohen, "Malaria and French Imperialism," 26. For the other points above, see the same article, 23, 25–26.

78. Curtin, *Disease and Empire*, 12.

79. On both canned goods and "eating French" in the colonies, see Furlough, "Une leçon des choses," 463; Peters, *Negotiating Power through Everyday Practices*, 140. On representations of colonial food, see Jennings, "L'Affaire Dreyfus et l'univers colonial français," 41–45. On the recognition in the colonial era that greater amounts of vegetables needed to be consumed by the colonizers, see Susanne Freidberg, "French Beans for the Masses," 449.

80. Bonnet, "Les coloniaux à Vichy," 305.

81. Ibid.

82. Cohen, "Malaria and French Imperialism," 26.

83. Ibid., 28.

84. Glénard, "Hépatisme colonial et crénothérapie," 148.

85. Montel, *Memento thérapeutique du praticien colonial*, 70.

86. Among the many "adjuvants" to a water cure, Jérôme Penez cites the electrical therapy practiced at Châtel-Guyon and Bourbonne-les-bains in the nineteenth century. Penez, *Histoire du thermalisme*, 174.

87. Vauthey, "Paludisme et accidents hépatiques de la thérapeutique arsenicale," 3–10.

88. Simon Hay, Jonathan Cox, David Rogers, Sarah Randolph, David Stern, Dennis Shanks, Monica Myers, and Robert Snow, "Climate Change and the Resurgence of Malaria in the East African Highlands," *Nature* 415 (February 2002): 905–9; Léong Pock Tsy et al., "Distribution of the Species of the *Anopheles gambiae* Complex and First Evidence of *Anopheles merus* as a Malaria Vector in Madagascar."

89. Eckstein-Ludwig et al., "Aremisinins Target the SERCA of *Plasmodium falciparum*," 957–61.

90. See above, chapter 1.

3. Highland Hydrotherapy in Guadeloupe

1. Cuzent, *Eau thermo-minérale de la Ravine-Chaude du Lamentin*, 13.

2. De Cassagnou, "Des différentes épidémies de fièvre jaune qui ont régné dans les hauteurs de la Guadeloupe," *Annales d'Hygiène et de Médecine Coloniales* (July–September

1904), 381; Abenon, *Petite histoire de la Guadeloupe*; Dubois, *A Colony of Citizens*; Régent, *Esclavage, Métissage, Liberté*; Adélaïde-Merlande, *Delgrès ou la Guadeloupe en 1802*.

3. Leroux, "Ressources climatiques et thermales d'une colonie française, la Guadeloupe," 2.

4. Labat, *Voyage aux Isles de l'Amérique* 1:270–71. For a comparison with hydrotherapy in Spanish colonies during the seventeenth and eighteenth centuries, see Pastrana, "Tradición y modernidad en la Nueva España: Esdudios sobre aguas minerales," 325–45.

5. Du Tertre, *Histoire générale des Antilles* 2:22.

6. Ibid.

7. Ibid.

8. Ibid.

9. Ibid., 1:81.

10. Philip Curtin makes the same point. Curtin, *Death by Migration*, 50.

11. On the same colonial spa phenomenon in Martinique, see Pope-Hennessy, *The Baths of Absalom*, and Conseil Général de la Martinique, *Le Site thermal d'Absalon*.

12. Londa Schiebinger has shown how Descourtilz advocated the use of local drugs for treating local ailments. His knowledge of these drugs apparently saved him during the Haitian Revolution. Schiebinger, *Plants and Empire*, 74.

13. Descourtilz, *Guide sanitaire des voyageurs aux colonies*, 89, 97, 105.

14. Levacher, *Guide Médical des Antilles et des régions intertropicales*, 93–95.

15. CAOM, DFC Guadeloupe, Mémoires, carton 31 # 663.

16. Ibid., # 664, December 19, 1823.

17. CAOM, DFC Guadeloupe, Mémoires, carton 31, # 718, May 27, 1826.

18. Ibid.

19. CAOM, DFC Guadeloupe, Mémoires, carton 31 # 785, April 29, 1829.

20. Ibid.

21. CAOM, DFC Guadeloupe, Mémoires, carton 32 # 823, "Rapport sur le projet d'établir un cantonnement sanitaire à l'habitation Dolé," March 9, 1832.

22. Ibid.

23. Ibid.

24. CAOM, DFC Guadeloupe, Mémoires, carton 32 # 829, Conseil privé, October 1831.

25. Kermorgant, "Eaux thermales et minérales des colonies françaises," 225.

26. Mackaman, *Leisure Settings*, 64.

27. Kermorgant, "Sanatoria et camps de dissémination de nos colonies," 347. For a recent study of Kermorgant, see Weiner and Flahaut, "Alexandre Kermorgant (1843–1921)," 267–74.

28. Kermorgant, "Sanatoria et camps de dissémination de nos colonies," 347.

29. Canquio, "La station d'altitude de Saint-Claude," 100, 103.

30. A present-day visitor to the French Caribbean will certainly be struck by the opulence of the highland administrative quarter, be it at Didier in Martinique or Saint-Claude in Guadeloupe.

31. Mackaman, *Leisure Settings*, 36–66.

32. Ibid., 68–72.

33. Taffin, "A propos d'une épidémie de choléra," 220. For a comparative perspective, see Kiple, "Cholera and Race in the Caribbean," 157–77.

34. Pichon, "Ressources sanitaires de la Guadeloupe," *La Guadeloupeénne*, January–February 1917, 18. For Pichon, see "Le docteur Pichon, mort," *Le Nouvelliste Quotidien* (Guadeloupe), January 18, 1923.

35. Anne Pérotin-Dumon has shown that the reputations of Grande Terre as noxious and Basse-Terre as healthful goes back at least to the eighteenth century. Pérotin-Dumon, *La ville aux îles*, 318.

36. Wilson, *Memoirs of West Indian Fever*, 134.

37. On St. Claude, see Lafleur, *St. Claude, histoire d'une commune de la Guadeloupe*.

38. Dryepont, *La question des sanatoria dans les colonies*, 84–85.

39. Kennedy, *The Magic Mountains*, 19.

40. Treille, *Principes d'hygiène coloniale*, 251.

41. Dryepont, *La question des sanatoria dans les colonies*, 42. On the French treatment of malaria, see Cohen, "Malaria and French Imperialism," 23–36.

42. Shortt, "The Occurrence of Malaria in a Hill Station," 771.

43. Jousset, *De l'acclimatement et de l'acclimatation*, 61.

44. Kermorgant, "Sanatoria et camps de dissémination . . . ," 346.

45. Drevon, "Morbidité et mortalité du personnel militaire de la Guadeloupe pendant l'année 1897," *Annales d'hygiène et de médecine coloniales* 1 (July 1898): 366.

46. Dryepont, *La question des sanatoria dans les colonies*, 73. On white morbidity in Jamaica, see Burnard, "The Countrie Continues Sicklie," 45–72.

47. Figures are drawn from Dryepont, *La question des sanatoria dans les colonies*, 74.

48. Chauleau, *La vie quotidienne aux Antilles françaises*, 264.

49. Drevon, "Morbidité et mortalité du personnel militaire de la Guadeloupe," 362.

50. R. Pichevin, "L'hygiène aux colonies d'Amérique," *La quinzaine coloniale*, December 25, 1907, 1097–1101.

51. M. Léger, "Quelques documents sur l'indice plasmodial du paludisme à la Guadeloupe," *Bulletin de Pathologie exotique* 3 (March 9, 1932): 214.

52. Cassagnou, "Des différentes épidémies de fièvre jaune qui ont régné dans les hauteurs de la Guadeloupe," *Annales d'hygiène et de médecine coloniales* (July–September 1904), 375–85 (quotation on 379–80).

53. Cazanove, "Histoire étiologique . . . ," 502. On slave use of this therapy, see Tardo-Dino, *Le collier de servitude*, 210.

54. Descourtilz, *Guide sanitaire des voyageurs aux colonies*, 92–93.

55. On this topic in the Americas more generally, see the chapter entitled "Reinventing America/Reinventing Europe: Creole Self-Fashioning," in Pratt, *Imperial Eyes*, 172–97.

56. Lafleur, *Gourbeyre, une commune de Guadeloupe*, 111.

57. C. le Dentu, "Dolé," *Le Nouvelliste de la Guadeloupe*, September 24, 1932, 2.

58. *La Guadeloupéenne*, September–October 1921.

59. On the mechanisms and urban planning involved in French colonial segregation, see Curtin, "Medical Knowledge and Urban Planning in Tropical Africa," 594–613; Wright, *The Politics of Design in French Colonial Urbanism*; Prochaska, *Making Algeria French*; Goerg, "From Hill Station (Freetown) to Downtown Conakry (First Ward)"; Coquery-Vidrovitch and Goerg, eds., *La Ville européenne outre-mers*.

60. Abenon, *Petite histoire de la Guadeloupe*, 109, 155, 173.

61. Animal discoveries of mineral springs constitute a recurring theme. A dog was also reputed to have found Karlsbad, for example. Hammarberg, "Spas *in Spe*."

62. As Jérôme Penez notes, nineteenth-century French hydrotherapeutic discourse is riddled with references to miracles. Penez, *Histoire du thermalisme*, 263.

63. "Les stations thermales des Antilles" *Le Nouvelliste quotidien* (Guadeloupe), February 23, 1924.

64. Thionville, *La Guadeloupe touristique*, 204–13.

65. Kermorgant, "Eaux thermales et minérales des colonies françaises; la Guadeloupe," *La Dépêche coloniale*, February 16, 1901, 2.

66. Banchelin, *Guide du touriste aux Antilles françaises*, 185–288. Cuzent, *Eau thermo-minérale de la Ravine-Chaude du Lamentin*, 3–14.

67. Pichon, "Le tourisme aux Antilles et à la Guyane," *La Guadeloupéenne*, January–February 1921, 7; Abbattucci and Matignon, *Le bréviaire thermal des coloniaux*, 129.

68. Kermorgant, "Eaux thermales et minérales des colonies françaises; la Guadeloupe," *La Dépêche coloniale*, February 16, 1901, 2.

69. Pascaline and Jeremie, *Les ressources hydrominérales et le thermalisme en Guadeloupe*, 35.

70. Cuzent, *Eau thermo-minérale de la Ravine-Chaude du Lamentin*, 35.

71. Leroux, "Ressources climatiques et thermales d'une colonie française, la Guadeloupe," 11.

72. Ibid.

73. "Le Skal-Club de la Guadeloupe: Eaux thermales à la Guadeloupe—extraits du rapport sur le thermalisme par le Dr. Edouard Chartol." Archives départementales de la Guadeloupe, document kindly made available by Ghislaine Bouchet, former director of Guadeloupe's archives.

74. Leroux, "Ressources climatiques et thermales d'une colonie française, la Guadeloupe," 15.

75. Kermorgant, "Eaux thermales et minérales des colonies françaises; la Guadeloupe," *La Dépêche coloniale*, February 16, 1901.

76. Tamby, "A propos des ressources hydro-minérales et du thermalisme en Guadeloupe," 31.

77. Pascaline, "Géochimie des roches et des eaux de sources chaudes du massif de la Soufrière, Guadeloupe," 96.

78. Leroux, "Ressources climatiques et thermales d'une colonie française, la Guadeloupe," 17.

79. Thionville, *La Guadeloupe touristique*, 193.

80. J. C. Pitat, "Dolé-les-Bains: historique et perspectives actuelles," *La Presse thermale et climatique* 129 (1992): 127–31.

81. Pichon, "Ressources sanitaires de la Guadeloupe," *La Guadeloupéenne*, January–February 1917, 16.

82. Pichon, "Le tourisme aux Antilles et à la Guyane," *La Guadeloupéenne*, January–February 1921, 7.

83. Abbatucci and Matignon, *Le bréviaire thermal des coloniaux*, 128.

84. Pichon, "Le tourisme aux Antilles et à la Guyane," *La Guadeloupéenne*, January–February 1921, 12.

85. Regarding the *excursionniste* in Guadeloupe, see Dumont, "*La Guadeloupe pittoresque* de Léon Le Boucher," 9–17.

86. Kermorgant, "Eaux thermales et minérales des colonies françaises," 221.

87. Kermorgant, "Eaux thermales et minérales des colonies françaises; la Guadeloupe," *La Dépêche coloniale*, February 16, 1901, 2.

88. Pascaline and Jeremie, *Les ressources hydrominérales et le thermalisme en Guadeloupe*, 43.

89. *L'Action* (Guadeloupe), December 15, 1920, 1.

90. Naraindas, "Poisons, Putrescence and the Weather," 33.

91. Carnot, preface of Abbatucci and Matignon, *Le bréviaire thermal des coloniaux*, x.

92. Leroux, "Ressources climatiques et thermales d'une colonie française, la Guadeloupe," 15.

93. ADG, 3N 118, Délibérations du Conseil Général, November 22, 1927, 91–99.

94. "Nos eaux thermales," *La Démocratie sociale* (Guadeloupe), January 30, 1944.

95. "La saison de Vichy, 1937" *Le Nouvelliste de la Guadeloupe*, May 26, 1937, 3.

96. On French Guyana's lethal reputation, see Curtin, *Death by Migration*, 25, and Redfield, *Space in the Tropics*.

97. "La Guyane et Dolé-les-Bains," *Le Nouvelliste quotidien* (Guadeloupe), July 28, 1924.

98. ADG, 3N 118, Délibérations du Conseil Général, November 22, 1927, 91–99.

99. C. Thionville, "Un hôtel touristique aux Bains Jaunes," *L'Action* (Guadeloupe), October 26, 1935, 2.

100. M. Laventure, "Dolé-les-Bains, l'offensive de St. Claude," *Le Nouvelliste quotidien*, May 13, 1933.

101. Kennedy, *Islands of White*.

102. Mackaman, *Leisure Settings*, 76–78.

103. "La Guyane et Dolé-les-Bains," *Le Nouvelliste quotidien*, July 28, 1924.

104. As the French government cuts back on thermal cure coverage (most notably for the treatment of rheumatism), it will be interesting to see whether Guadeloupean and metropolitan spas will be able once again to reinvent themselves. On cutbacks for thermal cures, see S. Thépot, "Les stations thermales défendent leurs cures," *Le Monde*, July 14, 1999, 11.

105. M. N. Blanquier, "Approche d'une mise en valeur diversifiée du patrimoine hydrominéral guadeloupéen," *La Presse thermale et climatique* 129 (1992): 132–34.

106. Ibid.

107. *Fodor's Guide to the Caribbean* (1999), 355.

4. The Spas of Réunion Island

1. Raphaël Barquissau, "Cilaos," in Barquissau, de Cordemoy, et al., *L'Ile de la Réunion*, 97.

2. Fuma, *L'esclavagisme à la Réunion*, 21.

3. This remark as well as the bulk of the information on Réunion's general history is derived from Combeau et al., *Histoire de la Réunion*, 14–48. The precise reference to nobility is from page 42.

4. Larson, "La diaspora malgache aux Mascareignes," 143–55.

5. Fuma, *L'esclavagisme à la Réunion*, 72.

6. Many would indeed settle on Bourbon island. Up until 1789, 11 percent of the island's nobles were of Protestant faith. Combeau et al., *Histoire de la Réunion*, 44.

7. Du Quesne, *Un projet de République à l'Ile Eden*, 74, 103.

8. Edwar Alpers, "The Idea of Marronage," in Alpers et al., *Slavery and Resistance in Africa and Asia*, 37.

9. M. Hermann, quoted by Mac-Auliffe, *Cilaos pittoresque et thermal*, 64.

10. As Pier Larson has shown, Malagasy served as the primary language among Réunion's slaves and even as a lingua franca among Réunionais slaves of non-Malagasy origin. Larson, "La diaspora malgache aux Mascareignes," 150, 155.

11. Mac-Auliffe, *Cilaos pittoresque et thermal*, 62–63.

12. Souffrin et al., *Salazie: histoire d'une commune*, 22.

13. M. Maillard, "Topographie de l'île de la Réunion," *Revue maritime et coloniale*, May 1862, 433. Maillard, a retired colonial engineer, states that the spring was discovered in 1831.

14. Souffrin et al., *Salazie: histoire d'une commune*, 43.

15. Lacaussade, *Les Salaziennes*, 55–56.

> Mais quel est ce piton dont le front sourcilleux
> Se dresse, monte et va se perdre dans les cieux ?
> Ce mont pyramidal, c'est le piton d'Anchaine.
> De l'esclave indompté brisant la lourde chaîne,
> C'est à ce mont inculte, inaccessible, affreux,
> Que dans son désespoir un nègre malheureux
> Est venu demander sa liberté ravie.
> Il féconda ces rocs et leur donna la vie ;
> Car, pliant son courage à d'utiles labeurs,
> Il arrosait le sol de ses libres sueurs.
> Il vivait de poissons, de chasse et de racines :
> Parfois, dans la forêt ou le creux des ravines,
> Aux abeilles des bois il ravissait leur miel,
> On prenait dans ses lacs le libre oiseau du ciel.
> Séparé dans ces lieux de toute créature,
> Se nourrissant des dons offerts par la nature,
> Africain exposé sur ces mornes déserts
> Aux mortelles rigueurs des plus rudes hivers,
> Il préférait sa vie incertaine et sauvage
> A des jours plus heureux coulés dans l'esclavage ;
> Et, debout sur ces monts qu'il prenait à témoin,
> Souvent il s'écriait : Je suis libre du moins !
> Cependant, comme l'aigle habitant des montagnes,
> Qui du trône des airs descend vers les campagnes,
> Sur la terre et les champs plane avec majesté,
> Et, s'approchant du sol par sa proie habité,
> La ravissant au ciel dans sa puissante serre,
> Reprend son vol royal et remonte à son aire ;
> Le noble fugitif, abandonnant les bois,
> De son mont escarpé descendait quelquefois ;
> Il parcourait les champs, butinait dans la plaine,
> Et revolant ensuite à son affreux domaine
> Par l'âpre aspérité d'un sentier rude et nu,
> Invisible aux regards et de lui seul connu,
> Il regagnait bientôt sa hutte solitaire.

16. All documents in this paragraph are drawn from ADR, 5 M 20, Salazie.

17. ADR, 20 305.

18. ADR, 5M 18, letter dated July 24, 1852. In French, "Le mal" signifies at once "the disease" and a much more ominous "evil."

19. Grove, *Green Imperialism*, 3.

20. Armand d'Avezac, *Iles de l'Afrique*, Vol. 3, 29.

21. Gaffarel, *Les colonies françaises*, 130–31.

22. Auber, *Bourbon Sanatorium*, 14.

23. Ibid., 38.

24. Ibid., 16, 82–86. Quote is from 82.

25. Mac-Auliffe, *Cilaos pittoresque et thermal*, 80–81.

26. Leal, *Voyage à la Réunion*, 65.

27. Auber, *Bourbon Sanatorium*, 86

28. As Alexandre Bourquin has shown, highland petits-blancs were also depicted as the victims of physical and moral degeneration—a point that harkens back to the Navarre-Virchow discrepancy I analyzed in chapter 1. Bourquin, *Histoire des Petits blancs de la Réunion*, 23.

29. Navarre, *Manuel d'hygiène coloniale*, 54.

30. Souffrin et al., *Salazie: histoire d'une commune*, 76.

31. De Cordemoy, "La vie et l'évolution économiques de l'île de la Réunion," in Barquissau et al., *L'Ile de la Réunion*, 211.

32. Lémure, *Madagascar, l'expédition au point de vue médical et hygiénique*, 56.

33. In November 1942, faced with a Free French attack on his island, the Pétainist governor fled to Hell-Bourg with his closest advisors. Victor de la Rodiére, *Les affaires de Saint-Denis*, 33.

34. De Cordemoy, *La médecine extra-médicale à l'Ile de la Réunion*, 15–16.

35. Mac-Auliffe, *Cilaos pittoresque et thermal*, 198–99.

36. Ibid., 200.

37. Gaudin, "De l'heureuse influence du climat de l'île de la Réunion et des eaux thermales de Salazie," Thèse de médecine, Université de Montpellier, December 17 1861, 9.

38. Merveilleux, "Réunion: Morbidité et mortalité à la Réunion en 1899," *Annales d'hygiène et de médecine coloniales* 3–4 (October–December 1900): 520–37.

39. Mac-Auliffe, *Cilaos pittoresque et thermal*, 212.

40. *Annales d'hygiène et de médecine coloniales*, July–September 1899, 356.

41. De Cordemoy, *Etude de l'Ile de la Réunion*, 39.

42. Gaudin, "De l'heureuse influence du climat de l'île de la Réunion et des eaux thermales de Salazie," 12.

43. Ibid., 41–42.

44. Ibid., 37.

45. Petit and Gaudin, *Guide hygiénique et médical des eaux de Salazie*, 20.

46. Ibid., 64.

47. Ibid., 96, case 16.

48. Ibid.

49. *Le Glaneur* (Réunion), August 25, 1895, 1.

50. ADR, 20 305, printed document, Saint-Denis, May 15, 1839 (produced by M. Azéma, notary in Saint-Denis).

51. ADR, 5M 18, St. Denis, July 24, 1852, handwritten letter to the Directeur de l'Intérieur.

52. *Vichy, Splendid-Guide* (1880), 64, and Mackaman, *Leisure Settings*, 55.

53. De Feuihade de Chauvin, ed., *La Réunion sous le Second Empire*, 30.

54. Ibid., 32, 35.

55. Ibid., 33, 35

56. Gaudin, "De l'heureuse influence du climat de l'île de la Réunion et des eaux thermales de Salazie," 9.

57. In the metropole, most spas (with the exception of the largest) limited their season to May through September. In Réunion and Madagascar — both in the Southern Hemisphere — the season reached its height in December. Penez, *Histoire du thermalisme*, 159.

58. *L'Industriel: Journal d'annonces (Réunion)*, October 3, 1885, 3.

59. ADR, 20 188, St. Louis, May 25, 1851.

60. Ibid.

61. *Vichy Thermal*, July 5, 1895, 2.

62. ADR, 20 305, Salazie, May 15, 1854.

63. Ibid., Governor of Réunion, June 10, 1854.

64. The same phenomenon occurred in metropolitan France, where the itinerant and concentrated nature of spa clienteles sometimes turned spa towns into hotbeds of contagious disease. See Murard and Zylberman, *L'Hygiène dans la république*, 315, 342.

65. Oliver, *Crags and Craters*, 39.

66. ADR, 5M 18, St. Denis, December 21, 1912.

67. *Journal officiel de la Réunion*, 1912, 583.

68. ADR, 20 305, March 19, 1839.

69. ADR, 5M 18, Letter to the Directeur de l'Intérieur, July 24, 1852.

70. ADR, 20 305, St. Denis, May 15, 1839.

71. De Cordemoy, *Etude de l'Ile de la Réunion*, 34.

72. Philippe Nun, doctoral thesis in progress at the University of Réunion.

73. ADR, 5M 18, Letter to the Directeur de l'Intérieur, July 24, 1852.

74. Bénard, *Guide pittoresque et historique de Cilaos*, 57.

75. ADR, 4T 47, "Complaints of Mauritians concerning Cilaos."

76. ADR, 4T 47, February 8, 1917, the president of the Syndicat d'Initiative to the Governor of Réunion.

77. ADR, 4T 48, note to the Governor of Réunion on "stations thermales and the question of tourism."

78. Ibid.

79. Souffrin et al., *Salazie: histoire d'une commune*, 65.

80. ADR, 2P 216, Salazie, November 16, 1864.

81. De Cordemoy, *Etude de l'Ile de la Réunion*, 40.

82. Leal, *Voyage à la Réunion*, 110.

83. Alexandre Bourquin suggests that hydrotherapy rarely enriched the "petits-blancs." Porters, for instance, saw their already meager purchasing power divided by five in the 1870s. Bourquin, *Histoire des Petits-Blancs de la Réunion*, 197.

84. ADR, 5M 18.

85. See Jennings, *French Anti-Slavery*.

86. Petit and Gaudin, *Guide hygiénique et médical des eaux de Salazie*, 11.

87. Mac-Auliffe, *Cilaos pittoresque et thermal*, 45. The first part, in Malagasy, reads, "Ah, Oh,

don't go there buffalo. Cilaos' path will kill us." The second part, in Creole, reads, "The Cilaos path will kill us."

88. Souffrin et al., *Salazie: histoire d'une commune*, 40, 79.

89. Oliver, *Crags and Craters*, 76.

90. Ibid., 80–82.

91. Mackaman, *Leisure Settings*, 87. On the sedan chair, also see 118.

92. For an interesting discussion of this practice and its representation both in Réunion and in metropolitan spas, see Voituret, "Genre, images, et représentations des loisirs de plein air à leur avènement à la Réunion," 105–6.

93. L. Simonin, "Voyage à l'île de la Réunion," *Le Tour du Monde: nouveau journal des voyages* (1862), 167.

94. Ibid., 97–99.

95. De Mahy, *Autour de Bourbon et de Madagascar*, 44.

96. Oliver, *Crags and Craters*, 43.

97. Ibid., 46.

98. Ibid., 35.

99. Ibid., 87–88.

100. Kermorgant, "Eaux thermales et minérales des colonies françaises," 232.

101. Ibid.

102. M. Réland, "Analyse élémentaire de quelques eaux minérales de l'île de la Réunion," *Annales d'hygiène et de médecine coloniales*, January–March 1904, 117.

103. Anonymous, *L'île de la Réunion: Guide illustré*, 20–27.

104. "Rencontre: André Rodier: L'homme qui capta les sources de Cilaos," *Le journal de l'île de la Réunion*, January 23, 2002.

105. Ribert, "A l'île de la Réunion: la station thermale de Cilaos," 84–85.

106. Brochure entitled "Thermes de Cilaos: les eaux de la forme."

107. The precise periodization of this shift is difficult to establish. Denis Voituret cites an article of the *Journal de l'Ile de la Réunion* from 1902, commenting on the virtual desertion of the island's beaches, to the great benefit of its spas. Voituret, "Genre, images, et représentations des loisirs de plein air à leur avènement à la Réunion," 109.

108. Duret and Augustini, "Sans l'imaginaire balnéaire, que reste-t-il de l'exotisme à la Réunion?" 439.

109. "Cilaos, capitale de l'eau," *Journal de l'île de la Réunion*, January 26, 2003.

5. Leisure and Power at the Spa of Antsirabe, Madagascar

1. Recent studies on French colonial tourism include Sherman, "Paradis à vendre"; Murray, "Le tourisme Citroën au Sahara"; Kahn, "Tahiti Intertwined"; Furlough, "Une leçon des choses"; and Jennings, "From *Indochine* to *Indochic*."

2. George Carle, the director of colonization services in colonial Madagascar, admitted in 1915 that "Antsirabe's thermal springs . . . had been known and used for a long time by natives." "Etudes et recherches pour la captation des eaux thermales d'Antsirabe," *Bulletin économique de Madagascar* (1915): 1, 93.

3. Chapus, *Antsirabe, passé, présent, avenir*, 15; "Antsirabe, Station hydro-thermale et climatique," *Madagascar, Bulletin d'Information*, July 15, 1942, 19.

4. J. T. Last, *The Field*, May 26, 1894, reprinted in *The Antananarivo Annual*, 1896, 186.

5. Bloch, *Ritual, History and Power*, 179.

6. Bloch, *From Blessing to Violence*; Bloch, "The Ritual of the Royal Bath in Madagascar," in Cannadine, ed., *Rituals of Royalty*.

7. Bloch, *Ritual, History and Power*, 195–97.

8. Rabenasolo, "La Station thermale d'Antsirabe," 18.

9. Moureu, "Rapport sur les études de quelques sources thermales de Madagascar," 25.

10. Grandidier, *Ethnographie de Madagascar* 3:343, 353–54.

11. James G. Mackay, "Some Notes on Native Medicine and Medical Customs, as Practiced by the Sihanaka," *Antananarivo Annual* 17 (Christmas 1893), 52. Note that Mackay claimed that this same treatment was common among the Merina (45).

12. Nyhagen Predelli, "Sexual Control and the Remaking of Gender," 81, 97.

13. "The Mineral Spring at Antsirabe," *The Antananarivo Annual and Madagascar Magazine*, 1891, 376.

14. Rosaas diary, NMSI. Box 470A, entry for 1879.

15. Rosaas diary, NMSI, Box 470A, entry for 1879. On June 29, 1879, Borchgrevink had written to the Malagasy prime minister that mineral waters could be effective where other medications had failed, adding that he thought it would be "good for [his son] to bathe there." NMSS, Antsirabe Mission (microfilm reel 19), letter 00357.

16. NMSS, Antsirabe Mission, (microfilm reel 19), letters 00972; 00976; 00977; 00985.

17. Rakotoarindrasata, "Rosaas et la ville d'Antsirabe, 1872–1896," 44.

18. Ibid.

19. NMSS, (microfilm reel 19), letter 00978.

20. An article from 1899 suggests that the precolonial Malagasy royal government had ordered the exploitation of Antsirabe's "calcite concretions" to extract lime that would be used for construction projects in Tananarive. Hérault, "Les eaux minérales de Madagascar," 248.

21. NMSS, Antsirabe Mission, (microfilm reel 19), letters 01013; 01074; 01122 (the latter dated 1894).

22. NMSS, Antsirabe Mission, (microfilm reel 19), letter 00359.

23. Rosaas diary, NMSI, Antananarivo, Madagascar, Box 470A, entry for 1880.

24. ANM, H (Santé), 14, 1911.

25. Ellis, *The Rising of the Red Shawls*.

26. "The Siege of Antsirabe: The Story of a Heroic Defense," translated from the French of Rev. Prof. Kruger by Rev. J. Sibree, *Antananarivo Annual* 20 (Christmas 1896): 485–89. Ellis, *The Rising of the Red Shawls*, 90–91, 148–49.

27. Rosaas diary, NMSI, Antananarivo, Madagascar, Box 470A.

28. Société des sciences médicales de Madagascar, séance du 28 mars 1939, in *Ny Bulletin Ny Société mutuelle du corps médical malgache*, January 1940, 57.

29. Kennedy, *The Magic Mountains*, 223.

30. Quoted in d'Escamps, *Histoire et géographie de Madagascar*, 603.

31. *Hova* strictly speaking referred to a class of Merina society. On the shifting meanings of the ethnonyms Merina and Hova, see Larson "Desperately Seeking the Merina," 541–60.

32. ANM, H (Santé) 5, "Rapport sur l'assistance médicale," 1904.

33. Descamps, *Histoire et Géographie de Madagascar*, 239.

34. Treille, "Questions d'hygiène coloniale," 228.

35. Lémure, *Madagascar, l'expédition au point de vue médical et hygiénique*, 89.

36. Treille, "Questions d'hygiène coloniale," 228.

37. Curtin, *Disease and Empire*, 180. This certainty stemmed at least in part from self-referencing. In his 1904 report, in which he puzzled over the rise of malaria in Imerina, Dr. Pin noted that "classic current texts, like Laveran's *Traité du paludisme* speak of the high plateaus as being relatively healthy. . . . Nor have ancient authors writing on Imerina, nor local annals, related murderous epidemics the likes of which we have been seeing in recent years." ANM, H (Santé) 5, "Rapport sur l'assistance médicale," 1904.

38. Paillard, "Les recherches démographiques sur Madagascar au début de l'époque coloniale," 38–39. Campbell "The State and Precolonial Demographic History," 415–45.

39. ANM, H (Santé) 5, "Rapport sur l'assistance médicale," 1904.

40. Paillard analyzes some French fantasies on Madagascar's previous colonization by ancient Greeks in "Visions mythiques d'une Afrique 'colonisable,' " 159–76.

41. Curtin, *Disease and Empire*, 177.

42. Reynaud, *Considérations sanitaires sur l'expédition de Madagascar*, 473.

43. Jacob, "Une expédition coloniale meurtrière: la campagne de Madagascar," 170.

44. Curtin, *Disease and Empire*, 76.

45. Information on Antsirabe's military camp can be found in CAOM, Madagascar 3D 19, dossier 34.

46. Gallieni, *Lettres de Madagacsar, 1895–1905*, 87.

47. *La quinzaine coloniale*, December 25, 1901, 743.

48. "Morbidité et mortalité à Madagascar pendant l'année 1897," *Annales d'Hygiène et de Médecine coloniales*, October–December 1898, 472–73.

49. CAOM, 64 MI 51, (2D 48) Antsirabé, rapport 1902.

50. ANM, H (Santé), 3, "Rapport sur le fonctionnement de l'assistance médicale à Madagascar en 1902," 29.

51. ANM, H (Santé), 8, "Rapport sur l'assistance médicale en 1906."

52. In 1936, the town's municipal council dedicated 300,000 F. to local malaria prevention. ANM, F 17, commission municipale, December 10, 1936.

53. Frenée, *Madagascar*, 171.

54. As Philip Curtin has noted, "The more significant question is not whether tropical medicine caused imperialism, but why European expeditionary armies profited so little from new medical knowledge." Curtin, *Disease and Empire*, 230.

55. "Madagascar," *La libre parole*, September 27, 1895, 3.

56. "Madagascar, l'état sanitaire," *La libre parole*, July 17, 1895, 2.

57. Lémure, *Madagascar, l'expédition au point de vue médical et hygiénique*, 52.

58. Reynaud, *Considérations sanitaires*, 406.

59. Ibid., 189–90.

60. Take, for instance, a report from 1905 on French troops on the island. It acknowledged that malaria was decimating troops that had freshly arrived in the high-altitude cities of Tananarive and Fianarantsoa, sometimes striking them within days of their arrival. But rather than recognizing that these areas were no longer healthy, the anonymous military doctor reached a two-part conclusion. First of all, most men must have contracted the disease in their port of arrival (Tamatave or Mananjary) or in the rain forest along the way (which is certainly possible, but the denial that any, let alone many, of the cases could have been locally contracted is striking). Second, soldiers were insufficiently versed in

colonial hygiene. ANM, H (Santé), 7, "Rapport sur le service médico-chirurgical et sur l'état sanitaire des troupes pendant l'année 1905."

61. Quoted in Hérault, "Les eaux minérales de Madagascar," 250.

62. These data are from 1903. ANM, D 290, meteorological reports from Antsirabe.

63. Léong Pock Tsy et al., "Distribution of the Species of the *Anopheles gambiae* Complex and First Evidence of *Anopheles merus* as a Malaria Vector in Madagascar," abstract.

64. Kennedy, *The Magic Mountains*, 37–38.

65. Hérault, "Les eaux minérales de Madagascar," 245.

66. Kermorgant, "Eaux thermales et minérales des colonies françaises," *La dépêche coloniale*, February 22, 1901, 2.

67. "Colonies françaises, Madagascar," *La dépêche coloniale*, June 23, 1901, 2.

68. Jacques Favreaux, "Le thermalisme à Madagascar," *Bulletin de Madagascar* 103 (1954): 1119.

69. Fressange, "Voyage à Madagascar en 1802–1803," 37.

70. Favreaux, "Le thermalisme à Madagascar," 1117.

71. CAOM, Madagascar 3D5, dossier 19, report from Fillon, July 30, 1918.

72. Pharmacist Réland, "Les eaux thermales et minérales d'Antsirabe," *Bulletin économique de Madagascar* (1905): 38.

73. CAOM, 64 MI 72 (2D 49), report from January 30, 1909.

74. "Etudes et recherches pour la captation des eaux thermales d'Antsirabe," *Bulletin économique de Madagascar* (1915): 1, 93.

75. Ibid., 110.

76. CAOM, Madagascar 3D5, dossier 19, report from Fillon, July 30, 1918.

77. See the *Guide annuaire de Madagascar* (1913): 241–42, and the *Annuaire Général de Madagascar* (1918): 282–83 for the contrast.

78. ANM, D 382, Antsirabe, November 1933 letter to Perrier de la Bathie.

79. Rabenasolo, "La Station thermale d'Antsirabe," 23.

80. Decree 3812 of September 5, 1941, *Journal Officiel de l'Etat Français*, 1941, 3811.

81. Grapin, *Madagascar, 1942*, 30, 100.

82. *Bulletin de l'Académie de Médecine*, February 11, 1902, 92.

83. Moureu, "Rapport sur les études de quelques sources thermales de Madagascar," 31.

84. M. Farinaud, "Indications et contre-indications de la cure thermale d'Antsirabe," *Bulletin de la Société de Pathologie Exotique* 32 (1939): 236–37.

85. M. Farinaud, "Traitement des Maladies du tube digestif et de ses annexes par les eaux d'Antsirabe," *Bulletin de la Société de Pathologie exotique* 30 (1937): 802–3.

86. M. Farinaud, "Indications et contre-indications de la cure thermale d'Antsirabe," *Gazette médicale de Madagascar*, January 1, 1939, 1.

87. Michael Vann has analyzed these everyday colonial health complaints in his dissertation on colonial Hanoi, "White City on the Red River." Vann notes some of the popular colonial terms ascribed to various "ills" in different parts of Indochina. On an empirewide scale, nagging tropical afflictions were sometimes grouped under the rubric *colonialites*.

88. *La femme coloniale* (Tananarive) November 1935, "Premières Chaleurs: Hygiène de Saison."

89. On cancer, see Gouzien, "A propos du *bréviaire thermal des coloniaux*." On the treatment of sterility, see Rajoelison-Ralalahariventiny, "Traitement de la stérilité au centre national de crénothérapie et de thermoclimatisme — Antsirabe."

90. Fontoynont, "Antsirabe, station thermale et climatique," 753.

91. Antelme, *Impressions de Voyage, 1915*, 29.

92. "Consultez le médecin," *Le Journal de Madagascar*, May 24, 1941, 1.

93. One such source explicitly compares "the similarities in the settings of the Massif Central of Madagascar and the Massif Central of France." "Antsirabe, le Vichy malgache," *La quinzaine coloniale*, July 10, 1934.

94. Hérault, "Les eaux minérales de Madagscar," 246.

95. Frenée, *Madagascar*, 170–71.

96. Scratton, *The Great Red Island*, 232–34. A very similar phenomenon can be detected in the hill stations of British India, where colonials wondered at "such beautiful *English* rain, such delicious *English* mud." Metcalf, *Ideologies of the Raj*, 84.

97. Chapus, "Une Ville de France sous les Tropiques, Antsirabe," 8.

98. Coze, "Le Vichy Malgache, Antsirabe," 32.

99. This is relationally reflexive because of the quotation marks around "real vegetables" but also because of the observation on the Parisian quest for exotic fruit. Again, this narrative of an acclimating ascension was in no way limited to Antsirabe. The above quote is worth comparing to George Orwell's account of a Burmese hill station, in, of all places, *Homage to Catalonia* (London: Penguin, 1989), 87:

> From Mandalay, in Upper Burma, you can travel by train to Maymyo, the principal hill-station of the province. . . . It is rather a queer experience. You start off in the typical atmosphere of an eastern city — the scorching sunlight, the dusty palms, the smells of fish and spices and garlic, the squashy tropical fruits, the swarming dark-faced human beings — and because you are so used to it you carry this atmosphere intact, so to speak, in your railway carriage. Mentally you are still in Mandalay when the train stops at Maymyo, four thousand feet above sea-level. But in stepping out of the carriage you step into a different hemisphere. Suddenly you are breathing cool sweet air that might be that of England, and all round you are green grass, bracken, fir-trees, and hill-women with pink cheeks selling baskets of strawberries.

100. Kennedy, *The Magic Mountains*, 16.

101. On the importance of "eating French" to French identity in the colonies, see Peters, "Negotiating Power through Everyday Practices in French Vietnam," 138–206.

102. On colonial nostalgia's treatment as a disease in itself, see Bullard, *Exile to Paradise*, chapter 7.

103. CAOM, 64 MI 72 (2D 49), Province du Vakinankaratra, rapports politiques et administratifs, 1904–26.

104. In 1914, the town counted one Japanese, one Algerian (hence nominally French at the time), one Greek, one British, and three "English subject" merchants. Of its six self-proclaimed entrepreneurs, two were Italian. Its sole hotelier was Greek, as was its one baker, and the sole primary school teacher Norwegian. Of its two silk producers, one was German. By 1918, it counted a Syrian industrialist, three Greek merchants, three British and one Luxembourgeois prospectors, and ten Norwegian missionaries. Save for one Algerian, all of its hoteliers in 1918 were "foreigners": one British and two Greek families operated the town's hotels and cafés. Based on *Guide annuaire de Madagascar* (1913): 241–42, *Annuaire général de Madagascar* (1918): 282–83.

105. Ann Stoler has noted, "Memoirs, contemporary press reports, period novels, and government archives display a discursive disjuncture between an emphasis on unity and a subjacent concern with social and political tensions among the European [settlers] themselves." Stoler, *Carnal Knowledge and Imperial Power*, 27.

106. CAOM, 64 MI 72 (2D 49), Province du Vakinankaratra, rapports politiques et administratifs, 1909 report.

107. The title of this section is from Kennedy, *The Magic Mountains*, 147.

108. FTM photo archives, Antananarivo, book 41, 108–10.

109. In colonial Indochina, conversely, prisons were deliberately "retrograde," eschewing modern methods of control for a "system," if one can speak of one, in which political, common law, and men, women, and children were lumped together. See Zinoman, *The Colonial Bastille*.

110. ANM, Travaux publics, D 2, "Plan de campagne de la province d'Antsirabe, 1903."

111. Chapus, "Une ville de France sous les tropiques," 3–16.

112. CAOM Agence FOM, Carton 788, Dossier 1779.

113. "Echos d'Antsirabe," *La Tribune de Madagascar*, January 22, 1931, 1.

114. "Antsirabe, le Vichy malgache," *La quinzaine coloniale*, July 10, 1934.

115. De Vogüé, "Madagascar," 691.

116. Hence, Madagascar was often described by colonial experimentors as a kind of "Far-West." See Feeley Harnik, *A Green Estate*.

117. "Solidarité intercoloniale: Cilaos et Antsirabe," *La Tribune de Madagascar*, January 31, 1931, 1.

118. Wright, *The Politics of Design in French Colonial Urbanism*, 278.

119. ANM, F 19, arrêté municipal # 15, June 1 1926, Antsirabe.

120. ANM, F 17, "Procès-verbal de la session du Conseil municipal d'Antsirabe, 28 février 1946." André Guillerme has noted how Antsirabe's Malagasy were essentially consigned to the "peripheral" or suburban neighborhoods west of the town. Guillerme, "Madagascar 1895–1960," in Culot and Thiveaud, eds., *Architectures françaises outre-mer*, 287.

121. Fontoynont, "Antsirabe, station thermale et climatique," 754.

122. Antelme, *Impressions de Voyage, 1915*, 28.

123. E. Desmaret, *Impressions de Madagascar*, brochure drawn from *La Presse médicale* 97 (December 4, 1935): 23.

124. Lenoble, "La station thermo-minérale d'Antsirabe," 27.

125. Interview with Jules Coré, Réunion Island, December 2003.

126. Cohen-Bessy, ed., *Le livre de Rakotovao*, 561.

127. *La quinzaine coloniale*, March 25, 1914, 225, refers to the "intensive recruitment of labor . . . for the railroad to Antsirabe." Also see "Chemin de fer de Tananarive à Antsirabe," *La quinzaine coloniale*, May 10, 1912, 341.

128. ANM, Travaux publics, D 2. "Plan de campagne de la province d'Antsirabe."

129. Ibid.

130. Kennedy, *The Magic Mountains*, 117–46.

131. ANM, F 17, "Internat," February 16, 1934.

132. "Le tourisme à Madagascar," *La Tribune de Madagascar*, February 27, 1929, 1.

133. *La quinzaine coloniale*, June 23, 1901, 2.

134. ANM, F 17.

135. Ibid.

136. In a case of history repeating itself, the current Malagasy government is once again trying to reorder Antsirabe's market.

137. Agence Anta, Madagascar, AI, photo 131.

138. ANM, F 17, September 14, 1941.

139. Interview with Jules Coré, Réunion Island, December 2003. On prostitution and French colonialism, see Taraud, *La prostitution coloniale*. On prostitution in another colonial context, see White, *The Comforts of Home*.

140. ANM, D 382, dossier "note sur l'organisation du tourisme à Madagascar," 1934.

141. CAOM, Madagascar 3D5, dossier 19, quoted in Fillon report of July 30, 1918.

142. ANM, D 381, "Organisation du tourisme colonial," February 2, 1924.

143. This and all other information on the Letcher incident and its consequences were found in the ANM, D 382, folder entitled "Tenue et discipline des porteurs dans les gares."

144. ANM, D 41, folder entitled "Déplacement de la capitale administrative à Antsirabe." Letter from Emile Delmotte, January 15, 1945.

145. ANM, D 41, unidentified dossier, Tananarive, October 3, 1944.

146. ANM, D 41, folder entitled "Déplacement de la capitale administrative à Antsirabe." Governor De Saint-Mart, October 3, 1944.

147. On these colonial massacres in 1947, see Tronchon, *L'insurrection malgache de 1947*; Arzalier and Suret-Canale, eds., *Madagascar 1947, la tragédie oubliée*; Raison-Jourde, "Une rébellion en quête de statut: 1947 à Madagascar," 24–32; Cole, *Forget Colonialism?*; and Benot, *Massacres coloniaux*, chapter 5.

148. ANM, D 41, folder entitled "Déplacement de la capitale administrative à Antsirabe."

149. Already in 1896, the French had chimerically presented their conquest as a liberation of coastal minorities from the control of the Merina.

150. ANM, D 41, folder entitled "Déplacement de la capitale administrative à Antsirabe." Tananarive December 31, 1946, from de Coppet to Minister of the Colonies. Emphasis mine.

151. ANM, D 41, folder entitled "Déplacement de la capitale administrative à Antsirabe" telegram 146, February 1, 1947.

152. ANM, D 41, folder entitled "Déplacement de la capitale administrative à Antsirabe."

6. Korbous, Tunisia: Negating the *Hammam*

1. Despois, *La Tunisie*, 24–26.

2. *Congrès international, Thermalisme et Climatisme, 14–16 octobre 1937*, 340–41.

3. Malinas, *Notice sur le groupe hydro-thermal de Korbous*, 10

4. National Archives of Vietnam, Hanoi. Gouvernement général I (52), 5724.

5. Alev Lytle Croutier, *Harem: The World behind the Veil*, 81.

6. Clancy-Smith, *Rebel and Saint*, 258.

7. Alexandropolous in Alexandropoulos and Cabanel, *La Tunisie Mosaïque*, 9.

8. Lorcin, "Rome and France in Algeria," 295–329.

9. In this instance at least, the Carthaginian past is equally elided.

10. ADN, Tunisie 1er versement (1933), 2052, undated: "La Côte du Soleil: Korbous, Tunisie."

11. Pamphlet, "La Côte du Soleil: Korbous, Tunisie. Station thermale et climatique d'hiver," no date.

12. ADN, Tunisie 2ème versement, carton 2460, dossier 346.

13. Carlier, "Les enjeux sociaux du corps: le hammam maghrébin," 1303–33; Saadaoui, "Les bains publics de Tunis à l'époque ottomane," 91–132.

14. Carlier, "Les enjeux sociaux du corps: le hammam maghrébin," 1305.

15. Ramond-Jurney, "Le Hammam dans *L'Enfant du sable* de Tahar Ben Jelloun et *Halfaouine: l'enfant des terrasses* de Ferid Boughedir," 1128–39.

16. Aldrich, *Colonialism and Homosexuality*, 329–30; Boone, "Vacation Cruises; or, The Homoerotics of Orientalism," 92.

17. Taraud, *La prostitution coloniale*, 223–25.

18. Croutier, *Harem*, 83, 89, 91.

19. In her history of medicine in Tunisia (from 1780 to 1900), Nancy Gallagher falls short of conflating mineral springs and hammams but does link them: "The hammams and the hot mineral springs located in various regions of Tunisia were frequently used for the treatment of disease." Gallagher, *Medicine and Power in Tunisia*, 16.

20. "Korbous, Source de Légendes" in *Tunisie, revue illustrée de l'actualité* 5 (December 31, 1932): 17.

21. Rajat, "Korbous, la Côte du Soleil," 8.

22. ADN, Tunisie 1er versement (1933), 2052, undated: "La Côte du Soleil: Korbous, Tunisie."

23. Geslin, "Korbous: histoire d'une station thermale d'Afrique," 58.

24. Weber, *Peasants into Frenchmen*, 27–28.

25. Gallagher, *Medicine and Power in Tunisia*, 9–10.

26. Geslin, "Korbous: histoire d'une station thermale d'Afrique," 54.

27. Arnaud, "Les eaux thermales de Korbous près de Tunis," 4–5.

28. Bastide, "Les eaux thermo-minérales d'Hammam Lif et d'Hammam Kourbès," 69.

29. Gitta Hammarberg has found much the same phenomenon at work in the Caucasus, where, under Peter the Great, folk medicine at once merged and competed with the latest "scientific" balneological cures. Hammarberg, "Spas *in Spe*: Russia Looks West."

30. See Fisher, *The First Indian Author in English*, 269–322.

31. Geslin, "Korbous: histoire d'une station thermale d'Afrique," 55.

32. Penez, *Histoire du thermalisme*, 161.

33. Malinas, *Notice sur le groupe hydrominéral de Korbous*, 9.

34. Geslin, "Korbous: histoire d'une station thermale d'Afrique," 59.

35. Cited ibid.

36. ADN, Tunisie 1er versement (1933), 2052, undated: "La Côte du Soleil: Korbous, Tunisie."

37. Bastide, "Les eaux thermo-minérales d'Hammam Lif et d'Hammam Kourbès," 61, 68. Although Bastide's thesis was published in 1888, his only trip to Korbous at that point had come in 1877.

38. Ibid., 69

39. Julia Clancy-Smith, *Migrations: The Trans-Mediterranean Peopling of Nineteenth-Century North Africa, 1880–1881*, forthcoming book.

40. Pyenson, *Civilizing Mission*, 130.

41. While the Napoleonic Egyptian missions have received ample attention, only recently have scholars turned to French scientific forays into Mexico in the 1860s. See Paul Edison's excellent study "Conquest Unrequited: French Expeditionary Science in Mexico."

42. ADN, Tunisie deuxième versement, carton 2460, dossier 346.

43. Malinas, *Les eaux de Korbous: communication à l'Institut de Carthage*, 3–4.

44. Geslin, "Korbous: histoire d'une station thermale d'Afrique," 61.

45. Bastide, "Les eaux thermo-minérales d'Hammam Lif et d'Hammam Kourbès," 61.

46. ADN, Tunisie 1er versement (1933), 2052, undated: "La Côte du Soleil: Korbous, Tunisie."

47. Geslin, "Korbous: histoire d'une station thermale d'Afrique," 63.

48. "Les eaux minérales de Korbous" in *La quinzaine coloniale*, September 25, 1909, 688.

49. *Annuaire médical des stations hydrominérales, climatiques et balnéaires de France* (1933).

50. Malinas, *Notice sur le groupe hydrominéral de Korbous*, 5, 15.

51. Pamphlet, "La Côte du Soleil: Korbous, Tunisie. Station thermale et climatique d'hiver," no date.

52. Schoull and Remlinger, *Les eaux thermo-minérales de Korbous*.

53. Corbin, "Le péril vénérien au début du siècle," 245–83.

54. Malinas, *Notice sur le groupe hydrominéral de Korbous*, 4.

55. Ibid., 5.

56. Anne-Marie Moulin shows how Institut Pasteur sources grudgingly recognized that cholera largely spared the Muslim, as well as European, middle classes. Moulin, "L'apprentissage pastorien de la mosaïque tunisienne," 380.

57. Malinas, *Notice sur le groupe hydrominéral de Korbous*, 14–15.

58. Pamphlet, "La Côte du Soleil: Korbous, Tunisie. Station thermale et climatique d'hiver," no date.

59. Geslin, "Korbous: histoire d'une station thermale d'Afrique," 55.

60. Pumonti to Benoît, March 29, 1901, ADN Tunisie deuxième versement, carton 2460, dossier 346.

61. Wright, *The Politics of Design in French Colonial Urbanism*; Lebovics, *True France: The Wars over Cultural Identity*; Celik, *Urban Forms and Colonial Confrontations*; Rabinow, *French Modern*.

62. Geslin, "Korbous: histoire d'une station thermale d'Afrique," 61.

63. ADN, Tunisie 1er versement (1933), 2052, undated: "La Côte du Soleil: Korbous, Tunisie."

64. Geslin, "Korbous: histoire d'une station thermale d'Afrique," 62.

65. Ibid.

66. ADN, Tunisie 2ème versement, carton 2460, dossier 346.

67. Ibid.

68. ADN, Tunisie 1er versement (1933), 2052, undated: "La Côte du Soleil: Korbous, Tunisie."

69. Ibid.

70. Ibid.

71. Charles Rearick interprets the growth of casinos at late-nineteenth-century French spas as a sign that leisure was now shared by more than an elite class. Rearick, *Pleasures of the Belle-Époque*, 29.

72. Birla, "Hedging Bets," 170–244.

73. Peters, "Negotiating Power through Everyday Practices in French Vietnam," 207–64.

74. ADN, Tunisie 2ème versement, carton 2460, dossier 346.

75. Ibid.

76. ADN, 2 MI 1791 "Tourisme, Tunisie, Cabinet technique, 1944–1949." Commissaire au Tourisme au Secrétaire général du Gouvernement tunisien, July 29, 1949.

77. Martin, *Histoire de la Tunisie contemporaine*, 161.

78. ADN, Tunisie 2ème versement, carton 2460, dossier 346.

79. Ibid.

80. Kallal and Djellouli, *ABC du thermalisme en Tunisie*, 40.

81. Ibid., 39.

82. Ibid., 38.

7. Vichy: Taking the Waters Back Home

1. "Fièvres quartes et tierces" in the original. The *Larousse* dictionary still today defines "fièvres tierces" and "quartes" as an "intermittent fever, observed especially in malaria, which recurs respectively every third or fourth day." *Petit Larousse illustré*, 2004, 431 (s.v. *fièvres*).

2. Fouet, *Nouveau sistème des bains et eaux minérales de Vichy*, 152.

3. Both the exact nature of the appropriation and its date remain uncertain. See Honigsbaum, *The Fever Trail*, 33.

4. In 1932, Raymond Durand-Fardel wrote, "An ancient tradition established empirically that Vichy exerted a particularly favorable action on malarial patients, whether they come from the colonies, or from metropolitan provinces where swamp fevers still reigned." R. Durand-Fardel, "Les Coloniaux à Vichy," 43.

5. Mackaman, *Leisure Settings*, 16.

6. Ibid., 44.

7. Merriman, *French Cities in the Nineteenth Century*, 24.

8. Chambriard, *Aux Sources de Vichy*, 113, 126.

9. Mackaman, *Leisure Settings*, 55. Chambriard, for his part, argues that the turning point for Vichy's affluence came with the opening of the Saint-Germain-des-Fosses train station in 1854. The statistics he presents (Chambriard, *Aux Sources de Vichy*, 126) seem to confirm this, showing a slight dip in summer visitors in 1848, followed by a sustained increase after 1854.

10. *Les stations françaises* 7 (1934): 8.

11. Anonymous, *Splendid-Guide, Vichy, Clermont, Royat, 1880*, 62.

12. On this duality, see Higgs, *Nobles in Nineteenth-Century France*, 212–13.

13. *L'Auvergne thermale et pittoresque* 2:9 (July 22, 1883): 2.

14. "La Saison de Vichy 1937," *Le Nouvelliste de la Guadeloupe* May 26, 1937, 3.

15. Chambriard, *Aux Sources de Vichy*, 138.

16. Alquier, quoted in *Le Bulletin de la Maison du missionnaire* 1 (1923–24): 29.

17. Raymond Durand-Fardel, "Les coloniaux à Vichy," 44.

18. Durand de Lunel, *Notice sur le mode d'action des eaux de Vichy*, 3,

19. Tamalet, "Les suites éloignées des affections des pays chauds et leur thérapeutique hydrominérale," 101.

20. Abbatucci and Matignon, *Le bréviaire thermal des coloniaux*, 59.

21. Bonnet, "Le traitement des paludéens à Vichy," 106.

22. Vidal, *Le paludisme chronique et son traitement par la cure de Vichy*.

23. Gandelin, *Vichy pour les Coloniaux et habitants des Pays chauds*, 5.

24. Bonnet, "Les Coloniaux à Vichy," 305.

25. *Vichy 1950* (Compagnie Fermiere, 1950), 24.

26. See note 14 of this chapter.

27. Shellshear, *Far from the Tamarind Tree: A Childhood Account of Indochine*, 153.

28. *Le Topo* (May 1934), 130.

29. Hilleret, "Vichy capitale thermale de la France d'outre-mer," 12.

30. Wirth, *Vichy 1860–1914*, 488.

31. J. Hilleret, "Vichy capitale thermale de la France d'outre-mer," 12.

32. Simpson-Fletcher, "Capital of the Colonies: Real and Imagined Boundaries between Metropole and Empire in 1920's Marseilles," 135–54.

33. Jamot, *Thermalisme et villes thermales en France*, 43–44.

34. *Les stations françaises*, special issue "France d'Outre-mer: Afrique du nord, les colonies" 7 (1934): 75.

35. Paul Jardet in *Bulletin de la Maison du missionnaire*, 1923–24, 28.

36. Soulier-Valbert, "Vichy Colonial" in *Bulletin de la Maison du missionnaire*, 1937–38, 98.

37. "Se reblanchir" in the original.

38. Glénard "Les maladies des pays chauds à Vichy," 156.

39. Ibid.

40. Anonymous, *Vichy, guide de l'étranger*, 86.

41. Simenon, *45 degrés à l'ombre*, 162–63.

42. AMV, 12, dossier 550.

43. *Ville de Vichy, liste officielle des étrangers, 1896*, June 17, 1896, 156.

44. Ibid., saison 1865.

45. Pascal Chambriand in his M.A. thesis estimated that 75 percent of the 191 colonials who visited Vichy in 1866 were from Algeria. Cited in Penez, *Histoire du thermalisme*, 73.

46. *Ville de Vichy, liste officielle des étrangers, 1899*, June through September.

47. Postcard, author's collection.

48. Tamalet, "Les suites éloignées des affections des pays chauds et leur thérapeutique hydro-minérale," 97.

49. Velten, "L'Hôpital militaire thermal de Vichy," 573–74. Hyacinthe Audiffred, *Un mois à Vichy: guide pittoresque et médical* (Paris: Davin et Fontaine, 1849), 62.

50. Velten, "L'Hôpital militaire thermal de Vichy," 573–74.

51. Ibid., 756–57.

52. *Vichy thermal*, 1899, quoted in Thierry Wirth, *Vichy, 1860–1914*, 258.

53. "La médaille coloniale," *Vichy Thermal*, June 11, 1895, 2.

54. ADR, 5M 17, "Rapport au sous-secrétaire d'état: création d'un hôpital colonial à Vichy," Paris, November 30, 1893, signed Billecocq.

55. ADR, 5M 17, "Circulaire: Création d'un hôpital colonial à Vichy," Paris, November 30, 1893, signed Delcassé.

56. Ibid.

57. ADR, 5M 17, "Rapport au sous-secrétaire d'état: création d'un hôpital colonial à Vichy," Paris, November 30, 1893, signed Billecocq.

58. Ibid.

59. Ibid.

60. Watthé, *La belle vie du missionnaire en Chine*, 218.

61. Watthé, "La maison du missionnaire à Vichy," cxxxii.

62. Watthé, *La belle vie du missionnaire en Chine*, 169, 212, 213.

63. Ibid., 212, 214.

64. Watthé, "La maison du missionnaire à Vichy," cxxxvi.

65. Bertin, "La maison du missionnaire de Vichy, 1922–1952," 19–25.

66. AMM, Dossier dons, letter from Father Jérôme, Congo, June 19, 1933.

67. Watthé, *La belle vie du missionnaire en Chine*, vi.

68. *Bulletin de la Maison du missionnaire*, 1923–24, 9.

69. Ibid., 6.

70. Watthé, "La maison du missionnaire à Vichy," cxxxix.

71. *Bulletin de la Maison du missionnaire*, 1923–24, 27.

72. On this point, see Eric Bertin, "La maison du missionnaire de Vichy, 1922–1952."

73. AMM Correspondance missionnaire, letter from J. Bousseau, October 23, 1931.

74. Daughton, "The Civilizing Mission: Missionaries, Colonialists and French Identity, 1885–1914," Ph.D. diss., University of California at Berkeley, 2002.

75. Watthé, "La maison du missionnaire à Vichy," cxxxviii.

76. Watthé noted in 1931 that that figure had been reduced to one-third. Ibid.

77. Ibid., cxxxvii.

78. AMM, Correspondance missionnaire, letter from Father Joulord, March 6, 1924.

79. AMM, Dossier dons, Tunisia, 22 February, no year indicated.

80. "Ils viennent maintenant de l'Inde et du Japon / De la Patagonie ainsi que du Gabon / Nos Apôtres de tous les points de l'horizon. / Ils accourent dans la moderne Béthanie / Sous le ciel bienfaisant de la Mère-Patrie / Retrouver à Vichy une nouvelle vie." *Bulletin de la Maison du missionnaire*, 1935–36, 79.

81. On missionary networks (like the Lyon connection) and on missionary sociability (songs, almanacs, etc.), see Daughton, *An Empire Divided*.

82. Bertin, "La maison du missionnaire de Vichy, 1922–1952," 52.

83. AMM, Dossier dons, letter from Father Portier, December 18, 1929.

84. AMM, Dossier dons, letter from Paulissen, Blitterswijck, no date.

85. AMM, Dossier dons, letter from Father Gabriel, London, December 21, 1929.

86. AMM, Correspondance missionnaire, letter from Father Guénolé Le Roux, August 1, 1933.

87. AMM, Dossier dons, letter from Father Le Bail, October 16, 1930.

88. AMM, Correspondance missionnaire, letter from Alfred Jarreau, April 2, 1922.

89. AMM, Correspondance missionnaire, letter from Langonnet, August 6, 1934.

90. *Bulletin de la Maison du missionaire*, 1935–36, 89.

91. AMM, Dossier dons, letter from Father Jérôme, June 19, 1933.

92. AMM, Dossier dons, letter from Hué, Annam, on September 4, 1925.

93. Durand-Fardel, "Les Coloniaux à Vichy," 44.

94. Wirth, *Vichy 1860–1914*, 260.

95. *Ville de Vichy: Liste officielle des étrangers*, 1899, 284–86.

96. The 1880 *Splendid-Guide* commented on the contrast between Vichy in season and out: "What is amazing about Vichy's rising prosperity, is that this tiny town, which takes on the aspect of a capital during one-third of the year, does not even have the attribution of a simple *chef-lieu de canton*." Anonymous, *Splendid-Guide*, 62.

97. Chambriard, *Aux Sources de Vichy*, 126–27.

98. Wirth, *Vichy 1860–1914*, 21; Mackaman, *Leisure Settings*, 55; Anonymous, *Splendid-Guide*, 84.

99. Aldrich, *Vestiges of the Colonial Empire in France*, 104.

100. Weber, *France, fin-de-siècle*, 183.
101. Weber, *Peasants into Frenchmen*. Weber's theory has been challenged, notably by James Lehning in *Peasant and French* and by a series of studies positing the concurrent and even complicit nature of regional and national identities. See, for example, Chanet, ed., *L'école républicaine et les petites patries*, and Anne-Marie Thiesse, "Les deux identités de la France," *Modern and Contemporary France* 9:1 (2001).
102. Boule et al., *Le Puy-de-Dôme et Vichy*, 137.
103. Anonymous, *Vichy, guide de l'étranger 1883*, 84.
104. *Anonymous, Vichy 1950*, 62–63.
105. Anonymous, *Splendid-Guide*, 90.
106. Chambriard, *Aux Sources de Vichy*, 53.
107. See www.toutsurlecaramel.free.fr.
108. Interestingly, these buildings are unproblematically described as colonial in present-day Vichy advertisements. The hydrotherapy website http://balneotherapie-spa.vichy-2 .thalasso-line.com/FR/hotel-balneo-auvergne.html reads, "[At Vichy] eras blend together, architectural styles vary widely. The town boasts an astonishing historical heritage, with buildings of colonial inspiration, of oriental inspiration, and the private dwellings of Napoleon III."
109. See Wright, *The Politics of Design in French Colonial Urbanism*; Rabinow, *French Modern*.
110. Chambriard, *Aux Sources de Vichy*, 83–84, 90.
111. See Dominique Jurrassé and Lise Grenier, "Les thermes," and Pierre Saddy, "Le casino," both in Grenier, ed., *Villes d'eaux en France*, 76, quote on 94.
112. On nineteenth-century advertising more generally, see Loeb, *Consuming Angels*, and Hahn, "Street Picturesque: Advertising in Paris, 1830–1914."
113. Glénard, "Les maladies des pays chauds à Vichy," 154.
114. Anonymous, "De l'usage des eaux minérales naturelles de Vichy dans l'Algérie . . . , 16–17.
115. Bottled mineral water became extremely popular in the late nineteenth century. As Eugen Weber has shown, in the 1890s the small spa of Vals-les-bains exported several million bottles of water a year, while Vichy exported eight to nine million. Weber, *France, fin de siècle*, 183.
116. Jennings, "L'Affaire Dreyfus et l'univers colonial français," 43.
117. Chambriard, *Aux Sources de Vichy*, 185–86.
118. Gaudilière, *Ciels d'Empire*, 111.
119. In fact, they insist that the regime be referred to properly as "régime de l'Etat français."
120. Adam Nossiter, whose book is entitled *The Algeria Hotel*, fails to discuss this glaring colonial connection. Instead, he evokes "a grotesque unconscious symmetry arising from the name of the hotel, its new function, and the regime's designation of the Jew as other, oriental, foreign." Nossiter, *The Algeria Hotel*, 179.
121. See Jennings, *Vichy in the Tropics*, 14; and Cointet, *Vichy capitale*, 146–47.

Conclusion

1. Furlough, "Une leçon des choses," 470.

Bibliography

Newspapers and Periodicals

L'Action (Guadeloupe)
Annales d'hygiène et de médecine coloniales
Annuaire du Ministère des Colonies
The Antananarivo Annual
L'Auvergne thermale et pittoresque
Le Bulletin de l'Académie de Médecine
Le Bulletin de la Société de Pathologie exotique
Le Bulletin de Madagascar
Le Bulletin du Missionnaire (Vichy)
Le Bulletin économique de Madagascar
La Dépêche coloniale
La Femme coloniale (Madagascar)
La Gazette médicale de Madagascar
La Guadeloupéenne
Le Journal de Madagascar
Le Journal officiel de l'Indochine française
La libre parole
Le Nouvelliste de la Guadeloupe
La Presse thermale et climatique
La quinzaine coloniale
La revue de Madagascar
Le Topo, Bulletin mensuel de l'association amicale du personnel des travaux publics de l'Indochine
La Tribune de Madagascar
Tunisie, revue illustrée de l'actualité
Vichy thermal
Ville de Vichy, liste officielle des étrangers

Other Primary Sources

Abbatucci, Serge. *Le parfum de la longue route*. Paris: Librairie L. Fournier, 1927.

Abbatucci, Serge, and J. J. Matignon. *Le bréviaire thermal des coloniaux*. Paris: Maloine, 1923.

L'Afrique du Nord illustrée, special issue "La France thermale et pittoresque" 159 (May 17, 1924).

Anonymous. *Annuaire médical des stations hydrominérales, climatiques et balnéaires de France*. 1933.

Anonymous. *De l'usage des eaux minerale naturelles de Vichy dans l'Algérie, la Grèce, le Levant et les Colonies*. Paris: Renou et Maulde, 1859.

Anonymous. *L'île de la Réunion: Guide illustré édité par le Syndicat d'initiative de la Réunion*. 1933.

Anonymous. *Précis sur la colonisation des bords de la Mana, à la Guyane française*. Paris: Imprimerie Royale, 1835.

Anonymous. *Splendid-Guide, Vichy, Clermont, Royat, 1880*. Paris, 1880.

Anonymous. *Vichy, guide de l'étranger*. Vichy: Wallon Imprimeur, 1883.

Anonymous. *Vichy 1950*. Vichy: Compagnie Fermière, 1950.

Antelme, G. *Impressions de Voyage, 1915*. Port Louis: General Printing and Stationery Co., 1919.

Arnaud, J. "Les eaux thermales de Korbous près de Tunis." *La Presse thermale*. Paris: Imprimerie Levé, 1912.

Auber, J. *Bourbon Sanatorium*. 1907 (ADR, PB 1807).

Barquissau, Raphaël, and Jacob de Cordemoy et al. *L'Ile de la Réunion (Ancienne Ile Bourbon)*. Paris: Librairie Emile Larose, 1925.

Bastide, Michel-Louis. "Les eaux thermo-minérales d'Hammam Lif et d'Hammam Kourbès." Medical doctorate, Université de Bordeaux, 1888–89 (# 82).

Beauperthuy, Louis-Daniel. "De la climatologie." Thesis, Faculté de médecine de Paris, 1837.

―――. *Travaux scientifiques*. Bordeaux: J. Gonzalex Font, 1891.

Bertillon, Alphonse. "Mésologie." *Dictionnaire encyclopédique des sciences médicales*. Paris: G. Masson, P. Asselin, 1873.

Bonnet, G. F. "Les coloniaux à Vichy." *Gazette médicale de France* (August 1945).

―――. "Le traitement des paludéens à Vichy." *Revue du paludisme et de médecine tropicale*, April 15, 1947.

Boule, M., P. G. Langeaud, G. Rouchon, A. Vernière. *Le Puy-de-Dôme et Vichy: Guide du Touriste, du Naturaliste et de l'Archéologue*. Paris: Masson et Cie., 1901.

Cazanove, Dr. "Histoire étiologique, expérimentale et thérapeutique de la fièvre jaune." *Outre-mer, revue générale de colonisation* 1 (December 1929).

Chapus, Georges. *Antsirabe, passé, présent, avenir*. Tananarive: Imprimerie luthérienne, 1951.

Chesterman, C. *Manuel du Dispensaire tropical*. London, 1938.

Cohen-Bessy, Annik, ed. *Le Livre de Rakotovao: 1829–1906*. Paris: L'Harmattan, 1991.

Congrès international, Thermalisme et Climatisme, 14–16 octobre 1937 au Palais du thermalisme et du climatisme à l'exposition. Paris: Fédération thermale et climatique française, 1937.

Coze, M. P. "Le Vichy Malgache, Antsirabe." *Section d'études et d'information des troupes coloniales*. November 1951.

Cuzent, G. *Eau thermo-minérale de la Ravine-Chaude du Lamentin*. Pointe-à-Pitre, 1864.

Dariste, Antoine Joseph. *Conseils aux Européens qui passent dans les pays chauds, et notamment aux Antilles*. Bordeaux: Lewalle Jeune et Neveu Libraires, 1824.

d'Avezac, Armand. *Iles de l'Afrique*. Paris: Firmin Didot Frères, 1848.

de Cordemoy, Jacob. *Etude de l'Ile de la Réunion: géographie physique, richesses naturelles, cultures et industries*. Marseille: Institut colonial, 1904.

————. *La médecine extra-médicale à l'Ile de la Réunion*. Saint Denis: Imprimerie Emile Delval, 1864.

de Feuihade de Chauvin, Tanneguy, ed. *La Réunion sous le Second Empire: Témoignage d'un gouverneur créole* (private correspondence of Henry Hubert de Lisle). Paris: Karthala, 1998.

de Mahy, François. *Autour de Bourbon et de Madagascar*. Paris: Alphonse Lemerre, 1891.

d'Escamps, Henry. *Histoire et géographie de Madagascar*. Paris: Firmin-Didot, 1884.

Descamps, Macé. *Histoire et Géographie de Madagascar*. Paris: P. Bertrand, 1846.

Descourtilz, Michel-Etienne. *Guide sanitaire des voyageurs aux colonies, ou conseils hygiéniques en faveur des Européens destinés à passer aux Îles; suivis d'une liste des médicaments dont on doit munir la pharmacie domestique à établir sur chaque habitation*. Paris, 1816.

Despois, Jean. *La Tunisie*. Paris: Librairie Larousse, 1930.

de Vogüé, Eugène-Melchior. "Madagascar." *La Revue des Deux Mondes*. December 1894.

Dobieszewski, Dr. "Sur le traitement par les eaux de Marienbad de la fièvre paludéenne (malaria)." Lu à la séance de la Société de médecine pratique de Paris, le 28 février 1889.

Drevon, Dr. "Morbidité et mortalité du personnel militaire de la Gaudeloupe pendant l'année 1897." *Annales d'hygiène et de médecine coloniales* 1 (July 1898).

Dryepont, Georges. *La question des sanatoria dans les colonies*. Bruxelles, 1900.

du Clos, Cottereau (Sieur). *Observation sur les eaux minérales de plusieurs provinces de France, faites en l'Académie royale des sciences en l'année 1670 et 1671*. Paris: Imprimerie royale, 1675.

du Quesne, Henri. *Un projet de République à l'Ile Eden (l'île Bourbon): réimpression d'un ouvrage disparu, publié en 1689, intitulé Recueil de quelques mémoirs servans d'instruction pour l'établissement de l'isle d'Eden*. Paris, Librairie ancienne et moderne de E. Dufossé, 1887.

Durand de Lunel, Auguste. *Traité dogmatique et pratique des fièvres intermittentes, suivi d'une notice sur le mode d'action des eaux de Vichy dans le traitement des affections consécutives à ces maladies*. Paris: F. Savy, Editeur, 1862.

Durand-Fardel, Max. *Traité Thérapeutique des Eaux minérales*. Paris, 1857.

Durand-Fardel, Raymond. "Les Coloniaux à Vichy." *Nutrition* 1 (1932).

du Tertre. *Histoire générale des Antilles*. Paris, 1667.

Duvivier, General. *Solution de la question de l'Algérie*. Paris: Librairie Gauthier, 1841.

Faure J. L., and A. Moll-Weiss, eds. *La vie aux colonies: préparation de la femme à la vie coloniale*. Paris: Larose, 1938.

Fleury, Louis. "Cours clinique d'hydrothérapie donné à l'Hôpital militaire de Bruxelles: conférences sur les fièvres intermittentes et leur traitement." *Archives médicales belges*, 1865.

Fontoynont, M. "Antsirabe, station thermale et climatique." *Bulletin de la Société de Pathologie Exotique* 26 (1933): 753.

Fouet, Claude. *Nouveau sistème des bains et eaux minérales de Vichy, fondé sur plusieurs belles experiences, et sur la doctrine de l'acide et de l'alcaly. . . .* Paris: Robert Pepie, 1686.

Frenée, M. *Madagascar*. Paris: Société d'éditions maritimes et coloniales, 1931.

Fressange, F. B. "Voyage à Madagascar en 1802–1803" in M. Malte-Brun, ed. *Annales des voyages, de la géographie, et de l'histoire*, Vol. 2, cahier 4. Paris: F. Busson, 1808.

Gaffarel, Paul. *Les colonies françaises*. Paris: Félix Alcan, 1888.

Gallieni, General. *Lettres de Madagascar, 1895–1905*. Paris: Société d'éditions géographiques, maritimes, et coloniales, 1928.

Gandelin, J. *Vichy pour les Coloniaux et habitants des Pays chauds*. Paris: A. Maloine, 1911.

Gaudilière, Commandant. *Ciels d'Empire*. Paris: Jean-Renard, 1942.

Gaudin, C. "De l'heureuse influence du climat de l'île de la Réunion et des eaux thermales de Salazie sur la guérison de la Cachexie paludéenne." M.D. thesis, Université de Montpellier, December 17, 1861.

Geslin, Louis. "Korbous: histoire d'une station thermale d'Afrique." Thesis, University of Paris, 1913.

Glénard, Roger. "Hépatisme colonial et crénothérapie." *La presse thermale et climatique* (March 1, 1927).

———. "Les maladies des pays chauds à Vichy." *Revue pratique des maladies des pays chauds* (May 1926).

Gouzien, Paul. "A propos du *bréviaire thermal des coloniaux*." *Académie des sciences coloniales, comptes-rendus des séances* 1 (1922–23).

Grapin, Henri J. M. *Madagascar, 1942*. Paris: La Pensée universelle, 1993.

Hérault, Philippe. "Les eaux minérales de Madagascar." *Revue de Madagascar* (October 1899).

Hilleret, J. "Vichy capitale thermale de la France d'outre-mer." *Nouvelle revue française d'outre-mer*, 1952.

Huillet, Dr. *Hygiène des Blancs, des Mixtes et des Indiens à Pondichéry*. Pondichéry: E. V. Géruzet, 1867.

Ingold, Général. *Veillons au salut de l'Empire*. Paris: SPES, 1945.

James, Constantin. *Guide pratique aux eaux minérales*. Paris: Victor Masson, 1851.

Jousset, Alfred. "De l'acclimatement et de l'acclimatation." *Archives de médecine navale* 40 (1883).

Just Navarre, P. *Manuel d'hygiène coloniale: guide de l'Européen dans les pays chauds*. Paris: Octave Doin, 1895.

Kallal and Djellouli, Drs. *ABC du thermalisme en Tunisie*. Tunis: Société d'action d'édition et de presse, 1966.

Kermorgant, Alexandre. "Eaux thermales et minérales des colonies françaises." *Annales d'hygiène et de médecine coloniales* 3–4 (April-June 1901): 210–48.

———. "Sanatoria et camps de dissémination de nos colonies." *Annales d'hygiène et de médecine coloniales* 2 (1899).

Labat, Jean-Baptiste. *Voyage aux Isles de l'Amérique (Antilles), 1693–1705*. Volume 1. Paris, 1931.

Lacaussade, Auguste. *Les Salaziennes*. 1839; reprint, ARS Terres Créoles, 1989.

Leal, Charles. *Voyage à la Réunion*. 1878; reprint, ARS Terres Créoles, 1990.

Leger, Marcel. "Le déterminisme de la guérison des paludéens: Relation possible avec le chimisme sanguin, climato et crénothérapie." *Bulletin de la société de pathologie exotique* 23 (1930).

Lémure, Jean. *Madagascar, l'expédition au point de vue médical et hygiénique: l'acclimatement et la colonisation*. Paris: Baillière et fils, 1896.

Leroux, Edouard. "Ressources climatiques et thermales d'une colonie française, la Guadeloupe." Ph.D. diss., Faculté de Médecine de Paris, 1926.

Levacher, M. G. *Guide Médical des Antilles et des régions intertropicales à l'usage de tous les habitans de ces contrées*. Paris, 1840.

Mac-Auliffe, Jean-Marie. *Cilaos pittoresque et thermal*. 1902; reprint, Grand océan, 1996.

Maillard, M. "Topographie de l'île de la Réunion." *Revue maritime et coloniale* (May 1862).

Malinas, Albert. *Les eaux de Korbous: communication à l'Institut de Carthage*. Tunis: Société anonyme de l'imprimerie rapide, 1910.

————. *Notice sur le groupe hydro-thermal de Korbous*. Tunis: Société anonyme de l'imprimerie rapide, 1909.

Montel, M. L. R. *Memento thérapeutique du praticien colonial*. Paris: Masson, 1945.

Montesquieu, Charles-Louis de Secondat, Baron de. *De l'Esprit des lois*. Paris, 1995.

Moureu, Charles. "Rapport sur les études de quelques sources thermales de Madagascar." *Bulletin économique de Madagascar* (1924).

Nicolas, Ad. Pietra Santa, Meugy, Monin, Moreau de Tours, eds. *Manuel d'Hygiène coloniale*. Paris: Félix Alcan, 1894.

Oliver, William Dudley. *Crags and Craters: Rambles in the Island of Réunion*. London: Longmans, Green, 1896.

Orgeas, Joseph Onésime. *Guide médical aux stations hivernales: climatologie, climatothérapie, hygiène*. Paris: Octave Doin, 1889.

————. *La pathologie des races humaines et le problème de la colonisation*. Paris: Octave Doin, 1886.

Petit, L. A., and C. Gaudin. *Guide hygiénique et médical des eaux de Salazie*. Réunion: Imprimerie de Vital Delval, 1857.

Pope-Hennessy, J. *The Baths of Absalom*. London, 1954.

Pretceille, Madeleine, and A. Levaré. *Le Confort aux colonies*. Paris: Larose, 1947.

Rajat, Henri. "Korbous, la Côte du Soleil." *Revue illustrée des colonies et protectorats* (February 1932).

Rakotozafiarison, Gabriel. *Encausse-les-Thermes, station des paludéens*. Thèse, Faculté de Médecine de Paris, 1967.

Reynaud, G. A. *Considérations sanitaires sur l'expédition de Madagascar*. Paris: L. Henry May, 1898.

Rochoux, J. A. *Recherches sur les différentes maladies qu'on appelle fièvre jaune*. Paris: Bechet Jeune, 1828.

Sainte-Luce Banchelin, Abel. *Guide du touriste aux Antilles françaises*. Paris, 1913.

Sambon, L. Westenra. "Acclimatization of Europeans in Tropical Lands." *Geographical Journal* 12:6 (December 1898).

Schoull and Remlinger, Drs. *Les eaux thermo-minérales de Korbous*. Tunis, 1903.

Scratton, Arthur. *The Great Red Island*. New York: Charles Scribner's Sons, 1964.

Shellshear, Iphigénie-Catherine. *Far from the Tamarind Tree: A Childhood Account of Indochine*. Double Bay, New South Wales: Longueville Books, 2003.

Shortt, Henry Edward. "The Occurrence of Malaria in a Hill Station." *Indian Journal of Medical Research* 11:3 (January 1924).

Les Stations françaises. Special issue "France d'Outre-mer: Afrique du nord, les colonies" 7 (1934).

Tamalet, M. "Les suites éloignées des affections des pays chauds et leur thérapeutique hydro-minérale." *Archives de médecine et de pharmacie militaires* 80 (1924).

Thibaut, Donatien. *Acclimatement et colonisation: Algérie et Colonies*. Paris: Just Rouvier, 1859.

Thionville, Camille. *La Guadeloupe touristique*. Paris, 1931.

Treille, George. *De l'acclimatation des Européens dans les pays chauds*. Paris: Octave Doin, 1888.

———. "Questions d'hygiène coloniale." *La quinzaine coloniale* (April 25, 1897).

Vaulthey, Max. "Paludisme et accidents hépatiques de la thérapeutique arsenicale: action de la cure de Vichy." *Revue générale de médecine et de chirurgie de l'Afrique du Nord et des Colonies françaises* (July 10, 1931): 3–10.

Velten, M. "L'Hôpital militaire thermal de Vichy." *Nutrition*. Special issue on "Séquelles tropicales" 1:5 (1931).

Verdalle, H. *La Bourboule, station thermale, station de climat*. Paris: Geisler, n.d.

Vichy, Guide de l'Etranger. Vichy: Wallon, 1883.

Vidal, Edmond. *Le paludisme chronique et son traitement par la cure de Vichy*. Algiers: Imprimerie Fontana, n.d.

Virchow, Rudolf. "L'acclimatement et les Européens aux colonies." *Revue Scientifique* 36 (December 12, 1885).

Watthé, Henry. "La maison du missionnaire à Vichy." *Nutrition*. Special issue on "séquelles tropicales" 1:5 (1931).

———. *La belle vie du missionnaire en Chine: Récits et croquis*. Vichy: Imprimerie Wallon, 1934.

Wilson, J. *Memoirs of West Indian Fever: Brief Notices Regarding the Treatment, Origin and Nature of the Disease Commonly Called Yellow Fever*. London, 1827.

Secondary Sources

Abenon, Lucien-René. *Petite histoire de la Guadeloupe*. Paris: L'Harmattan, 1992.

Ackerknecht, Erwin. *Rudolf Virchow*. New York, 1981.

Adélaïde-Merlande, Jacques. *Delgrès, ou la Guadeloupe en 1802*. Paris: Karthala, 1986.

Adler, Laure. *Marguerite Duras*. Paris: Gallimard, 1998.

Aiken, Robert. "Early Penang Hill Station." *Geographical Review* 77 (1987): 421–39.

———. *Imperial Belvederes: The Hill Stations of Malaya*. Oxford: Oxford University Press, 1994.

Aldrich, Robert. *Colonialism and Homosexuality*. London: Routledge, 2003.

———. *Greater France: A History of French Overseas Expansion*. New York: St. Martin's Press, 1996.

———. *Vestiges of the Colonial Empire in France: Monuments, Museums and Colonial Memories*. London: Palgrave, 2005.

Alexandropoulos, Jacques, and Patrick Cabanel, eds. *La Tunisie mosaïque*. Toulouse: Presses universitaires du Mirail, 2000.

Alpers, Edward A., Gwyn Campbell, and Michael Salman, eds. *Slavery and Resistance in Africa and Asia*. London and New York: Routledge, 2005.

Anderson, Warwick. "Climates of Opinion: Acclimatization in Nineteenth-Century France and England." *Victorian Studies* 35 (1992): 2–24.

———. *The Cultivation of Whiteness: Science, Health, and Racial Destiny in Australia*. Melbourne: Melbourne University Press, 2002.

———. "Disease, Race, and Empire." *Bulletin of the History of Medicine* 70:1 (1996): 62–67.

Appel, Toby. *The Cuvier-Geoffroy Debate: French Biology in the Decades before Darwin*. Oxford: Oxford University Press, 1987.

Arnold, David. "'An Ancient Race Outworn': Malaria and Race in Colonial India, 1860–1930." In Waltraud Ernst and Bernard Harris, eds., *Race, Science and Medicine, 1700–1960*. London: Routledge, 1999.

———. *Colonizing the Body: State Medicine and Epidemic Disease in Nineteenth-Century India*. Berkeley: University of California Press, 1993.

———. *Warm Climates and Western Medicine*. Amsterdam: Rodopi, 1996.

Arzalier, Francis, and Jean Suret-Canale, eds. *Madagascar 1947, la tragédie oubliée*. Paris: Le temps des cerises, 1999.

Bénard, Jules. *Guide pittoresque et historique de Cilaos*. Saint-Denis: Azalées éditions, 1996.

Benot, Yves. *Massacres coloniaux*. Paris: La Découverte, 1994.

Bertin, Eric. "La maison du missionnaire de Vichy, 1922–1952." Mémoire de maîtrise, under the supervision of Prof. Olivier Faure, 1993–94.

Bewell, Alan. *Romanticism and Colonial Disease*. Baltimore: Johns Hopkins University Press, 1999.

Bhasin, Raja. *Simla, the Summer Capital of British India*. London: Penguin, 1992.

Birla, Ritu. "Hedging Bets: The Politics of Commercial Ethics in Late Colonial India." Ph.D. diss., Columbia University, 1999.

Bloch, Maurice. "The Ritual of the Royal Bath in Madagascar: The Dissolution of Death, Birth and Fertility into Authority." In Philip Cannadine, ed., *Rituals of Royalty: Power and Ceremonial in Traditional Societies*. Cambridge: Cambridge University Press, 1987.

———. *From Blessing to Violence: History and Ideology of the Circumcision Ritual of the Merina of Madagascar*. Cambridge: Cambridge University Press, 1986.

———. *Ritual, History and Power: Selected Papers in Anthropology*. London: Athlone, 1989.

Bonneuil, Christophe. *Des savants pour l'empire: la structuration des recherches coloniales au temps de la 'mise en valeur' des colonies françaises, 1917–1945*. Paris: ORSTOM, 1991.

Boone, Joseph. "Vacation Cruises; or, The Homoerotics of Orientalism." *PMLA*. Special issue on "Colonialism and the Postcolonial Condition" (January 1995): 110:1.

Bourquin, Alexandre. *Histoire des Petits-Blancs de la Réunion, xixème-début xxème siècles*. Paris: Karthala, 2005.

Boyd, B. *Rudolf Virchow: The Scientist as Citizen*. New York, 1991.

Brechtken, Magnus. *Madagaskar für die Juden: Antisemitsche Idee und politische Praxis, 1885–1945*. Munich: R. Oldenbourg Verlag, 1997.

Bullard, Alice. *Exile to Paradise: Savagery and Civilization in Paris and the South Pacific*. Stanford: Stanford University Press, 2000.

Burnard, Trevor. "The Countrie Continues Sicklie: White Mortality in Jamaica, 1655–1780." *Social History of Medicine* 12 (1999): 45–72.

Bynum, W. F., and Caroline Overy. *The Beast in the Mosquito: The Correspondence of Ronald Ross and Patrick Manson*. Amsterdam: Rodopi, 1998.

Campbell, Gwyn. "The State and Precolonial Demographic History: The Case of Nineteenth-Century Madagascar." *Journal of African History* 32:3 (1991): 415–45.

Canquio, Germain. "La station d'altitude de Saint-Claude, Guadeloupe." Research paper, Institut de géographie alpine de Grenoble, 1975.

Carlier, Omar. "Les enjeux sociaux du corps: le hammam maghrébin, lieu pérenne, menacé ou recréé." *Annales, Histoire, Société* 6 (November-December, 2000): 1303–33.

Çelik, Zeynep. *Urban Forms and Colonial Confrontations: Algiers under French Rule*. Berkeley: University of California Press, 1997.

Chambriard, Pascal. *Aux Sources de Vichy: Naissance et développement d'un bassin thermal, XIXe–XXe siècles*. Saint-Pourçain-sur-Sioule: Bleu autour, 1999.

Chamley, Paul. "The Conflict Between Montesquieu and Hume: A Study of the Origins of Adam Smith's Universalism." In Andrew Skinner and Thomas Wilson, eds., *Essays on Adam Smith*. Oxford: Clarendon Press, 1975.

Chanet, Jean-François, ed. *L'école républicaine et les petites patries*. Paris: Aubier, 1996.

Chapus, G. S. "Une Ville de France sous les Tropiques, Antsirabe." *Bulletin de Madagascar* 84 (July 1953): 3–16.

Chauleau, Liliane. *La vie quotidienne aux Antilles françaises au temps de Victor Schoelcher*. Paris: Hachette, 1979.

Cheney, Paul. "The History and Science of Commerce in the Century of Enlightenment: France, 1915–1789." Ph.D. diss., Columbia University, 2002.

Clancy-Smith, Julia. *Rebel and Saint: Muslim Notables, Populist Protest, Colonial Encounters (Algeria and Tunisia, 1800–1904)*. Berkeley: University of California Press, 1994.

Cohen, William B. *The French Encounter with Africans: White Response to Blacks, 1530–1880*. Bloomington: Indiana University Press, 1980.

———. "Malaria and French Imperialism." *Journal of African History* 24:1 (1983).

Cohn, Bernard. *Colonialism and Its Forms of Knowledge: The British in India*. Princeton: Princeton University Press, 1996.

Cointet, Michèle. *Vichy capitale*. Paris: Perrin, 1993.

Cole, Jennifer. *Forget Colonialism? Sacrifice and the Art of Memory in Madagascar*. Berkeley: University of California Press, 2001.

Combeau, Yvan, Prosper Eve, Sudel Fuma, and Edmond Maestri. *Histoire de la Réunion*. Paris: SEDES, 2001.

Conklin, Alice. *A Mission to Civilize: The Republican Idea of Empire in France and West Africa, 1895–1930*. Stanford: Stanford University Press, 1997.

———. "What is Colonial Science? Interwar Ethnologie in France." Paper presented at Oberlin College workshop, December 2005.

Conseil Général de la Martinique. *Le Site thermal d'Absalon*. Fort-de-France, 1989.

Coquery-Vidrovitch, Catherine, and Odile Goerg, eds. *La Ville européenne outre-mers: un modèle conquérant?* Paris: L'Harmattan, 1996.

Corbin, Alain. *L'avènement des loisirs, 1850–1960*. Paris: Aubier, 1995.

———. *The Lure of the Sea: The Discovery of the Seaside in the Western World*. New York: Polity, 1994.

———. "Le péril vénérien au début du siècle: prophylaxie sanitaire et prophylaxie morale." *Recherches* 29 (1977): 245–83.

Crossette, Barbara. *The Great Hill Stations of Asia*. New York: Westview, 1998.

Croutier, Alev Lytle. *Harem: The World behind the Veil*. New York: Abbeville Press, 1989.

Curtin, Philip. "Medical Knowledge and Urban Planning in Tropical Africa." *American Historical Review* 90 (1985): 594–613.

———. *Death by Migration: Europe's Encounter with the Tropical World in the Nineteenth Century*. Cambridge: Cambridge University Press, 1989.

———. *Disease and Empire: The Health of Euorpean Troops in the Conquest of Africa*. Cambridge: Cambridge University Press, 1998.

Daughton, James Patrick. "The Civilizing Mission: Missionaries, Colonialists and French Identity, 1885–1914." Ph.D. diss., University of California at Berkeley, 2002.

———. *An Empire Divided: Religion, Republicanism, and the Making of French Colonialism.* Oxford: Oxford University Press, 2006, forthcoming.

de Certeau, Michel. *The Practice of Everyday Life.* Berkeley: University of California Press, 2002.

de la Rodiére, Victor. *Les affaires de Saint-Denis.* Saint Deis: Librairie Gérard, 1977.

Dubois, Laurent. *A Colony of Citizens: Revolution and Slave Emancipation in the French Caribbean, 1787–1804.* Chapel Hill: University of North Carolina Press, 2004.

Dumont, J. "*La Guadeloupe pittoresque* de Léon Le Boucher: naissance de l'excursion." *Bulletin de la société d'histoire de la Guadeloupe* 112–13 (1997): 9–17.

Duret, Pascal, and Muriel Augustini. "Sans l'imaginaire balnéaire, que reste-t-il de l'exotisme à la Réunion?" *Ethnologie française* 32:3 (2002).

Eckart, Wolfgang. *Medizin und Kolonial imperialismus: Deutschland 1884–1945.* Paderborn: Ferdinand Schöningh, 1997.

Eckstein-Ludwig, U. R. J. Webb, I. D. A. Van Geothem, J. M. East, A. G. Lee, M. Kumira, P. M. O'Neill, P. G. Bray, S. A. Ward, and S. Krishna. "Aremisinins Target the SERCA of *Plasmodium falciparum*." *Nature* 424 (August 2003): 957–61.

Edison, Paul. "Conquest Unrequited: French Expeditionary Science in Mexico, 1864–1867." *French Historical Studies* 26:3 (Summer 2003): 459–96.

Edwards, Penny. "Restyling Colonial Cambodia: French Dressing, Indigenous Custom and National Costume." *Fashion Theory* 5:4 (2001): 389–416.

Ehrard, Jean. *L'Idée de nature en France dans la première moitié du xviième siècle.* Paris: SEVPEN, 1963.

Ellis, Stephen. *The Rising of the Red Shawls: A Revolt in Madagascar, 1895–1899.* Cambridge: Cambridge University Press, 1985.

Fallope, Josette. *Esclaves et citoyens: les Noirs à la Guadeloupe au xixème siècle.* Basse-Terre: Société d'histoire de la Guadeloupe, 1992.

Feeley Harnik, Gilian. *A Green Estate: Restoring Independence in Madagascar.* Washington: Smithsonian Institution Press, 1991.

Fisher, Michael. *The First Indian Author in English: Dean Mahomed (1759–1851) in India, Ireland, and England.* New Delhi: Oxford University press, 1996.

Freidberg, Susanne. "French Beans for the Masses: A Modern Geography of Food in Burkina Faso." *Journal of Historical Geography* 29:3 (2003): 445–63.

Fuma, Sudel. *L'esclavagisme à la Réunion.* Paris: L'Harmattan,1992.

Furlough, Ellen. "Une leçon des choses: Tourism, Empire, and the Nation in Interwar France." *French Historical Studies* 25:3 (2002): 441–74.

Furlough, Ellen, and Shelly Baranowski, eds. *Being Elsewhere: Tourism, Consumer Culture and Identity in Modern Europe and North America.* Ann Arbor: University of Michigan Press, 2001.

Gallagher, Nancy Elizabeth. *Medicine and Power in Tunisia.* Cambridge: Cambridge University Press, 1983.

Gilman, Sander. *The Jew's Body.* New York: Routledge, 1991.

Giraudier, Vincent, ed. *Histoire de Vals-les-bains.* Vals-les-bains: Office de tourisme, 2000.

Goerg, Odile. "From Hill Station (Freetown) to Downtown Conakry (First Ward): Comparing French and British Approaches to Segregation in Colonial Cities at the Beginning of the Twentieth Century." *Canadian Journal of African Studies* 32:1 (1998): 1–31.

Gregory, Derek. "(Post)Colonialism and the Production of Nature." In Noel Castree and Bruce Braun, *Social Nature: Theory, Practice and Politics*. Oxford: Blackwell, 2001.

Grenier, Lise, ed. *Villes d'eaux en France*. Paris: Institut français d'Architecture, 1985.

Grosse, Pascal. "Turning Native? Anthropology, German Colonialism, and the Paradoxes of the Acclimatization Question, 1885–1914." In Glenn Penny and Matti Bunzl, *Worldly Provincialism: German Anthropology in the Age of Empire*. Ann Arbor: University of Michigan Press, 2003.

Grove, Richard. *Green Imperialism: Colonial Expansion, Tropical Island Edens, and the Origins of Environmentalism, 1600–1860*. Cambridge: Cambridge University Press, 1995.

Guillerme, André. "Madagascar 1895–1960." In Maurice Culot and Jean-Marie Thiveaud, eds., *Architectures françaises outre-mer*. Paris: Mardaga, 1992.

Hahn, Hazel. "Street Picturesque: Advertising in Paris, 1830–1914." Ph.D. diss., University of California at Berkeley, 1997.

Hammarberg, Gitta. "Spas *in Spe*: Russia Looks West." Paper delivered at the annual meeting of the Modern Language Association, Philadelphia, December 2004.

Harp, Stephen. *Marketing Michelin: Advertising and Cultural Identity in Twentieth-Century France*. Baltimore: Johns Hopkins University Press, 2001.

Harrison, Mark. " 'The Tender Frame of Man': Disease, Climate and Racial Difference in India and the West Indies, 1760–1860." *Bulletin of the History of Medicine* 70 (1996): 68–93.

―――. *Climates and Constitutions: Health, Race, Environment and British Imperialism in India, 1600–1850*. Oxford: Oxford University Press, 1999.

Harvey, Joy. "Races Specified, Evolution Transformed: The Social Contest of Scientific Debates Originating in the Société d'anthropologie in Paris." Ph.D. diss., Harvard University, 1983.

Higgs, David. *Nobles in Nineteenth-Century France: The Practice of Inegalitarianism*. Baltimore: Johns Hopkins University Press, 1987.

Honigsbaum, Mark. *The Fever Trail: The Hunt for the Cure for Malaria*. London: Macmillan, 2001.

Jacob, Guy. "Une expédition coloniale meurtrière: la campagne de Madagascar." In Marc Michel and Yvan Paillard, eds., *Australes: Etudes historiques aixoises sur l'Afrique australe et l'Océan indien occidental*. Paris: L'Harmattan, 1996.

Jacquart, Jean, ed. *Villes d'eaux: histoire du thermalisme*. Paris: Editions du CTHS, 1994.

Jamot, Christian. *Thermalisme et villes thermales en France*. Clermont-Ferrand: Université de Clermont-Ferrand, 1988.

Jennings, Eric. "L'Affaire Dreyfus et l'univers colonial français." *Les cahiers naturalistes* 49 (numéro hors série: "Zola l'homme-récit"), 2002.

―――. "From *Indochine* to *Indochic*: The Lang Bian/Dalat Palace Hotel and French Colonial Leisure, Power and Culture." *Modern Asian Studies* 37:1 (February 2003): 159–94.

―――. *Vichy in the Tropics: Pétain's National Revolution in Madagascar, Guadeloupe and Indochina*. Stanford: Stanford University Press, 2001.

Jennings, Lawrence. *French Anti-Slavery: The Movement for the Abolition of Slavery in France*. Cambridge: Cambridge University Press, 2000.

Kahn, Miriam. "Tahiti Intertwined: Ancestral Land, Tourist Postcard, and Nuclear Test Site." *American Anthropologist* 102:1 (2000): 7–26.

Kanwar, Pamela. "The Changing Profile of the Summer Capital of British India: Simla, 1864–1947." *Modern Asian Studies* 18 (1984): 215–36.

Kennedy, Dane. *Islands of White: Settler Society and Culture in Southern Rhodesia*. Durham: Duke University Press, 1987.

———. *The Magic Mountains: Hill Stations of the British Raj*. Berkeley: University of California Press, 1996.

———. "The Perils of the Midday Sun: Climatic Anxieties in the Colonial Tropics." In John Mackenzie, ed., *Imperialism and the Natural World*. Manchester: University of Manchester Press, 1990.

Kenny, Judith. "Climate, Race and Imperial Authority: The Symbolic Landscape of the British Hill Station in India." *Annals of the Association of American Geographers* 85 (1995): 694–714.

———. "Constructing an Imperial Hill Station: The Representation of British Authority in Ootacamund." Ph.D. diss., Syracuse University, 1990.

Kiple, Kenneth. "Cholera and Race in the Caribbean." *Journal of Latin American Studies* 17 (1985): 157–77.

Koshar, Rudi, ed. *Histories of Leisure*. Oxford: Berg, 2002.

Kupperman, Karen. "Fear of Hot Climates in the Anglo-American Colonial Experience." *William and Mary Quarterly*, 3rd. ser., 41 (1984): 213–40.

Lafleur, Gérard. *Gourbeyre, une commune de Guadeloupe*. Paris: Karthala, 1997.

———. *St. Claude, histoire d'une commune de la Guadeloupe*. Paris: Karthala, 1993.

Larson, Pier. "Desperately Seeking the Merina: Reading Ethnonyms and Their Semantic Fields in African Identity Histories." *Journal of Southern African Studies* 22:4 (1996): 541–60.

———. "La diaspora malgache aux Mascareignes (xviiième–xixème siècles: notes sur la démographie et la langue." *Revue d'histoire de l'Océan indien* (2005): 143–55.

Latour, Bruno. *The Pasteurization of France*. Cambridge, Mass.: Harvard University Press, 1988.

Lebovics, Herman. *True France: The Wars over Cultural Identity, 1900–1945*. Ithaca: Cornell University Press, 1992.

Lehning, James. *Peasant and French: Cultural Contact in Rural France during the Nineteenth Century*. New York: Cambridge University Press, 1995.

Lenoble, André. "La station thermo-minérale d'Antsirabe." *Revue de Madagascar*, July 1946.

Léong Pock Tsy, Jean-Michel, Jean-Bernard Duchemin, Laurence Marrama, Patrick Rabarison, Gilbert Le Goff, Voahirana Rajaonarivelo, and Vincent Robert. "Distribution of the Species of the *Anopheles gambiae* Complex and First Evidence of *Anopheles merus* as a Malaria Vector in Madagascar." *Malaria Journal* 2:33 (October 2003).

Livingstone, David. "Human Acclimatization: Perspectives on a Contested Field of Enquiry in Science, Medicine and Geography." *History of Science* 15 (1987): 359–94.

———. "Race, Space and Moral Climatology: Notes Toward a Genealogy." *Journal of Historical Geography* 28:2 (2002): 159–80.

———. "'Tropical Climate and Moral Hygiene': The Anatomy of a Victorian Debate." *British Journal for the History of Science* 32 (1999): 93–110.

Loeb, Lori. *Consuming Angels: Advertising and Victorian Women*. Oxford: Oxford University Press, 1994.

Lorcin, Patricia. "Rome and France in Algeria: Recovering Colonial Algeria's Latin Past." *French Historical Studies* 25:2 (Spring 2002): 295–329.

Mackaman, Douglas. *Leisure Settings: Bourgeois Culture, Medicine and the Spa in Modern France*. Chicago: University of Chicago Press, 1998.

Mangin, Nathalie. "Les relations franco-allemandes et les bains mondains d'outre-Rhin." *Histoire, Economie et Société* 13:4 (1994): 649–75.

Martin, Jean-François. *Histoire de la Tunisie contemporaine*. Paris: L'Harmattan, 1993.

Massin, Benoist. "From Virchow to Fischer: Physical Anthropology and 'Modern Race Theories' in Wilhelmine Germany." In George Stocking, Jr., ed., *Volksgeist as Method and Ethic: Essays on Boasian Ethnography and the German Anthropological Tradition*. Madison: University of Wisconsin Press, 1996.

McLintock Anne. *Imperial Leather: Race, Gender and Sexuality in the Colonial Contest*. New York: Routledge, 1995.

McNeely, Ian. *Medicine on a Grand Scale: Rudolf Virchow, Liberalism and Public Health*. London: Wellcome Institute, 2002.

Merriman, John. *French Cities in the Nineteenth Century*. London: Hutchinson, 1982.

Metcalf, Thomas. *Ideologies of the Raj*. Cambridge: Cambridge University Press, 1995.

Mitchell, Nora. *The Indian Hill-Station: Kodaikanal*. Chicago: University of Chicago Geography Department, 1972.

Mitchell, Timothy. *Rule of Experts: Egypt, Techno-politics, Modernity*. Berkeley: University of California Press, 2002.

Mosse, George. *Toward the Final Solution: A History of European Racism*. New York: Howard Fertig, 1978.

Moulin, Anne-Marie. "L'Apprentissage pastorien de la mosaïque Tunisie." In Jacques Alexandropoulos and Patrick Cabanel, eds., *La Tunisie mosaïque*. Toulouse: Presses universitaires du Mirail, 2000.

———. "Expatriés français sous les tropiques: cent ans d'histoire de la santé." *Bulletin de la Société de Pathologie exotique* 90:4 (1997): 221–28.

———. "Tropical without Tropics: The Turning Point of Pastorian Medicine in North Africa." In David Arnold, ed., *Warm Climates and Western Medicine: The Emergence of Tropical Medicine, 1500–1900*. Amsterdam: Rodopi, 1996.

Murard, Lion, and Patrick Zylberman. *L'Hygiène dans la république: santé publique en France ou l'utopie contrariée, 1870–1918*. Paris: Fayard, 1996.

Murray, Alison. "Le tourisme Citroën au Sahara, 1924–1925." *Vingtième Siècle, Revue d'Histoire* 68 (October-December 2000): 95–107.

Musée de la Corse. *Corse-colonies: actes du colloque (Corte), 19–20 septembre 2002*. Ajaccio: A. Piazzola, 2004.

Naraindas, Harish. "Poisons, Putrescence and the Weather: A Genealogy of the Advent of Tropical Medicine." In Anne-Marie Moulin, ed., *Les Sciences hors d'occident au xxème siècle*. Volume 4: "Médecines et Santé," 1995.

Neill, Deborah. "Transnationalism in the Colonies: Rivalry and race in German and French Tropical Medicine, 1880–1930." Ph.D. diss., University of Toronto, 2005.

Nossiter, Adam. *The Algeria Hotel: France, Memory and the Second World War*. Boston: Houghton Mifflin, 2001.

Nyhagen Predelli, Line. "Sexual Control and the Remaking of Gender: The Attempt of Nineteenth-Century Protestant Norwegian Women to Export Western Domesticity to Madagascar." *Journal of Women's History* 12:2 (Summer 2000): 81–103.

Orsenna, Erik. *L'Exposition coloniale*. Paris: Le Seuil, 1988.

Osborne, Michael. "Acclimatizing the World: A History of the Paradigmatic Colonial Science." *Osiris* 15 (2000): 135–51.

———. *Nature, the Exotic and the Science of French Colonialism*. Bloomington: Indiana University Press, 1994.

Pagden, Anthony. *European Encounters with the New World, from the Renaissance to Romanticism*. New Haven: Yale University Press, 1993.

Paillard, Yvan-Georges. "Les recherches démographiques sur Madagascar au début de l'époque coloniale et les documents de l'AMI." *Cahiers d'études africaines* 27 (1987): 17–42.

———. "Visions mythiques d'une Afrique 'colonisable': Madagascar et les fantasmes européens à la fin du 19ème siècle." *Revue française d'histoire d'outre-mer* 77 (1990): 159–76.

Pascaline, Hélène. "Géochimie des roches et des eaux de sources chaudes du massif de la Souffrière, Guadeloupe." Ph.D. diss., Université Paris-Sud, Orsay, 1980.

Pascaline, Hélène, and J. J. Jeremie. *Les ressources hydrominérales et le thermalisme en Guadeloupe et en Martinique*. Pointe-à-Pitre, 1992.

Pastrana, P. A. "Tradición y modernidad en la Nueva España: Estudios sobre aguas minerales (S. XVII–XVIII)." *Llull* 19 (1996): 325–45.

Paul, Harry. *From Knowledge to Power: The Rise of the Science Empire in France, 1860–1939*. Cambridge: Cambridge University Press, 1985.

———. *Bacchic Medicine: Wine and Alcohol Therapies from Napoleon to the French Paradox*. New York: Rodopi, 2001.

Payne, Stanley. *A History of Fascism*. Madison: University of Wisconsin Press, 1995.

Peabody, Sue, and Tyler Stovall. *The Color of Liberty: Histories of Race in France*. Durham: Duke University Press, 2003.

Pellan, Marie-Laure. *Encausse-les-Thermes hier et aujourd'hui*. Aspet: Editions Catherine de Coarraze, 1997.

Penez, Jérôme. *Histoire du thrmalisme en France au XIXème Siècle: Eau, médecine, loisirs*. Paris: Economica, 2005.

Pérotin-Dumon, Anne. *La Ville aux îles, la ville dans l'île: Basse-Terre et Pante-à-Pitre, Guadeloupe, 1650–1820*. Paris: Karthala, 2000.

Peters, Erica. "Negotiating Power through Everyday Practices in French Vietnam, 1880–1924." Ph.D. diss., University of Chicago, 2000.

Pick, Daniel. *Faces of Degeneration: A European Disorder, 1848–1918*. Cambridge: Cambridge University Press, 1989.

Porter, Roy, ed. *The Medical History of Waters and Spas*. London: Wellcome Institute for the History of Medicine, 1990.

Pratt, Mary-Louise. *Imperial Eyes: Travel Writing and Transculturation*. New York: Routledge, 1992.

Price, R. "Hydrotherapy in England, 1840–1870." *Medical History* 25 (1981): 269–80.

Prochaska, David. *Making Algeria French: Colonialism in Bône, 1870–1920*. New York: Oxford University Press, 1990.

Pyenson, Lewis. *Civilizing Mission: Exact Sciences and French Overseas Expansion, 1830–1940*. Baltimore: Johns Hopkins University Press, 1993.

Rabenasolo, K. V. "La Station thermale d'Antsirabe." Medical thesis, University of Antananarivo, 1981.

Rabinow, Paul. *French Modern: Norms and Forms of the Social Environment*. Chicago: University of Chicago Press, 1995.

Raison-Jourde, Françoise. "Une rébellion en quête de statut: 1947 à Madagascar." *Revue de la Bibliothèque nationale* 34 (1989): 24–32.

Rajoelison-Ralalahariventiny, Lila. "Traitement de la stérilité au centre national de crénothérapie et de thermoclimatisme — Antsirabe." Medical thesis, University of Antananarivo, 1981.

Rakotoarindrasata, Richard Claude. Mémoire de Capes, Université d'Antananarivo, Ecole normale, Histoire-Géographie, July 1990. "Rosaas et la ville d'Antsirabe, 1872–1896."

Ramond-Jurney, Florence. "Le Hammam dans *L'Enfant du sable* de Tahar Ben Jelloun et *Halfaouine: l'enfant des terrasses* de Ferid Boughedir." *French Review* 77:6 (May 2004): 1128–39.

Rearick, Charles. *Pleasures of the Belle-Époque*. New Haven: Yale University Press, 1985.

Redfield, Peter. *Space in the Tropics: From Convicts to Rockets in French Guiana*. Berkeley: University of California Press, 2000.

Reed, Robert. "The Colonial Genesis of Hill Stations: The Genting Exception." *Geographical Review* 69 (October 1979): 463–68.

Régent, Frédéric. *Esclavage, Métissage, Liberté: La Révolution française à la Guadeloupe (1789–1802)*. Paris: Grasset, 2004.

Ribert, Hervé-Claude. "A l'île de la Réunion: la station thermale de Cilaos." *Revue d'histoire de la pharmacie* 36 (1989).

Rockel, Ian. *Taking the Waters: Early Spas in New Zealand*. Wellington: Government Printing Office, 1986.

Ross, Kristen. *Fast Cars, Clean Bodies: Decolonization and the Reordering of French Culture*. Cambridge: MIT Press, 1995.

Saadaoui, Ahmed. "Les bains publics de Tunis à l'époque ottomane." *Revue tunisienne de sciences sociales* 124 (2003): 91–132.

Said, Edward. *Culture and Imperialism*. New York: Vintage, 1993.

Schiebinger, Londa. *Plants and Empire: Colonial Bioprospecting in the Atlantic World*. Cambridge, Mass.: Harvard University Press, 2004.

Sherman, Daniel. "Paradis à vendre: Tourisme et imitation en Polynésie française, 1958–1971." *Terrain* 44 (March 2005), 39–56.

Simenon, Georges. *45 degrés à l'ombre*. Paris: Gallimard, 1936.

Simpson-Fletcher, Yael. "Capital of the Colonies: Real and Imagined Boundaries Between Metropole and Empire in 1920's Marseilles." In Felix Driver and David Gilbert, eds., *Imperial Cities: Landscape, Display and Identity*. Manchester: Manchester University Press, 1999.

Slavin, David Henry. *Colonial Cinema and Imperial France: White Blind Spots, Male Fantasies, Settler Myths*. Baltimore: Johns Hopkins University Press, 2001.

Société des Sciences médicales de Vichy. *Index médical de Vichy*. Vichy: Imprimerie Wallon, 1965.

Souffrin, Emmanuel, et al. *Salazie: histoire d'une commune*. Sainte Marie: Editions Azalées, 2000.

Staum, Martin. *Labeling People: French Scholars on Society, Race, and Empire, 1815–1848*. Kingston: McGill-Queen's University Press, 2003.

Stewart, Mary. "Climate, Race, and Cultural Distinctiveness." In Mikulas Teich, Roy Porter, and Bo Gustafsson, eds., *Nature and Society in Historical Context*. Cambridge: Cambridge University Press, 1997.

Stoler, Ann. *Carnal Knowledge and Imperial Power: Race and the Intimate in Colonial Rule*. Berkeley: University of California Press, 2002.

———. *Race and the Education of Desire*. Durham: Duke University Press, 2000.

———. "Rethinking Colonial Categories: European Communities and the Boundaries of Rule." *Comparative Studies in Society and History* 31 (1989).

Taffin, Dominique. "A propos d'une épidémie de choléra: science médicale, société créole et pouvoir colonial à la Guadeloupe, 1865–66." *Asclepio* 44 (1992).

Tamarozzi, Federica. "Retour aux sources: Flux et reflux du tourisme thermal à Salsomaggiore." *Ethnologie française* 32:2 (2002).

Tamby, P. "A propos des ressources hydro-minérales et du thermalisme en Guadeloupe." Ph.D. diss., Université de Bordeaux II, 1986.

Taraud, Christelle. *La prostitution coloniale: Algérie, Tunisie, Maroc*. Paris: Payot, 2003.

Tardo-Dino, Frantz. *Le collier de servitude: la condition sanitaire des esclaves aux Antilles françaises du xviième au xixème siècle*. Paris: Editions caribéennes, 1985.

Tronchon, Jacques. *L'insurrection malgache de 1947*. Paris: Karthala, 1986.

Vann, Michael. "Of le Cafard and Other Tropical Threats: Disease and White Colonial Culture in Indochina." In Kathryn Robson and Jennifer Yee, eds. *France and Indochina, Cultural Representations*. Lanham, Va.: Lexington Books, 2005.

———. "White City on the Red River: Race, Power and Culture in French Colonial Hanoi, 1872–1954." Ph.D. diss., University of California, Santa Cruz, 1999.

Vaughan, Megan. *Curing Their Ills: Colonial Power and African Illness*. Stanford: Stanford University Press, 1991.

Vigarello, Georges. *Le propre et le sale: L'hygiène du corps depuis le Moyen Age*. Paris: Le Seuil, 1985.

Voituret, Denis. "Genre, images, et représentations des loisirs de plein air à leur avènement à la Réunion, 1870–1930." In Evelyne Combeau-Mari, ed., *Spors et loisirs dans les colonies*. Paris: Sedes, 2004.

Weber, Eugen. *France fin-de-siècle*. Cambridge, Mass.: Harvard University Press, 1986.

———. *Peasants into Frenchmen: The Modernization of Rural France, 1870–1914*. Stanford: Stanford University Press, 1976.

Weiner, B., and J. Flahaut. "Alexandre Kermorgant (1843–1921), témoin de l'état sanitaire des anciennes colonies françaises." *Histoire des Sciences médicales* 33 (1999): 267–74.

Weisz, George. "Spas, Mineral Waters and Hydrological Science in Twentieth-Century France." *Isis* 92:3 (September 2001): 451–83.

———. "Water Cures and Science: The French Academy of Medicine and Mineral Waters in the Nineteenth Century." *Bulletin of the History of Medicine* 64:3 (1990): 393–416.

White, Luise. *The Comforts of Home: Prostitution in Colonial Nairobi*. Chicago: University of Chicago Press, 1990.

———. *Speaking with Vampires: Rumor and History in Colonial Africa*. Berkeley: University of California Press, 2000.

White, Owen. "The Decivilizing Mission: Auguste Dupuis-Yakouba and French Timbuktu." *French Historical Studies* 27:3 (Summer 2004): 541–68.

Williams, Elizabeth. "The Science of Man: Anthropological Thought and Institutions in Nineteenth-Century France." Ph.D. diss., Indiana University, 1983.

Wirth, Thierry. *Vichy 1860–1914, ou la jeunesse de la reine des villes d'eaux*. Vichy: Thierry Wirth, 2000.

Wright, Gwendolyn. *The Politics of Design in French Colonial Urbanism*. Chicago: University of Chicago Press, 1991.

Young, Robert. *Colonial Desire: Hybridity in Theory, Race and Culture*. London: Routledge, 1995.

Zinoman, Peter. *The Colonial Bastille: A History of Imprisonment in Vietnam, 1862–1940*. Berkeley: University of California Press, 2000.

Index

Pichon, A., 73, 82. *See also* Dolé-les-Bains; Guadeloupe

Pilgrimage. *See* Religion

Plombières, 2, 48, 51, 55, 57

Pointe-à-Pitre (Guadeloupe), 73–74. *See also* Guadeloupe

Polish refugees, 56

Polygenism, 13; polygenists and, 20, 28

Pondichery (India), 189

Porters: as former Malagasy slaves, 111; homesickness of, 112; in off-season, 105; profession of, 108, 110–12, 233 n.83; on trains, 149

Prostitution: in Antsirabe, 147; in hammam, 160; in Vichy, 105

Québec, 25

Quinine: Fouet on, 178, 213; as prophylactic, 60; as treatment for malaria, 45, 59, 60, 100, 130

Quinquina. *See* Quinine

Race: anti-acclimatization and, 26–32; Cilaos and the conditioning of, 98; decline of, 17; defining and debating, 11–13, 219 n.20, 221–22 n.104; European, 37–38, 74–75; role of climate in producing, 21–22, 219 n.27; segregation in baths by, 145–46; Thibaut on, 24; Watthé and Barrès on the French, 196

Racism, 49. *See also* Anti-Semitism; Race

Radioactivity, 49, 139

Raj. *See* India

Rajat, Henri, 162, 164

Rakotovao, 146

Ranavalona II, 122, 124–25, 145

Ravine-Chaude (Le Lamentin), 80–84, 86, 88–89

Régent, Frédéric, 65

Religion: Korbous and, 160–65, 176–77; Lourdes and, 41, 162, 195; *menalamba* insurrection and, 125; mineral water and hydrotherapy and, 6, 41–42, 222 n.123; missionaries and Maison du missionnaire (Vichy), 195–98; pilgrimages and, 139,

161, 177, 180, 184; Vichy catering to, 189. *See also* Missionaries

Respiratory system. *See* Body

Réunion Island: disorder and disease on, 105–6; "highland Creoles" of, 30, 97–100; history of, 91–93, 95; maroon practices on, 6, 93–94, 212; popularity of spas on, 104–5, 233 n.57; porters of, 110–13; presence of malaria on, 100–102, 129; region and springs of, 90–91, 93, 95–97; Salazie military sanatorium on, 102–4; spa drinking waters of, 115–16; spa tax exemption request on, 58; as symbol of French colonial power, 2, 3; tourists and, 106–10, 113. *See also* Cilaos; Hell-Bourg; Salazie

Rheumatism: Antsirabe water as treatment for, 49, 120, 123, 138; Cilaos water as treatment for, 116; Korbous water as treatment for, 157, 165, 168; River-Chaude water as treatment for, 80, 230 n.104

Rochoux, J. A., 24

Roman baths, 151, 157–60, 166, 179, 202, 213

Rosaas, Pastor, 122–26

Ross, Kristin, 5

Ross, Sir Ronald, 32–33, 47, 63, 132, 224 n.24

Royal bath (Madagascar), 121

Royat, 57, 65, 84

Rules and regulations governing spas, 55–58

Saadaoui, Ahmed, 159

Said, Edward, 3

Saint-Claude (Guadeloupe), 69, 71–74, 76–77, 79, 81, 88

Saint-Denis (Réunion), 102–4, 108, 110

Saint Domingue (Haiti), 68

Saint-François (Réunion), 103, 113

Saint-Gilles (Réunion), 117

Saint-Hilaire, Isidore Geoffroy, 15

Saint-Louis (Réunion), 105, 108, 110

Saint-Mart, Pierre de, 150–51

Saint-Pierre, Bernardin de, 14, 95–96

Salazie (Réunion): climate and springs of, 98–102; disorder at, 105–6; drinking waters at, 115–16; foreign tourists and, 107–9; history and settlement of, 94–96;

Vichy regime, 189, 203, 209
Vidal, Edmond, 47, 182–83
Vietnam. *See* Indochina
Vigarello, Georges, 5, 48
Virchow, Rudolf, 11, 28–31, 33–37, 98–99,
 221 n.103, 221–22 n.104, 222 n.106
Virey, Julien Joseph, 11
Vittel, 2, 43, 50, 54–55, 142

Water cures. *See* Hydrotherapy
Watthé, Henry, 194–97. *See also* Missionaries
Weisz, George, 39, 43, 44, 223 n.141, 225 n.62
Wilson, John, 73–74

Wood, Sir Richard, 165–66
World War I, 55, 83, 135, 142, 148, 203
World War II, 38, 136
Wright, Gwendolyn, 144, 171

Yellow fever: altitude as cure for, 75–77,
 altitudinal immunity from, 38, 62, 69;
 Beauperthuy on, 20–21; Dariste's guide
 on, 15–16; Dolé-les-Bains as treatment
 for, 70–71; evasive action against, 34; in
 Guadeloupe, 69, 73–74; heat as cause of,
 68; "mulatress' treatment" for, 78–79,
 212

Eric T. Jennings is an associate professor in the Department of History at the University of Toronto. He is the author of *Vichy in the Tropics: Pétain's National Revolution in Madagascar, Guadeloupe, and Indochina, 1940–1944* (2001) and coeditor of *L'Empire colonial sous Vichy* (2004).

Library of Congress Cataloging-in-Publication Data
Jennings, Eric Thomas.
Curing the colonizers : hydrotherapy, climatology, and French colonial spas /
Eric T. Jennings.
p. cm.
Includes bibliographical references and index.
ISBN-13: 978-0-8223-3808-6 (cloth : alk. paper)
ISBN-10: 0-8223-3808-4 (cloth : alk. paper)
ISBN-13: 978-0-8223-3822-2 (pbk. : alk. paper)
ISBN-10: 0-8223-3822-x (pbk. : alk. paper)
1. Hydrotherapy—French colonies—History. 2. Health resorts—French colonies—History.
I. Title.
RM813.J46 2006
615.8'53—dc22   2006010438